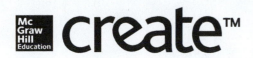

Taking Sides: Clashing Views
in Food and Nutrition, 3/e

Janet M. Colson

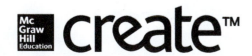

http://create.mheducation.com

ISBN-10: 1259661636   ISBN-13: 9781259661631

Contents

Detailed Table of Contents

Unit 1: The *Dietary Guidelines for Americans 2015*

Issue: Will the Government's Dietary Guidance Improve Health?
YES: 2015 Dietary Guidelines Advisory Committee, from "Executive Summary," *Scientific Report of the 2015 Dietary Guidelines Advisory Committee* (2015)
NO: Adele Hite, from "Healthy Nation Coalition's Letter to the Secretaries of Health and Human Services and the United States Department of Agriculture Regarding the *Scientific Report of the 2015 Dietary Guidelines Advisory Committee*," Healthy Nation Coalition (2015)

The 2015 DGAC committee acknowledges that the average American has not followed dietary recommendations to reduce consumption of saturated fat, sodium and sugar and continues to recommend for reductions in the three nutrients to improve health in Americans. They also stress the importance of eating an overall healthy diet and support food-based dietary guidelines with emphasis on fruits, vegetables, and whole grains. Adele Hite and The Healthy Nation Coalition believe that the DGAC report will "perpetuate the same ineffective federal nutrition guidance that has persisted for nearly four decades, but has not achieved positive health outcomes for the American public." They cite studies that claim reductions in saturated fat, cholesterol and sodium while increasing starch and vegetable oils actually increase the risk for chronic diseases. The Coalition claims that, "Millions of taxpayer dollars are spent on policies and practices related to guidance whose scientific foundation has yet to be established."

Issue: Are the 2015 *Dietary Guidelines* Based on Sound Science?
YES: Barbara E. Millen, from "Part C: Methodology" and "Appendix E-4: NHANES Data Used in DGAC Data Analyses," *Scientific Report of the 2015 Dietary Guidelines Advisory Committee* (2015)
NO: Edward Archer, Gregory A. Hand, and Steven N. Blair, from, "Validity of U.S. Nutritional Surveillance: National Health and Nutrition Examination Survey Caloric Energy Intake Data, 1971–2010" *PLOS ONE* (2013)

The 2015 DGAC titled their report as being "Scientific" yet acknowledge that most food and nutrient intakes used to formulate the report are based on 24-hour recalls from the NHANES and WWEIA data. The DGAC also point out that the "strengths and shortcomings of these dietary assessment methods have been discussed over time and that no assessment method is perfect." Archer and colleagues criticize the methods used by NHANES to collect dietary data and question the validity of the data collected using the 24-hour recall method. They validated the self-reported energy intakes of over 60,000 NHANES participants and found that the majority of people underreport energy intake and consider the NHANES energy intake data physically implausible.

Issue: Should We Eat Less Saturated Fat?
YES: Barbara E Millen, from "Part D. Chapter 6: Cross-Cutting Topics of Public Health Importance: Saturated Fat," *Scientific Report of the 2015 Dietary Guidelines Advisory Committee* (2015)
NO: Richard A. Passwater, from "An Interview with Professor Fred A. Kummerow, Ph.D., Cholesterol and Saturated Fats Won't Kill You, but Trans Fat May (Parts 1 and 2)," *WholeFoods Magazine* (2014)

The DGAC, led by Barbara E. Millen, followed the lead of the American Heart Association and the American College of Cardiology and recommend eating less saturated fat. It concludes there is "strong and consistent" evidence that replacing saturated fat with polyunsaturated fat reduces risk of cardiovascular disease and coronary mortality and only "limited evidence" that replacing saturated with monounsaturated fats is beneficial. Richard A. Passwater interviews biochemist Fred Kummerow, who at 100 years of age reports that he eats one egg, uses real butter, and drinks three glasses of whole milk each day. He says that "saturated fats are heart neutral and have no effect on cholesterol/HDL ratio or heart disease. They do provide calories, though, and should not be overdone in terms of daily calories."

Issue: Should We Eat Less Added Sugars?
YES: Barbara E Millen, from "Part D. Chapter 6: Cross-Cutting Topics of Public Health Importance: Added Sugars and Low-Calorie Sweeteners," *Scientific Report of the 2015 Dietary Guidelines Advisory Committee* (2015)
NO: Andrew C. Briscoe III and P. Courtney Gaine, from "The Sugar Association's Letter Written in Response to *Scientific Report of the 2015 Dietary Guidelines Advisory Committee*," *The Sugar Association* (2015)

The DGAC concludes that there is strong evidence that diets high in added sugars are associated with overweight, obesity, and type 2 diabetes and moderate evidence that sugars are linked to dental caries, hypertension, stroke, and cardiovascular disease. They call for an upper limit (UL) of 10 percent of energy to come from added sugars in the diet. They also recommend that additional studies need to be conducted on the roles of sugars and various health conditions. The Sugar Association, whose mission is to "monitor nutrition science . . . to provide science-based information . . . and to ensure that Federal nutrition and food policy regarding sugar is based on the preponderance of scientific evidence," asks the Secretaries of HHS and USDA to continue the same advice about added sugars that was in the *2010 DGA*. The 2010 advice is to simply reduce intake of calories from added sugars and limit refined grains that contain added sugars, without a specific upper limit recommendation based on the percent of energy.

Unit 2: Nutrition and Health

Issue: Can an Overemphasis on Eating Healthy Become Unhealthy?
YES: Lindsey Getz, from "Orthorexia: When Eating Healthy Becomes an Unhealthy Obsession," *Today's Dietitian* (2009)
NO: Chris Woolston, from "What's Wrong with the American Diet?" *Consumer Health Interactive* (2009)

Writer Lindsey Getz describes "orthorexia" as the condition that makes a person strive for a perfect diet. People with orthorexia avoid sugar, *trans* fat, cholesterol, sodium, and anything they believe is "unhealthy" and take pride in being in total control of the foods they eat. Health and medical writer Chris Woolston believes the typical American diet is excessive in calories, fat, and sugar. He says we would be much healthier if we ate more "fish, poultry, cruciferous vegetables (i.e. cabbage and broccoli), greens, tomatoes, legumes, fresh fruits, and whole grains." He also believes we should "skimp on fatty or calorie-rich foods such as red meats, eggs, high-fat dairy products, French fries, pizza, mayonnaise, candy, and desserts."

Issue: Does a Diet High in Fructose Increase Body Fat?
YES: Joseph Mercola, from "This Harmful Food Product Is Changing Its Name—Don't Get Swindled," *Mercola* (2010)
NO: Corn Refiners Association, from "Questions & Answers About High Fructose Corn Syrup," *Sweet Surprise* (2008)

Osteopathic physician Joseph Mercola considers that HFCS is more deadly than sugar and explains how the body converts fructose to fat. He accuses the Corn Refiners Association of trying to convince us that their product is equal to table sugar. The Corn Refiners Association claims that HFCS has no adverse health effect and is the same as sucrose and honey. They also include the many benefits that HFCS provides to food.

Issue: Do Americans Need Vitamin D Supplements?
YES: Jane Brody, from "What Do You Lack? Probably Vitamin D," *The New York Times* (2010)
NO: Institute of Medicine, from "Dietary Reference Intakes for Calcium and Vitamin D," *The National Academies Press* (2010)

Best-selling author Jane Brody says that a huge part of the population is deficient in vitamin D and studies indicate that deficiency increases risk of cancer, heart disease, arthritis, and a host of other conditions. She also reports that the "experts" recommend a supplement of 1000 to 2000 IU each day. The 14-member committee appointed by the Institute of Medicine (IOM) of the National Academy of Sciences to establish the Recommended Dietary Allowance (RDA) disagrees. After reviewing over 1000 studies and listening to testimonies from scientists and other stakeholders, the committee set the RDA for people up to age 70 years at 600 IU and at 800 IU for those over age 70. They conclude that few people are deficient in vitamin D and the only health benefit is the vitamin's role in bone health.

Issue: Does Coconut Oil Provide Health Benefits?
YES: The Coconut Research Center, from "The Coconut Oil Miracle: Where Is the Evidence?" Coconut Research Center (2015)
NO: William A. Correll, from, "FDA Warning Letter to Carrington Farms," Food and Drug Administration (2015)

Authors of the Coconut Research Center website boast of the various health benefits of coconut oil related to seizures, dementia, ALS, and cardiovascular disease. They describe the number of studies available through a PubMed search that support the health benefits of coconut oil and the medium-chain fatty acids found in the oil. After reviewing claims that Carrington Farms includes on the labels of coconut oil, William Correll, FDA Director Office of Compliance, Center for Food Safety and Applied Nutrition, issues a warning letter to the company pointing out the therapeutic claims on their website about coconut oil classify it as a drug, not a food, and points out other violations on the labels.

Issue: Should Physicians Use BMI to Assess Overall Health?
YES: Jeremy Singer-Vine, from "Beyond BMI: Why Doctors Won't Stop Using an Outdated Measure for Obesity," *Slate* (2009)
NO: Keith Devlin, from "Do You Believe in Fairies, Unicorns, or the BMI?" *Devlin's Angle* (2009)

Journalist Jeremy Singer-Vine points out "the circumference around a person's waist provides a much more accurate reading of his or her abdominal fat and risk for disease than BMI." He also acknowledges that waist measurements require slightly more time and training than it takes to record a BMI, however, because BMI is cheap and easy to use, physicians and the medical community will continue using it. Mathematician Keith Devlin, whose is labeled as "overweight" by his physician because his BMI is 25.1, despite his 32 inch waist, considers that BMI is "numerological nonsense." While he applauds the knowledge that physicians have about the human body and health issues, he feels that the mathematics behind the BMI calculations are used irresponsibly and says BMI should not be used in medical practice. He calls for mathematicians to demand responsible use of math.

Unit 3: Our Food Supply

In June 2015, the FDA issued the final determination that partially hydrogenated oils (PHOs) are no longer on the GRAS list because they are not "generally considered as safe." In effect, this means that *trans* fats are banned from foods because PHOs are the main source of *trans* fat. FDA announced that PHOs must be removed from processed foods by June 2018. The Grocery Manufacturers Association filed a detailed petition outlining the safety of PHOs and requesting that low levels of PHOs be allowed in certain processed foods.

Ed Hamer and Mark Anslow indicate that organically produced foods use less energy, water, and pesticides and produce less pollution while producing foods that taste better and contain more nutrients. Mark Bittman says that eating organically offers no guarantee of eating well, healthfully, sanely, even ethically. He points out that people may feel better about eating an organic Oreo than a conventional Oreo, and sides with Marion Nestle who says "Organic junk food is still junk food."

William Saletan defends biotechnology used in genetically modifying foods and believes they bring many advantages and help ensure a safe food supply. He says the case AGAINST genetic modification is full of errors, fallacies, misconceptions, misrepresentations, and lies. *GMWatch* editor Claire Robinson, and co-author of the free online book *GM Myths and Truths*, points out the fallacies of Saletan's defense of GM foods in her rebuttal to his article. She grades his "critical thinking in which Saletan gets a big "F" for "Fail."

Journalist Anneli Rufus describes how chemicals added to today's food supply destroy the good bacteria (probiotics) and various ways to restore the bacteria to the body. She also encourages us to start looking for prebiotic-fortified foods, because it is hard to get an adequate amount from foods. Matt Wood discusses what the scientific studies show about the two biotics but points out some negative effects of prebiotics and the short list of probiotics shown to actually be beneficial to health.

Kris Gunnars claims that there are profound genetic changes in modern wheat and that it is processed differently than wheat grown in earlier times. He describes how the new wheat is the root of a variety of health problems. Cereal chemist Donald

Kasarda reports that today's wheat has the same level of protein and gluten it had hundreds of years ago and believes modern wheat is not the cause of celiac disease or gluten sensitivity.

Issue: Should Infant Formulas Contain Synthetic ARA and DHA?
YES: Haley C. Stevens and Mardi K. Mountford, from "Infant Formula and DHA/ARA," International Formula Council (IFC) (2008)
NO: Ari LeVaux, from "Dangerous Hype: Infant Formula Companies Claim They Can Make Babies 'Smarter,'" *AlterNet* (2009)

Haley Stevens and Mardi Mountford, representing the International Formula Council (IFC), point out "the available evidence strongly supports benefits of adding DHA and ARA to infant formula." They point out that "a large database exists concerning not only the safety but also the efficacy of infant formula containing both ARA and DHA. These facts, together, support the addition of both ARA and DHA when LC-PUFAs [long-chain polyunsaturated fatty acids] are added to formula." Ari LeVaux is more skeptical. He says the oils are produced from lab-grown algae and fungi and extracted with the neurotoxin hexane. He also is concerned that some "parents and medical professionals believe these additives are causing severe reactions in some babies, and it has been repeatedly shown that taking affected babies off DHA/ARA formula makes the problems go away almost immediately."

Unit 4: Nutrition and Food Policy

Issue: Should Government Control Sodium Levels in the Food Supply?
YES: Institute of Medicine, from "Strategies to Reduce Sodium Intake in the United States: Brief Report," *The National Academies Press* (2010)
NO: Michael Moss, from "The Hard Sell on Salt," *The New York Times* (2010)

The Institute of Medicine's report on sodium recommends for the FDA to set mandatory national standards for the sodium content of foods and require the food industry (including manufacturers and restaurants) to gradually lower the amount of sodium they add to processed foods and prepared meals. Writer Michael Moss describes the numerous problems that food giants such as Kellogg, Frito-Lay, and Kraft claim to face if they attempt to lower sodium in the foods they make.

Issue: Should Government Levy a "Fat Tax"?
YES: Kelly D. Brownell, et al., from "The Public Health and Economic Benefits of Taxing Sugar-Sweetened Beverages" *The New England Journal of Medicine* (2009)
NO: Daniel Engber, from "Let Them Drink Water! What a Fat Tax Really Means for America," *Slate* (2009)

Kelly Brownell and colleagues propose a "fat tax" targeting sugar-sweetened beverages. They feel a tax will decrease the amount of sugary drinks people consume and ultimately help reduce obesity. They also suggest that the tax has the "potential to generate substantial revenue" to help fund health-related initiatives. Daniel Engber disagrees with a fat tax on sugary beverages since it will impact poor, nonwhite people most severely and they would be deprived of the pleasures of palatable foods. He says that the poor would be forced to "drink from the faucet" while the more affluent will sip exotic beverages such as POM Wonderful, at about $5 a pop.

Issue: Can Michelle Obama's "Let's Move!" Initiative Halt Childhood Obesity?
YES: White House Press Release, from "First Lady Michelle Obama Launches *Let's Move*: America's Move to Raise a Healthier Generation of Kids," (2010)
NO: Michele Simon, from "Michelle Obama's *Let's Move*—Will It Move Industry?" *AlterNet* (2010)

First Lady Michelle Obama says that the Let's Move! campaign can correct the health problems of the upcoming generation and realizes that the problem cannot be solved overnight. She thinks that "with everyone working together, it can be solved." The "first ever" Task Force on Childhood Obesity was formed to help implement the campaign. Public health attorney Michelle Simon claims that Let's Move! is just another task force and there is more talk than action. She questions if it's realistic to be able to reverse the nation's childhood obesity epidemic in a generation.

Issue: Do Pesticides Cause Birth Defects and Other Health Problems?
YES: Christopher Pala, from "Pesticides in Paradise: Hawaii's Spike in Birth Defects Puts Focus on GM Crops," *The Guardian* (2015)
NO: Environmental Protection Agency, from "Food and Pesticides," (2015)

Christopher Pala reports an increase in birth defects and pediatric morbidity in areas of Hawaii where high levels of pesticides are used for testing growth of GMO corn. He also describes the steps some Hawaiians are taking to restrict the testing of pesticides in Hawaii. The EPA claims that American agricultural products are rigorously tested and the pesticide residue levels cause no health problems, especially among children.

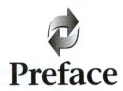

Preface

As humans, we must eat to live. However, determining what to eat has become very perplexing for many of us. We are bombarded with advertisements for newly formulated products that claim to be healthier than the foods humans have thrived on for years. Reports of the latest scientific studies cast doubt on many things we have always considered to be wholesome. Controversy continues when the nutrient content of foods are considered. Nutrition researchers throughout the world continue to investigate the effects that specific nutrients have on health, and each discovery leads to another question. One thing they have agreed about is what we consume does influence health. But is that influence positive, negative, or neutral?

The purpose of this book is to present some of the most hotly debated current issues on food and nutrition as related to health. The issues are presented as yes/no questions. For each question, two previously published selections that present clashing views on the topic are included; one selection says "yes" to the question and the second one supports the negative position. *Taking Sides: Clashing Views in Food and Nutrition* is designed to challenge students to do just that—decide if they agree with one of the views or to think beyond the two sides to formulate another opinion. A class of 30 students may yield 30 different opinions on the same issue.

Each issue begins with background information that provides the foundation for the topic. Learning objectives are included at the beginning of the issues and review questions are at the conclusion; instructors may assign these as a written assignment for submission or simply use them as a springboard for in-class debate and discussion.

Acknowledgments

Many thanks to my colleagues and students at Middle Tennessee State University for all their helpful suggestions. A very special thanks goes to Mary Foust for her patience, guidance, and support. Without the editorial staff at McGraw-Hill Contemporary Learning Series, this book would not exist. And, of course, I owe everything to my wonderful children, Beau and Heather, and precious grandchildren, Bray and Jennings. Without them, my world would not exist.

Editor of This Volume

JANET M. COLSON has served on the faculty in the Nutrition and Food Science (NFS) Program at Middle Tennessee State University (MTSU) since 1990 and currently holds the rank of professor. She earned the BS and MS degrees in home economics education from Mississippi College and the University of Southern Mississippi, respectively. Her PhD is in NFS with a gerontology concentration from Florida State University. In addition to serving as coordinator for the NFS program at MTSU, she teaches the maternal/child, introductory, and advanced nutrition courses.

Academic Advisory Board Members

Members of the Academic Advisory Board are instrumental in the final selection of articles for the Taking Sides series. Their review of the articles for content, level, and appropriateness provides critical direction to the editor(s) and staff. We think that you will find their careful consideration reflected in this book.

Patricia Abraham
Arkansas State University

Bernice Adeleye
University of Louisiana, Lafayette

Paul Arciero
Skidmore College

RoseAnn Benson
Utah Valley University

Ruth Bindler
Washington State University

C. Ann Blakey
Ball State University

Jack Brook
Mt. Hood Community College

Paula Brown
Los Angeles Harbor College

Elaine Bryan
Georgia Perimeter College

Sharon Bullock
UNC Charlotte

Joanne Burke
University of New Hampshire

Prithiva Chanmugam
Louisiana State University

Lakshmi Chilukuri
University of California, San Diego

Brian Coble
Carroll College

Sheri Colberg-Ochs
Old Dominion University

Margaret Craig-Schmidt
Auburn University

Leslie Cunningham-Sabo
Colorado State University

Noemi Custodia-Lora
Northern Essex Community College

Ruth Davies
Edison State College

Jonathan Deutsch
Goodwin College

Joannie Dobbs
University of Hawaii, Manoa

Kelly Eichmann
State Center Community College District

Marie Emerson
Washington County Community College

Brad Engeldinger
Sierra College

Mary Flynn
Brown University

Amy Frith
Ithaca College

Bernard Frye
University of Texas, Arlington

Joe Giacalone
Regis University

Wynn Gillan
Southeastern Louisiana University

Elizabeth Greene
Blinn College

Stacy Hastey
Connors State College

Lori Jones
Saint Louis University

Phillip Jones
Erie Community College

Marcy Jung
Fort Lewis College

Kendra Kattelmann
South Dakota State University

Younghee Kim
Bowling Green State University

Linda Lamont
University of Rhode Island

Julie Lee
Western Kentucky University

Mary Lyons
El Camino College

Julie McCullough
University of Southern Indiana

Glen McNeil
Fort Hays State University

Monica Meadows
University of Texas

Katherine Mellen
University of Iowa

Craig Meservey
NH Technical Institute

Regina Munster
California State University, Chico

Mary Murimi
Louisiana Tech University

Lisa Nicholson
California Polytechnic State University

Martha Olson
Iowa Lakes Community College

Felicia Omick
Southside Virginia Community College

Susan Quinn
Southeastern Louisiana University

Elizabeth Quintana
West Virginia University

Wendy Repovich
Eastern Washington University

Robin R. Roach
University of Memphis

Jeffrey Ruterbusch
Central Michigan University

Joshua Searcy
Central State University

Reginald Smith
West Virginia University Institute of Technology

Mary Ellen Smith
Butler County Community College

Marsha Spence
University of Tennessee, Knoxville

Theresa Tiso
Stony Brook University

Barbara Utendorf
Wilmington College

Debra Vinci
University of West Florida

Audrey Weaver
Northwestern State University of Louisiana

LaVern Whisenton-Davidson
Millersville University

Aleida Whittaker-Gordon
California State Polytechnic University, Pomona

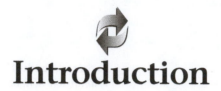

Introduction

When I was growing up in rural Mississippi during the 1960s, eating was very simple. Summer meals consisted of vegetables from my father's garden served with meat or fish. My father kept the freezer filled with beef or pork that he had slaughtered from his farm and fish from the river. We had three meals a day with the entire family sitting around the kitchen table. And for snacks, my mother very patiently taught us to use a knife to peel oranges, making sure the rind stayed in one continuous coil. Winter meals consisted of hot vegetables, the product of hours spent picking and freezing produce harvested during the warmer months. School lunches consisted of "meat and three" cooked from scratch by some of the best cooks in the county. The only beverages available in school were plain white milk and water from the fountain. The first time I saw pizza, tacos, chicken nuggets, and chocolate milk in a school cafeteria was when I had lunch with my daughter in the 1980s.

So what has happened over the last 50 years? Most people don't have time or space for a family garden, so we rely on what the local grocer decides to stock. Some of us, including many college students, opt for whatever is on sale. And eating out, especially at fast food restaurants, can actually be cheaper and easier than cooking at home. Most of us are aware that the substances we consume will eventually affect our health. But what will the effect be? Will it contribute positively to health or be a detriment and result in obesity, type 2 diabetes, hypertension, or other degenerative disease? This is where the confusion, controversy, and discussion begin.

Each year, thousands of articles appear in professional journals, magazines, newspapers, and blogs about the latest discoveries and claims about food as related to health, beauty, athletic abilities, intelligence, etc. In most instances, if you read three articles on the same topic, you'll get three different opinions. The authors may agree on some aspects, but vary on others. Not only is it mind-boggling to the general public, but health and nutrition professionals are often confused on whom to believe. This book presents a variety of the most current and debated issues about food and nutrition, and challenges the reader to analyze each issue and form his or her own opinion. The issues are designed to help the reader work through the process of thinking analytically and critically—to compare, analyze, critique, and justify.

Our Food Supply

As humans, we must eat food to stay alive. Fortunately, our food supply is plentiful. In 2015, a Food Marketing Institute report shows that the average grocery store carries 42,214 different items. While the immense number of products gives us vast variety, it also makes selecting food very confusing. Many people base their food choices on the claims they see in food advertisements, or what is written on food labels. Virtually all advertisements promote the beneficial aspects of the food they are promoting and these ads do influence our decision to buy the product. The Nutrition Facts on food labels also influences many people's choices. The Food and Drug Administration (FDA) has tracked food label use since 1982. Based on results of their 2008 Health and Diet Survey, 54 percent of Americans report they read food labels, compared to only 44 percent in 2004. Most are looking at calories, fat, or salt content. Additionally, the FDA study found more Americans say they know about the heart-health benefits of omega-3 fatty acids and negative aspects of *trans* fats than in earlier years. However, less people recognize the relationships between fruits and vegetables and heart disease. This could be related to less advertising by the vegetable and fruit industry compared to the billions spent by the processed food and beverage industry.

Our food supply is changing and becoming very complex. Because of the advances in food chemistry, hundreds of natural chemicals in foods have been identified. They include nutrients—proteins, carbohydrates, fats, vitamin, and minerals—plus live microorganisms and hundreds of phytochemicals. Nutrition scientists investigate the effect that these natural substances have on health status. Results of their investigations influence our diets in two ways. First, the food industry promotes the health benefits of the foods that contain these substances, which increase sales. Second, food manufacturers extract the substances from its natural source, and add it to newly created products. Some food manufacturers use synthetically produced versions of the nutrients. After products are developed, the manufacturer spends millions marketing the new food to the public.

Debate begins when people question the safety and benefit of extracting nutrients or other substances from food, and creating a new food or supplement. And many people question the safety of how the synthetic versions are made and speculate that fake versions may be harmful to humans.

Complexities of Our Diets

If foods we eat are complex, our diets are even more so. Southerners have a totally different diet than people from New York or California. And what we eat varies based on the season; most of us eat more fresh fruits and vegetables in the summer months and more candy and other sweets beginning at Halloween continuing until New Year's Day. Culture, traditions, and religion also influence our diets. As the world's population becomes more transient, dietary practices change. Not only do immigrants bring their native foods and dietary preferences to the new country, they also adopt dietary practices of the culture. USDA has evaluated acculturation of immigrants to the United States and found that dietary quality decreases as immigrants become more "Americanized" and give up their native lifestyles. Religion also affects the diet. Some of the healthiest populations are those with strict religious dietary practices. For example, Seventh Day Adventists (SDA) who follow vegetarian diets are healthier than the general population. According to a recent SDA Academy of Nutrition and Dietetics report:

> SDAs in general, have 50% less risk of heart disease, certain types of cancers, strokes, and diabetes. More specifically, recent data suggests that vegetarian men under 40 can expect to live more than eight years longer and women more than seven years longer than the general population. SDA vegetarian men live more than three years longer than SDA men who eat meat.
>
> Researchers believe this added length of life and quality of health is due in particular to the consumption of whole grains, fruits and vegetables as well as the avoidance of meat, alcohol, coffee and tobacco.

Our diets are composed of foods that contain hundreds of nutrients and other chemicals. However, many studies that examine the influence of nutrition on health focus on a single nutrient. For example, many reports suggest that eating fructose increases triglyceride levels in the body. Researchers may base this observation on laboratory animals that are fed high levels of plain fructose, then become obese, and ultimately develop obesity-related diseases. But few of us have a diet that is predominately fructose. Do our bodies handle free fructose differently than natural fructose found in fruits and vegetables? Or is fructose that is eaten with other foods handled differently than pure fructose? Some people say "yes" to both of these, whereas others claim there are no differences. Many people believe that the total diet should be considered instead of focusing on a single food or a single nutrient.

Who Writes about Food and Nutrition

The issues presented in this book fit into one of two general categories. Some deal with the recommendations about food, or specific nutrients in food, and the influence they have on health. Others focus on policies and practices that affect our food supply. Each of the issues begins with an introduction, which sets the stage for the debate, and provides historical context for the issue. For each selection, the affiliation and education of the author or authors are included. Consider who the authors are and their stakes in the issue as you critique what they write. Question their positions on the issue and if they may profit from their opinions or is their position totally altruistic. Ask yourself:

> *"What does the author (or who pays the author) stand to benefit from his or her position?"*

Authors of the selections represent one of five main groups. Each of the groups has a different stake in the issue; be sure to consider the authors' backgrounds as you read and analyze each of the selections. The five groups are described below.

1. Food, Nutrition, and Health Professionals

Professionals in this category include people who have the academic training and credentials to interpret the scientific evidence behind nutrition recommendations. They include professions such as dietitians, physicians, chiropractors, nurses, and food and nutrition researchers. Some of the professionals work directly with the public and have first-hand experience with dietary needs of the general population, whereas others work in research. Some of their research is laboratory-based and other research may be with large clinical trials. Some of the selections are written by registered dietitians/nutritionists (RDNs) who describe their experiences advising the public about nutrition. Other selections are written by food and nutrition researchers, many of them are the leading authorities in the nation.

2. Representatives of Government Agencies

The two main U.S. agencies that publish reports, policies, and recommendations related to food and nutrition are the United States Department of Agriculture (USDA) and the Department of Health and Human Services (HHS). The two agencies work together to develop the *Dietary Guidelines for Americans*, but have specific functions in other areas. The main responsibility of USDA is to promote the sale and consumption of American agricultural products, but it also houses units that work on nutrition policies and advise the public about diet and health such as MyPyramid. Interestingly, one section of USDA promotes agricultural products such as beef, pork, eggs, dairy products, and oils made from soy beans, peanuts, and corn, while another section recommends to limit saturated fats (found in meats, eggs, and dairy) and total fat intake. This different functions can and do generate debate. USDA also oversees the following food and nutrition assistance programs: the Supplemental Nutrition Assistance Program (SNAP, formerly Food Stamps); the Supplemental Nutrition Program for Women, Infants, and Children (WIC), and the National School Lunch Program.

The HHS consists of several sub-agencies; several deal with food, nutrition, and health. The Food and Drug Administration (FDA) regulates the safety and labeling of the food supply. The Centers for Disease Control and Prevention (CDC) conducts research and sponsors programs to prevent diet-related diseases. CDC tracks the health status of the nation including National Health and Nutrition Examination Survey (NHANES) and sponsor Healthy People 2020. The National Institutes of Health (NIH) conducts and sponsors research on many areas of nutrition and health. NIH consists of 20 institutes such as the National Cancer Institute, National Heart, Lung, and Blood Institute, and the National Institute on Drug Abuse.

Several other government, or government-sponsored, agencies investigate food and nutrition matters. For example, the General Accounting Office conducts research in response to congressional queries. In 2010, it investigated the safety of herbal dietary supplements and provided the report to Congress. The Institute of Medicine (IOM) of the National Academies is a private, nonprofit group; the government contracts with that to conduct research related to health.

3. Representatives from the Food Industry

The food industry is the term that describes any group involved in growing, harvesting, processing, transport, and sale of food and beverages. It has the biggest impact on what we eat. According to the Food Industry Center of the University of Minnesota, "Few industries reach as many consumers on a daily basis or are as fundamental to their lives as the food industry. Americans spend more than $1 trillion annually for food, accounting for nearly 10 percent of our Gross Domestic Product (GDP). The food system employs over 16.5 million people. . . . " We must eat, therefore the food industry affects everyone. Food must be produced, processed, distributed, and prepared before we eat it, and each stage is represented by its own segment of the food industry with its own special interests in influencing dietary advice and government regulations. Advice to avoid a particular food, or component in a food, can decrease sale of the item, and results in loss of profit for that segment of the food industry. Therefore, the food industry hires food and nutrition researchers, either paid directly or through grants, to conduct studies that support the benefits of their products. They also hire lobbyists to make sure laws and government regulations do not interfere with use of their products.

4. Advocacy Groups and Individuals

Advocacy may come from an individual or by an advocacy group such as the Center for Science in the Public Interest (CSPI) or from national organizations such as the American Heart Association (AHA) or the American Cancer Society. Groups such as these attempt to promote the nutritional health of the public, and sometimes point out problems of the food industry or petition the government to strengthen policies. Advocacy can also take the form of media campaigns, public speaking, commissioning and publishing research or polls, or filing law suits.

For example, in 1993 the CSPI recommended that the *trans* fat content should be included on food labels after it had recognized that *trans* fats are linked to elevated blood cholesterol. However, it took 13 years until FDA agreed to require *trans* fat content on the nutrition facts label of processed foods. In 2003, California attorney Stephen Joseph filled a law suit ordering Nabisco to stop selling Oreo Cookies to children in California, because the cookies were high in *trans* fat. The suit did not actually go to trial because Nabisco agreed to reformulate their Oreos. Joseph dropped the suit. More recently, the AHA suggested to USDA that the sodium intake recommendation should be lowered to 1500 mg of sodium each day. Authors of the *Dietary Guidelines for Americans* for 2010 and 2015 agreed to include the lower sodium recommendation for the entire adult population, based, in part, on the strong recommendation from AHA.

Some people advocate against pesticide use and genetic modification to seeds, whereas others question the safety of man-made products such as high-fructose corn syrup, synthetically manipulated fats, and many other food processing practices. And many individuals and groups who advocate for healthier food get results.

5. Journalists Who Write about Food and Nutrition Issues

Many of the selections are written by journalists who write about other people's opinions on the topic or simply report results of recent developments related to food and nutrition. Some of the journalists have academic training in food and nutrition; however, others have developed expertise through personal interest. Journalists are often criticized about what they write; some people accuse journalists of sensationalizing the story. Stories about controversial issues attract readers and enhance the careers of journalists as well as of the researchers or groups that they write about. Research about the effects of food, nutrients, or agricultural practices on health often grabs front-page attention, and many leading journalists issue press releases on studies likely to gain attention. Reporters writing about food and nutrition issues of unusual interest win prizes and book contracts for their work. Because controversy makes news, media attention tends to focus on the differences rather than the similarities in points of view.

Ruth Kava, Director of Nutrition at the American Council on Science and Health, warns journalists about "Good Stories, Bad Science: A Guide for Journalists to the Health Claims of 'Consumer Activist' Groups." She stresses the need for journalists to be skeptical of reporting information from consumer activist groups about the alleged hazards in our food supply. She concludes:

Often these claims are coupled with suggestions for specific actions to reduce the purported risk of disease or premature death by avoiding or reducing exposure to the allegedly harmful substance. . . . Supposedly, the public claims and warnings that these activist groups make are based on scientific evidence. But in general, there is no independent peer review of their claims or recommendations. The groups publish the reports themselves, often via press release or paid advertisements. Often, the claims are extrapolations from small studies or animal studies, and lack strong supporting evidence. This is not the way mainstream science works.

Therefore, journalists must be very careful about what they report and must understand the science behind the nutrition or health claims. Additionally, they must use reliable resources for the content of their articles.

In some instances, an author's affiliation may fit into two or more of these categories. For example, many times a food, nutrition, or health professional will be employed by a government agency or in the food industry. Professionals must promote the interest of their employer, whether they agree with it or not. And some work as freelance journalists or begin their own blogs on nutrition and health issues in an effort to voice their own opinions. Other professionals work for advocacy groups, or are simply very vocal in their opinions.

Unit 1

UNIT

The *Dietary Guideline for Americans* 2015

Nutrient deficiencies, such as rickets and pellagra, and other forms of undernutrition were common throughout the first half of the twentieth century in the United States. During the 1950s and 1960s, as the nation's food supply increased and processed foods became the norm, the classical deficiency diseases became almost nonexistent, whereas conditions caused by nutrient excesses, such as heart disease, diabetes, and obesity, were on the rise.

In 1968, the U.S. Senate Select Committee on Nutrition and Human Needs was formed, headed by Senator George McGovern. The committee's first major accomplishment was establishment of the free food stamps program in 1970; the committee was also instrumental in establishing the WIC program and expansions in the school lunch program. Beginning in 1974, the Committee switched gears and began investigating the roles of dietary excesses on the nation's health. They sought a small group of physicians with nutrition expertise to assist in preparation of a report about nutrition and health. On January 14, 1977, the Committee introduced the first report of the *Dietary Goals for the United States* which consisted of six dietary recommendations. In the press conference to announce the *Goals*, Senator McGovern explained why the nation needed such a report:

> I should note from the onset that this is the first comprehensive statement by any branch of the Federal Government on risk factors in the American Diet.
>
> The simple fact is that our diets have changed radically within the last 50 years, with great and often very harmful effects on our health. These dietary changes represent as great a threat to the public health as smoking. Too much fat, too much sugar or salt, can be and are linked directly to heart disease, cancer, obesity and stroke, among other killer diseases. In all, six of the leading causes of death in the United States have been linked to our diet.
>
> Those of us within Government have an obligation to acknowledge this. The public wants some guidance, wants to know the truth, and hopefully today we can lay the cornerstone for the building of better health for all Americans, through better nutrition.

Two of the physicians who advised the senators also gave statements at the press conference. Perhaps the most controversial was Harvard's Dr. Mark Hegsted whose words angered the beef industry:

> The diet of the American people has become rich—rich in meat, other sources of saturated fat and cholesterol, and sugar. . . . It should be emphasized that the diet which affluent people generally consume is generally associated with a similar disease pattern—high rates of ischemic heart disease, certain forms of cancer, diabetes, and obesity . . . .
>
> [Our diets] are related to our affluence, the productivity of our farmers and the activities of the food industry. The question to be asked, therefore, is not why should we change our diet, but why not? What are the risks associated with eating less meat, less fat, less saturated fat, less cholesterol, less sugar, less salt, and more fruits, vegetables, unsaturated fats, and cereal products—especially whole grains. . . .
>
> We have an obligation to inform the public of the correct state of knowledge and to assist the public in making the correct food choices. To do less is to avoid our responsibility.

The recommendations to reduce meat, fat, saturated fat, and cholesterol translate into people not only eating less beef, but cutting back on eggs and most dairy products. Therefore, the farmers and ranchers of America bitterly objected to the *Dietary Goals*. Eating less sugar and salt means limiting soft drinks, candy, cookies, and most processed foods. Harvard-educated Dr. Beverly Winikoff's statement at the press conference describes the government's role in the nation's food:

What people eat is affected not only by what scientists know, or by what doctors tell them or even by what they themselves understand. It is affected by Government decisions in the area of agriculture policy, economic and tax policy, export and import policy, and involves questions of good production, transportation, processing, marketing, consumer choice, income and education; as well as food availability and palatability. Nutrition, then, is the end result of pushes and pulls in many directions, a response to the multiple forces creating the "national nutrition environment."

The original edition of the *Dietary Goals* met with bitter criticism, which continues today. In 1980, the *Dietary Goals* were replaced by the *Dietary Guidelines for Americans*. Following the protocol used to develop the *Dietary Goals*, every five years an advisory committee of health and nutrition experts are selected to review new scientific studies published since the previous edition and formulate a technical report based on their review. The committee submits the technical report to the secretaries of Health and Human Services and U.S. Department of Agriculture, which is known as the *Scientific Report of the Dietary Guidelines Committee*. The report is posted on a government website followed by a "public comment period," which is the time that the public is invited to express their opinions on the report. The secretaries and their staff review the technical report and the public's comments, and then write the actual *Dietary Guidelines for Americans* publication. According the 2010 edition, the *Guidelines* are intended to be:

> . . . used in developing educational materials and aiding policymakers in designing and carrying out nutrition-related programs, including Federal nutrition assistance and education programs. The *Dietary Guidelines* also serve as the basis for nutrition messages and consumer materials developed by nutrition educators and health professionals for the general public and specific audiences, such as children.

The issues in this unit consist of excerpts from the *Scientific Report of the 2015 Dietary Guidelines Advisory Committee* paired by either a comment letter about the recommendations from a health organization or food industry group, or from an article that disagrees with the recommendations in the *Scientific Report*.

The timeline below provides a summation of the changes in the *Dietary Goals for the United States* and the *Dietary Guidelines for Americans* over the last four decades.

Chronology of the *Dietary Goals and Guidelines for Americans*

(Adapted from the *Scientific Report of the 2015 Dietary Guidelines Advisory Committee*, 2015 with the 2015/2016 information from the health.gov/dietaryguidelineswebsite.)

1977 In January, the first edition of the *Dietary Goals for the United States* (the "McGovern Report") was issued by the U.S. Senate Select Committee on Nutrition and Human Needs. The *Goals* reflected a shift in focus from obtaining adequate nutrients to avoiding excessive intake of food components linked to chronic disease. The *Goals* were controversial among some nutritionists and others concerned with food, nutrition, and health. A second edition of the *Dietary Goals* was published in December.

1979 The American Society for Clinical Nutrition formed a panel to study the relationship between dietary practices and health outcomes. The findings were reflected in *Healthy People: The Surgeon General's Report on Health Promotion and Disease Prevention*.

1980 Seven principles for a healthful diet were jointly issued in response to the public's desire for authoritative, consistent guidelines on diet and health. These principles became the first edition of *Nutrition and Your Health: Dietary Guidelines for Americans*. The *Guidelines* generated some concern among consumer, commodity, and food industry groups, as well as some nutrition scientists, who questioned the causal relationship between certain guidelines and health.

1983 An external federal advisory committee of nine nutrition scientists was convened to review and make recommendations in a report to the secretaries of USDA and HHS about the first (1980) edition of the *Dietary Guidelines*.

1985 USDA and HHS jointly issued the second edition of *Nutrition and Your Health: Dietary Guidelines for Americans*. This edition was nearly identical to the first, retaining the seven guidelines from the 1980 edition. Some changes were made for clarity, while others reflected advances in scientific knowledge of the associations between diet and chronic diseases. The second edition received wide acceptance and was used as the basis for dietary guidance for the general public as well as a framework for developing consumer education messages.

1989 USDA and HHS established a second federal advisory committee of nine members, which considered whether revisions to the *1985 Dietary Guidelines* were needed and made recommendations for revision in a report to the secretaries. The *1988 Surgeon General's Report on Nutrition and Health* and the 1989 National Research Council's report *Diet and Health: Implications for Reducing Chronic Disease Risk* were key resources used by the Committee.

1990 USDA and HHS jointly released the third edition of *Nutrition and Your Health: Dietary Guidelines for Americans*. The basic tenets of the *1985 Dietary Guidelines* were reaffirmed, with additional refinements made to reflect increased understanding of the science of nutrition and how best to communicate the science to consumers. The language of the new *Dietary Guidelines* was positive, was oriented toward the total diet, and provided specific information regarding food selection. For the first time, quantitative recommendations made for intakes of dietary total fat (<30% of energy) and saturated fat (<10% of energy) were included in the *Dietary Guidelines*.

1990 The 1990 National Nutrition Monitoring and Related Research Act (Section 301 of Public Law 101–445, 7 USC 5341, Title III) directed the secretaries of USDA and HHS to jointly issue at least every 5 years a report entitled *Dietary Guidelines for Americans*. This legislation also required USDA and HHS to review all federal publications containing dietary advice for the general public.

1995 The first official Dietary Guidelines Advisory Committee (DGAC) submitted its technical report to the secretaries of HHS and USDA, who used the DGAC report to jointly develop and release the fourth edition of *Nutrition and Your Health: Dietary Guidelines for Americans*. This edition continued to support the concepts from earlier editions. New information included the Food Guide Pyramid, Nutrition Facts label, boxes highlighting good food sources of key nutrients, and a chart illustrating three weight ranges in relation to height.

1998 An 11-member DGAC was appointed by the secretaries of USDA and HHS to review the fourth edition of the *Dietary Guidelines* to determine whether changes were needed and, if so, to recommend suggestions for revision.

2000 President Bill Clinton spoke of the *Dietary Guidelines* in his radio address after USDA and HHS jointly issued the fifth edition of *Nutrition and Your Health: Dietary Guidelines for Americans*. Earlier versions of the *Guidelines* included seven statements. This version included 10—created by breaking out physical activity from the weight guideline, splitting the grains and fruits/vegetables recommendations for greater emphasis, and adding a new guideline on safe food handling.

2003 A 13-member DGAC was appointed by the secretaries of HHS and USDA to review the fifth edition of the *Dietary Guidelines* to determine whether changes were needed and, if so, to recommend suggestions for revision.

2003–2004 The DGAC used a modified "systematic approach" to review the scientific literature and develop its recommendations. Committee members initially posed approximately 40 specific research questions that were answered using an extensive search and review of the scientific literature. Issues relating diet and physical activity to health promotion and chronic disease prevention were included in the Committee's evidence review. Other major sources of evidence used were the Dietary Reference Intake (DRI) reports prepared by expert committees convened by the Institute of Medicine (IOM) as well as various Agency for Healthcare Research and Quality (AHRQ) and World Health Organization (WHO) reports. In addition, USDA completed numerous food intake pattern modeling analyses and the Committee analyzed various national data sets and sought advice from invited experts.

2004 The DGAC submitted its technical report to the secretaries of HHS and USDA (HHS/USDA, 2004). This 364-page report contained a detailed analysis of the science and was accompanied by many pages of evidence-based tables that were made available electronically. After dropping some questions because of incomplete or inconclusive data, the DGAC wrote conclusions and comprehensive rationales for 34 of the 40 original questions.

2005 Using the DGAC's technical report as a basis, HHS and USDA jointly prepared and issued the sixth edition of *Dietary Guidelines for Americans* in January 2005. This 80-page policy document was the first policy document that was intended primarily for use by policymakers, health care professionals, nutritionists, and nutrition educators. The content of this document included nine major *Dietary Guidelines* messages that resulted in 41 Key Recommendations, of which 23 were for the U.S. population overall and 18 for specific population groups. The policy document highlighted the USDA Food Guide and the DASH Eating Plan as two examples of eating patterns that exemplify the *Dietary Guidelines* recommendations. Shortly thereafter, USDA released the MyPyramid Food Guidance System, an update of the Food Guide Pyramid, which included more detailed advice for consumers to help them follow the *Dietary Guidelines*.

2008 A 13-member DGAC was appointed by the secretaries of USDA and HHS to review the sixth edition of *Dietary Guidelines for Americans* to determine whether changes were needed and, if so, to recommend suggestions for revision.

2008–2009 USDA's Center for Nutrition Policy and Promotion established the Nutrition Evidence Library (NEL) to conduct systematic reviews to help inform federal nutrition policy and programs. The NEL supported the DGAC in answering approximately 130 of the total 180 diet and health-related questions posed. This was the most rigorous and comprehensive approach used to date for reviewing the science in order to develop nutrition-related recommendations for the public. Other sources of evidence for answering scientific questions included modeling analyses of USDA's Food Patterns, review of reports from various data analyses, as well as other available authoritative reports (e.g., 2005 DGAC Report and IOM reports). An elaborate web-based public comments database was developed and provided a successful mechanism for the public to provide comments and thereby participate in the Committee's evidence review process. The database also allowed the public to read other comments that were submitted.

2010 The DGAC submitted its technical report to the secretaries of USDA and HHS (USDA/HHS, 2010). This 445-page report contained a detailed analysis of the science and was accompanied by an additional 230 pages of Food Pattern modeling appendices made available electronically at www .DietaryGuidelines.gov.

2011 Using the Committee's technical report as the basis, HHS and USDA jointly prepared and published the seventh edition of *Dietary Guidelines for Americans* released publicly in January 2011 (USDA/HHS, 2011). The 95-page policy document encompassed the overarching concepts of maintaining calorie balance over time to achieve and sustain a healthy weight, and consuming nutrient-dense foods and beverages. The policy document included 23 key recommendations for the general population and 6 additional key recommendations for specific populations. To assist individuals to build a healthy diet based on the *Dietary Guidelines*, the USDA Food Patterns were updated and new vegetarian adaptations were included. The DASH Eating Plan also was included as an example of a healthy dietary pattern. This publication will serve as the basis for federal nutrition policy until the next policy document is released. In June, USDA released MyPlate, a new visual icon, and the ChooseMyPlate.gov website that provides tools to help consumers of all ages, educators, and health professionals learn about and follow the *Dietary Guidelines*.

2013 A 15-member DGAC was appointed by the secretaries of USDA and HHS to review the seventh edition of *Dietary Guidelines for Americans* and recommend suggestions for revision. One member resigned due to professional obligations within the first three months after appointment; 14 members served the remainder of the two-year charter. The DGAC also added three consultant subcommittee members during its work to address specific issues; these members participated in discussions and decision at the subcommittee level but were not members of the full Committee.

The first committee meeting was held in June.

Beginning on May 29, the public Federal Register notices alerted the public to DGAC meetings held in person and allowed the public to view them via the web; the public comment process was open to allow the public to provide their comments to the DGAC. The first DGAC meeting was held in June 2013.

2014 Committee meetings were held in January, March, July, September, October, November, and December. A total of 912 relevant public comments were submitted to the DGAC from May 29, 2013 to December 30, 2014.

2015 The Committee submitted its technical *Scientific Report of the 2015 Dietary Guidelines Advisory Committee* to the secretaries of USDA and HHS on January 28, 2015. This 571-page report contains a detailed analysis of the science and was accompanied by substantial documentation of the process made available electronically at www.DietaryGuidelines.gov. The public comment period opened in February and had planned to remain open for 45 days; however, due to numerous requests for the public, the comment period was extended to 75 days and closed on May 8 with over 29,000 comments.

Selected, Edited, and with Issue Framing Material by:
Janet M. Colson, *Middle Tennessee State University*

ISSUE

Will the Government's Dietary Guidance Improve Health?

YES: 2015 Dietary Guidelines Advisory Committee, from "Executive Summary," *Scientific Report of the 2015 Dietary Guidelines Advisory Committee* (2015)

NO: Adele Hite, from "Healthy Nation Coalition's Letter to the Secretaries of Health and Human Services and the United States Department of Agriculture Regarding the *Scientific Report of the 2015 Dietary Guidelines Advisory Committee*," http://health.gov/dietaryguidelines/dga2015/comments/readComments.aspx (Comment ID #22858) (2015)

Learning Outcomes
After reading this issue, you will be able to:
• Describe the health and nutritional status of Americans as reported by the Dietary Guidelines Advisory Committee (DGAC) and their recommendations.
• Identify the roles that the government and society must play to improve the nutritional status of Americans.
• Outline the accusations that the Healthy Nation Coalition makes about the DGAC's report related to chronic diseases, adequate nutrition, diversity of Americans, and strength of the scientific evidence.

ISSUE SUMMARY

YES: The 2015 DGAC acknowledges that the average American has not followed dietary recommendations to reduce consumption of saturated fat, sodium, and sugar and continues to recommend for reductions in the three nutrients to improve health in Americans. They also stress the importance of eating an overall healthy diet and support food-based dietary guidelines with emphasis on fruits, vegetables, and whole grains.

NO: Adele Hite believes that the DGAC report will "perpetuate the same ineffective federal nutrition guidance that has persisted for nearly four decades, but has not achieved positive health outcomes for the American public." He cites studies that claim reductions in saturated fat, cholesterol, and sodium, while increasing starch and vegetable oils actually increase the risk for chronic diseases. Hite, the Healthy Nation Coalition director and co-founder, claims that "Millions of taxpayer dollars are spent on policies and practices related to guidance whose scientific foundation has yet to be established."

In 1787, a small group of statesmen spent several weeks drafting the Constitution of the United States. The document begins with the Preamble, "We the People of the United States, in Order to form a more perfect Union, establish Justice, ensure domestic Tranquility, provide for the common defence, promote the general Welfare, and secure the Blessings of Liberty to ourselves and our Posterity . . ."

Although the terms "diet" and "health" are not included in the original document, many aspects of the government's commitments to us relate to our physical well-being; perhaps the most obvious is to promote our "general welfare." Even though the direct reference to perfection, justice, tranquility, and defense was related to problems of that era, our forefathers penned the document for guidance for themselves and their posterity—and we are their posterity.

Today, the government still strives to perfect the nation and many of their efforts focus on the nation's health and the foods we consume. Governmental awareness about the role that nutrition has on health began in the 1960s, spearheaded by Senator George McGovern, Chair of the U.S. Senate Select Committee on Nutrition and Human Needs. McGovern recruited a few of the country's "leading thinkers in the area of nutritional health" to assist the committee with the scientific basis of nutritional studies. The Committee, with the aid of the scientists, introduced the first *Dietary Goals for the United States* in January 1977. McGovern's introduction to the report called the Federal Government to action:

> *The purpose of this report is to point out that the eating practices of this century* represent as critical a public health concern as any now before us.
>
> We must acknowledge and recognize that the public is confused about what to eat to maximize health. If we as a Government want to reduce health costs and maximize the quality of life for all Americans, we have an obligation to provide practical guides to the individual consumer as well as set national dietary goals for the country as a whole.

The purpose of the goals was to improve the health of Americans with emphasis on reducing heart disease, diabetes, obesity, and certain cancers. The six original goals include six nutrient-specific recommendations with seven suggestions for food selection and preparation. The original nutrient goals are as follows:

1. Increase carbohydrate consumption to account for 55 to 60 percent energy (caloric) intake.
2. Reduce overall fat consumption from approximately 40 to 30 percent energy intake.
3. Reduce saturated fat intake consumption to account for about 10 percent of total energy intake, and balance that with polyunsaturated and monounsaturated fats, which should account for about 10 percent of energy intake each.
4. Reduce cholesterol consumption to about 300 milligrams a day.

5. Reduce sugar consumption by about 40 percent to account for about 15 percent of total energy intake.
6. Reduce salt consumption by about 50 to 85 percent to approximately 3 grams a day.

The report also lists the following specific suggestions for changes in food selection and preparation:

1. Increase consumption of fruits and vegetables and whole grains.
2. Decrease consumption of meat and increase consumption of poultry and fish.
3. Decrease consumption of foods high in fat and partially substitute polyunsaturated fat for saturated fat.
4. Substitute non-fat milk for whole milk.
5. Decrease consumption of butterfat, eggs, and other high cholesterol sources.
6. Decrease consumption of sugar and foods high in sugar content.
7. Decrease consumption of salt and foods high in salt content.

Because the original *Dietary Goals* were not well-accepted by the beef, dairy, and egg industries, and criticized by some health organizations, the Committee revised them and published a second set in December 1977. The revised *Dietary Goals* for the United States adjusted some of the advice by "easing the cholesterol goal for premenopausal women, young children and the elderly in order to obtain the nutritional benefits of eggs in the diet." They also suggested to "choose meats, poultry and fish which will reduce saturated fat intake" and included that low-fat dairy products are acceptable. (The original goals only recommended non-fat milk.) They clarified the recommendation about sugar by specifying "refined and processed sugars be reduced to 10 percent [the original one said 15 percent] of total energy intake" while easing up on the salt recommendation from 3 grams to 5 grams per day. Two additional sections were added regarding obesity and alcohol.

In the Preface to the second edition of the *Dietary Goals*, Senator Charles Percy, ranking minority member of the Committee, and two colleagues were very critical of the recommendations. They pointed out that there is no consensus among health professionals that modifications in diet will improve health and suggest that "the failure of dietary change remains controversial and that science cannot at this time ensure that an altered diet will provide improved protection from certain killer diseases such as heart disease and cancer."

By 1980, the title *Dietary Goals for the United States* was changed to *Dietary Guidelines for Americans (DGA)*. Instead of a Senate Committee being in charge of the *DGA*, the responsibility was transferred to the Department of Health and Human Services (HHS) whose mission is "to enhance the health and well-being" of the nation, and the United States Department of Agriculture (USDA), whose mission is broader and includes providing "leadership on food, agriculture, natural resources, rural development, nutrition, and related issues." Both HHS and USDA support science-based research related to either health or our food supply and are the logical government departments to provide dietary advice for Americans.

Every five years, HHS and USDA follow Senator McGovern's lead and assemble a group of "leading thinkers in the area of nutritional health" to review the scientific evidence and either continue with the existing nutritional guidance or recommend revisions to the *DGA*. In 1977, McGovern reported that "six of the leading causes of death in the United States have been linked to our diet" and acknowledged that the government has an obligation to "lay the cornerstone for the building of better health for all Americans, through better nutrition." Almost four decades later, the leading causes of death are still linked to diet. All seven editions of *DGA* have included similar recommendations about limiting added sugar, saturated fat, and salt, moderation in alcohol consumption, and losing weight.

For the *2015 DGA*, an advisory committee of 15 "leading thinkers" began work in 2013 to review the scientific evidence about health and diet and wrote a technical report to the Secretaries of HHS and USDA. Throughout the process, the public was allowed to watch the advisory committee via webcam. The committee submitted their technical, 571-page *Scientific Report of the 2015 Dietary Guidelines Advisory Committee to the Secretaries* in January 2015. In their letter to the secretaries, the DGAC acknowledges that "few improvements in consumers' food choices have occurred in recent decades." The report points out that U.S. diets are still "low in vegetables, fruit, and whole grains and too high in calories, saturated fat, sodium, refined grains, and added sugars."

Over 29,000 comment letters were submitted to the secretaries of HHS and USDA during the 75-day public comment period that ended in May 2015. One of the strongest letters was from the Healthy Nation Coalition, who believe that the committee has developed a report that will "perpetuate the same ineffective federal nutrition guidance that has persisted for nearly four decades."

Is the government succeeding in building better health for all Americans and providing the basic rights to the people promised in the Constitution? Are HHS and USDA fulfilling their missions of using the best available scientific evidence for improving the health of Americans or are the accusations of the Healthy Nation Coalition justified? The two selections on the following pages present both sides of this issue.

YES ↵

Executive Summary

The 2015 Dietary Guidelines Advisory Committee (DGAC) was established jointly by the Secretaries of the U.S. Department of Health and Human Services (HHS) and the U.S. Department of Agriculture (USDA). The Committee was charged with examining the *Dietary Guidelines for Americans*, 2010 to determine topics for which new scientific evidence was likely to be available with the potential to inform the next edition of the Guidelines and to place its primary emphasis on the development of food-based recommendations that are of public health importance for Americans ages 2 years and older published since the last DGAC deliberations.

The 2015 DGAC's work was guided by two fundamental realities. First, about half of all American adults—117 million individuals—have one or more preventable, chronic diseases, and about two-thirds of U.S. adults—nearly 155 million individuals—are overweight or obese. These conditions have been highly prevalent for more than two decades. Poor dietary patterns, overconsumption of calories, and physical inactivity directly contribute to these disorders. Second, individual nutrition and physical activity behaviors and other health-related lifestyle behaviors are strongly influenced by personal, social, organizational, and environmental contexts and systems. Positive changes in individual diet and physical activity behaviors, and in the environmental contexts and systems that affect them, could substantially improve health outcomes.

Recognizing these realities, the Committee developed a conceptual model based on socio-ecological frameworks to guide its work and organized its evidence review to examine current status and trends in food and nutrient intakes, dietary patterns and health outcomes, individual lifestyle behavior change, food and physical activity environments and settings, and food sustainability and safety.

Topic-Specific Findings and Conclusions

Food and Nutrient Intakes, and Health: Current Status and Trends

The DGAC conducted data analyses to address a series of questions related to the current status and trends in the Nation's dietary intake. The questions focused on: intake of specific nutrients and food groups; food categories (i.e., foods as consumed) that contribute to intake; eating behaviors; and the composition of various dietary patterns shown to have health benefits. These topics were addressed using data from the What We Eat in America dietary survey, which is the dietary intake component of the ongoing National Health and Nutrition Examination Survey. Food pattern modeling using the USDA Food Pattern food groups also was used to address some questions. In addition, the DGAC examined the prevalence and trends of health conditions that may have a nutritional origin, or where the course of disease may be influenced by diet.

The DGAC found that several nutrients are underconsumed relative to the Estimated Average Requirement or Adequate Intake levels set by the Institute of Medicine (IOM) and the Committee characterized these as shortfall nutrients: vitamin A, vitamin D, vitamin E, vitamin C, folate, calcium, magnesium, fiber, and potassium. For adolescent and premenopausal females, iron also is a shortfall nutrient. Of the shortfall nutrients, calcium, vitamin D, fiber, and potassium also are classified as nutrients of public health concern because their underconsumption has been linked in the scientific literature to adverse health outcomes. Iron is included as a shortfall nutrient of public health concern for adolescent females and adult females who are premenopausal due to the increased risk of iron-deficiency in these groups. The DGAC also found that two nutrients—sodium and saturated fat—are overconsumed by the U.S. population relative to the Tolerable Upper Intake Level set by the IOM or other maximal standard and that the overconsumption poses health risks.

In comparison to recommended amounts in the USDA Food Patterns, the majority of the U.S. population has low intakes of key food groups that are important sources of the shortfall nutrients, including vegetables, fruits, whole grains, and dairy. Furthermore, population intake is too high for refined grains and added sugars. The data suggest cautious optimism about dietary intake of the youngest members of the U.S. population because many young children ages 2 to 5 years consume recommended amounts of fruit and dairy. However, a better understanding is needed on how to maintain and encourage good habits that are started early in life. Analysis of data on food categories, such as burgers, sandwiches, mixed dishes, desserts, and beverages, shows that the composition of many of these items could be improved so as to increase population intake of vegetables, whole grains, and other underconsumed food groups and to lower population intake of the nutrients sodium and saturated fat, and the food component refined grains. Improved beverage selections that limit or remove sugar-sweetened beverages and place limits on sweets and desserts would help lower intakes of the food component, added sugars.

The U.S. population purchases its food in a variety of locations, including supermarkets, convenience stores, schools, and the workplace. The DGAC found that although diet quality varies somewhat by the setting where food is obtained, overall, no matter where the food is obtained, the diet quality of the U.S. population does not meet recommendations for vegetables, fruit, dairy, or whole grains, and exceeds recommendations, leading to overconsumption, for the nutrients sodium and saturated fat and the food components refined grains, solid fats, and added sugars.

Obesity and many other health conditions with a nutritional origin are highly prevalent. The Nation must accelerate progress toward reducing the incidence and prevalence of overweight and obesity and chronic disease risk across the U.S. population throughout the lifespan and reduce the disparities in obesity and chronic disease rates that exist in the United States for certain ethnic and racial groups and for those with lower incomes.

The DGAC had enough descriptive information from existing research and data to model three dietary patterns and to examine their nutritional adequacy. These patterns are the Healthy U.S.-style Pattern, the Healthy Mediterranean-style Pattern, and the Healthy Vegetarian Pattern. These patterns include the components of a dietary pattern associated with health benefits.

Dietary Patterns, Foods and Nutrients, and Health Outcomes

A major goal of the DGAC was to describe the common characteristics of healthy diets, and the Committee focused on research examining dietary patterns because the totality of diet—the combinations and quantities in which foods and nutrients are consumed—may have synergistic and cumulative effects on health and disease. The Committee focused on providing a qualitative description of healthy dietary patterns based on scientific evidence for several health outcomes.

The DGAC found remarkable consistency in the findings and implications across its conclusion statements for the questions examining dietary patterns and various health outcomes. When reviewing the evidence, the Committee attempted to adhere to the language used by the study authors in describing food groupings. There was variability across the food groupings, and this was particularly apparent in the meat group. For example, "total meat" may have been defined as "meat, sausage, fish, and eggs," "red meat, processed meat, and poultry," or various other combinations of meat. Similarly, "vegetables" seemed to most often exclude potatoes, but some studies included potatoes, yet those that mentioned potatoes rarely provided information on how the potatoes were consumed (e.g., fried versus baked). When reported in the studies, the Committee considered these definitions in their review. However, the Committee provided a general label for the food groupings in its conclusion statements.

The overall body of evidence examined by the 2015 DGAC identifies that a healthy dietary pattern is higher in vegetables, fruits, whole grains, low- or non-fat dairy, seafood, legumes, and nuts; moderate in alcohol (among adults); lower in red and processed meat; and low in sugar-sweetened foods and drinks and refined grains. Vegetables and fruit are the only characteristics of the diet that were consistently identified in every conclusion statement across the health outcomes. Whole grains were identified slightly less consistently compared to vegetables and fruits, but were identified in every conclusion with moderate to strong evidence. For studies with limited evidence, grains were not as consistently defined and/or they were not identified as a key characteristic. Low- or non-fat dairy, seafood, legumes, nuts, and alcohol were identified as beneficial characteristics of the diet for some, but not all, outcomes. For conclusions with moderate to strong evidence, higher intake of red and processed meats was identified as detrimental compared to lower intake. Higher consumption of sugar-sweetened foods and beverages as well as refined grains was identified as detrimental in almost all conclusion statements with moderate to strong evidence.

Regarding alcohol, the Committee confirmed several conclusions of the 2010 DGAC, including that moderate alcohol intake can be a component of a healthy dietary pattern, and that if alcohol is consumed, it should be consumed in moderation and only by adults. However, it is not recommended that anyone begin drinking or drink more frequently on the basis of potential health benefits, because moderate alcohol intake also is associated with increased risk of violence, drowning, and injuries from falls and motor vehicle crashes. Women should be aware of a moderately increased risk of breast cancer even with moderate alcohol intake. In addition, there are many circumstances in which people should not drink alcohol, including during pregnancy. Because of the substantial evidence clearly demonstrating the health benefits of breastfeeding, occasionally consuming an alcoholic drink does not warrant stopping breastfeeding. However, women who are breastfeeding should be very cautious about drinking alcohol, if they choose to drink at all.

Following a dietary pattern associated with reduced risk of CVD, overweight, and obesity also will have positive health benefits beyond these categories of health outcomes. Thus, the U.S. population should be encouraged and guided to consume dietary patterns that are rich in vegetables, fruit, whole grains, seafood, legumes, and nuts; moderate in low- and non-fat dairy products and alcohol (among adults); lower in red and processed meat; and low in sugar-sweetened foods and beverages and refined grains. These dietary patterns can be achieved in many ways and should be tailored to the individual's biological and medical needs as well as socio-cultural preferences.

The dietary pattern characteristics being recommended by the 2015 DGAC reaffirm the dietary pattern characteristics recommended by the 2010 DGAC. Additionally, these characteristics align with recommendations from other groups, including the American Institute for Cancer Research (AICR) and the American Heart Association (AHA). The majority of evidence considered by the Committee focused on dietary patterns consumed in adulthood. Very little evidence examined dietary patterns during childhood. However, the healthy dietary pattern components described above also apply to children and

are reaffirmed with the USDA Food Patterns, which are designed to meet nutrient needs across the lifespan.

Individual Diet and Physical Activity Behavior Change

The individual is at the innermost core of the social-ecological model. In order for policy recommendations such as the *Dietary Guidelines for Americans* to be fully implemented, motivating and facilitating behavioral change at the individual level is required. This chapter suggests a number of promising behavior change strategies that can be used to favorably affect a range of health-related outcomes and to enhance the effectiveness of interventions. These include reducing screen time, reducing the frequency of eating out at fast food restaurants, increasing frequency of family shared meals, and self-monitoring of diet and body weight as well as effective food labeling to target healthy food choices. These strategies complement comprehensive lifestyle interventions and nutrition counseling by qualified nutrition professionals.

For this approach to work, it will be essential that the food environments in communities available to the U.S. population, particularly to low-income individuals, facilitate access to healthy and affordable food choices that respect their cultural preferences. Similarly, food and calorie label education should be designed to be understood by audiences with low health literacy, some of which may have additional English language fluency limitations. Although viable approaches are available now, additional research is necessary to improve the scientific foundation for more effective guidelines on individual-level behavior change for all individuals living in the United States, taking into account the social, economic, and cultural environments in which they live.

The evidence reviewed in this chapter also indicates that the social, economic, and cultural context in which individuals live may facilitate or hinder their ability to choose and consume dietary patterns that are consistent with the Dietary Guidelines. Specifically, household food insecurity hinders the access to healthy diets for millions of Americans. In addition, immigrants are at high risk of losing the healthier dietary patterns characteristic of their cultural background as they acculturate into mainstream America. Furthermore, preventive nutrition services that take into account the social determinants of health are largely unavailable in the U.S. health system to systematically address nutrition-related health problems, including overweight and obesity, cardiovascular disease, type 2 diabetes, and other health outcomes.

This chapter calls for: a) stronger Federal policies to help prevent household food insecurity and to help families to cope with food insecurity if it develops, b) food and nutrition assistance programs to take into account the risk that immigrants have of giving up their healthier dietary habits soon after arriving in the United States, and c) efforts to provide all individuals living in the United States with the environments, knowledge, and tools needed to implement effective individual- or family-level behavioral change strategies to improve the quality of their diets and reduce sedentary behaviors. These goals will require changes at all levels of the social-ecological model through coordinated efforts among health care and social and food systems from the national to the local level.

Food Environment and Settings

Environmental and policy approaches are needed to complement individual-based efforts to improve diet and reduce obesity and other diet-related chronic diseases. These approaches have the potential for broad and sustained impact at the population level because they can become incorporated into organizational structures and systems and lead to alterations in sociocultural and societal norms. Both policy and environmental changes also can help reduce disparities by improving access to and availability of healthy food in underserved neighborhoods and communities. Federal nutrition assistance programs, in particular, play a vital role in achieving this objective through access to affordable foods that help millions of Americans meet Dietary Guidelines recommendations.

The DGAC focused on physical environments (settings) in which food is available. Its aim was to better understand the impact of the food environment to promote or hinder healthy eating in these settings and to identify the most effective evidence-based diet-related approaches and policies to improve diet and weight status. The DGAC focused on four settings—community food access, child care, schools and worksites—and their relationships to dietary intake and quality and weight status.

The DGAC found moderate and promising evidence that multi-component obesity prevention approaches implemented in child care settings, schools, and worksites improve weight-related outcomes; strong to moderate evidence that school and worksite policies are associated with improved dietary intake; and moderate evidence that multi-component school-based and worksite approaches increase vegetable and fruit consumption. For the questions on community food access addressing the relationship between food retail settings and dietary intake and quality and weight status, the evidence was too limited or insufficient to assign grades. To reduce the disparity gaps that currently exist in low resource and underserved communities, more solution-oriented strategies need to be implemented and evaluated on ways to increase access to and procurement of healthy affordable foods and beverages, and also to reduce access to energy-dense, nutrient-poor foods and beverages. Although several innovative approaches are taking place now throughout the country, they generally lack adequate evaluation efforts.

The Committee's findings revealed the power of multi-component approaches over single component interventions. For obesity prevention, effective multi-component interventions incorporated both nutrition and physical activity using a variety of strategies, such as environmental policies to improve the availability and provision of healthy foods and beverages; increasing opportunities for physical activity; increased parent engagement (in child care and school settings); and educational approaches, such as a school nutrition curriculum. For multi-component dietary interventions (e.g., to increase consumption of vegetables and fruit) the most effective strategies included nutrition education, parent engagement (in school and child care settings) and environmental modifications (e.g., policies for nutrition standards, food service changes, point of purchase information).

Collaborative partnerships and strategic efforts are needed to translate this evidence into action. Further work on restructuring the environment to facilitate healthy eating and physical activity, especially in high risk populations, is needed to advance evidence-based solutions that can be scaled up.

Food Sustainability and Safety

Access to sufficient, nutritious, and safe food is an essential element of food security for the U.S. population. A sustainable diet ensures this access for both the current population and future generations.

The major findings regarding sustainable diets were that a diet higher in plant-based foods, such as vegetables, fruits, whole grains, legumes, nuts, and seeds, and lower in calories and animal-based foods, is more health promoting and is associated with less environmental impact than is the current U.S. diet. This pattern of eating can be achieved through a variety of dietary patterns, including the Healthy U.S.-style Pattern, the Healthy Mediterranean-style Pattern, and the Healthy Vegetarian Pattern. All of these dietary patterns are aligned with lower environmental impacts and provide options that can be adopted by the U.S. population. Current evidence shows that the average U.S. diet has a larger environmental impact in terms of increased greenhouse gas emissions, land use, water use, and energy use, compared to the above dietary patterns.

This is because the current U.S. population intake of animal-based foods is higher and plant-based foods are lower, than proposed in these three dietary patterns. Of note is that no food groups need to be eliminated completely to improve sustainability outcomes over the current status.

A moderate amount of seafood is an important component of two of three of these dietary patterns, and has demonstrated health benefits. The seafood industry is in the midst of rapid expansion to meet worldwide demand. The collapse of some fisheries due to overfishing in the past decades has raised concern about the ability to produce a safe and affordable supply. In addition, concern has been raised about the safety and nutrient content of farm-raised versus wild-caught seafood. To supply enough seafood to support meeting dietary recommendations, both farm-raised and wild caught seafood will be needed. The review of the evidence demonstrated, in the species evaluated, that farm-raised seafood has as much or more EPA and DHA per serving as wild caught. It should be noted that low-trophic seafood, such as catfish and crawfish, regardless of whether wild caught or farm-raised seafood, have less EPA and DHA per serving than high-trophic seafood, such as salmon and trout.

Regarding contaminants, for the majority of wild caught and farmed species, neither the risks of mercury nor organic pollutants outweigh the health benefits of seafood consumption. Consistent evidence demonstrated that wild caught fisheries that have been managed sustainably have remained stable over the past several decades; however, wild caught fisheries are fully exploited and their continuing productivity will require careful management nationally and internationally to avoid long-term collapse. Expanded supply of seafood nationally and internationally will depend upon the increase of farm-raised seafood worldwide.

The impact of food production, processing, and consumption on environmental sustainability is an area of research that is rapidly evolving. As further research is conducted and best practices are evaluated, additional evidence will inform both supply-side participants and consumers on how best to shift behaviors locally, nationally, and globally to support sustainable diets. Linking health, dietary guidance, and the environment will promote human health and the sustainability of natural resources and ensure current and long-term food security.

In regard to food safety, updated and previously unexamined areas of food safety were studied. Currently, strong evidence shows that consumption of coffee within the moderate range (3 to 5 cups per day or up to 400 mg/d

caffeine) is not associated with increased long-term health risks among healthy individuals. In fact, consistent evidence indicates that coffee consumption is associated with reduced risk of type 2 diabetes and cardiovascular disease in adults. Moreover, moderate evidence shows a protective association between caffeine intake and risk of Parkinson's disease. Therefore, moderate coffee consumption can be incorporated into a healthy dietary pattern, along with other healthful behaviors. However, it should be noted that coffee as it is normally consumed can contain added calories from cream, milk, and added sugars. Care should be taken to minimize the amount of calories from added sugars and high-fat dairy or dairy substitutes added to coffee.

The marketing and availability of high-caffeine beverages and products is on the rise. Unfortunately, only limited evidence is currently available to ascertain the safety of high caffeine intake (greater than 400 mg/day for adults and undetermined for children and adolescents) that may occur with rapid consumption of large-sized energy drinks. Limited data suggest adverse health outcomes, such as caffeine toxicity and cardiovascular events. Concern is heightened when caffeine is combined with alcoholic beverages. Limited or no consumption of high-caffeine drinks, or other products with high amounts of caffeine, is advised for children and adolescents. Energy drinks with high levels of caffeine and alcoholic beverages should not be consumed together, either mixed together or consumed at the same sitting.

The DGAC also examined the food additive aspartame. At the level that the U.S. population consumes aspartame, it appears to be safe. However, some uncertainty continues about increased risk of hematopoietic cancer in men, indicating a need for more research.

Individual behaviors along with sound government policies and responsible private sector practices are all needed to reduce foodborne illnesses. To that end, the DGAC updated the established recommendations for handling foods at home.

Cross-cutting Topics of Public Health Importance

The *2010 Dietary Guidelines* included guidance on sodium, saturated fat, and added sugars, and the 2015 DGAC determined that a reexamination of the evidence on these topics was necessary to determine whether revisions to the guidance were warranted. These topics were considered to be of public health importance because each has been associated with negative health outcomes when overconsumed. Additionally, the Committee acknowledged that a potential unintended consequence of a recommendation on added sugars might be that consumers and manufacturers replace added sugars with low-calorie sweeteners. As a result, the Committee also examined evidence on low-calorie sweeteners to inform statements on this topic.

The DGAC encourages the consumption of healthy dietary patterns that are low in saturated fat, added sugars, and sodium. The goals for the general population are: less than 2,300 mg dietary sodium per day (or age-appropriate Dietary Reference Intake amount), less than 10 percent of total calories from saturated fat per day, and a maximum of 10 percent of total calories from added sugars per day.

Sodium, saturated fat, and added sugars are not intended to be reduced in isolation, but as a part of a healthy dietary pattern that is balanced, as appropriate, in calories. Rather than focusing purely on reduction, emphasis should also be placed on replacement and shifts in food intake and eating patterns. Sources of saturated fat should be replaced with unsaturated fat, particularly polyunsaturated fatty acids. Similarly, added sugars should be reduced in the diet and not replaced with low-calorie sweeteners, but rather with healthy options, such as water in place of sugar-sweetened beverages. For sodium, emphasis should be placed on expanding industry efforts to reduce the sodium content of foods and helping consumers understand how to flavor unsalted foods with spices and herbs.

Reducing sodium, saturated fat, and added sugars can be accomplished and is more attainable by eating a healthy dietary pattern. For all three of these components of the diet, policies and programs at local, state, and national levels in both the private and public sector are necessary to support reduction efforts. Similarly, the Committee supports efforts in labeling and other campaigns to increase consumer awareness and understanding of sodium, saturated fats, and added sugars in foods and beverages. The Committee encourages the food industry to continue reformulating and making changes to certain foods to improve their nutrition profile. Examples of such actions include lowering sodium and added sugars content, achieving better saturated fat to polyunsaturated fat ratio, and reducing portion sizes in retail settings (restaurants, food outlets, and public venues, such as professional sports stadiums and arenas). The Committee also encourages the food industry to market these improved products to consumers.

Physical Activity

This chapter provides strong evidence supporting the importance of regular physical activity for health promotion and disease prevention in the U.S. population. Physical activity is important for all people—children, adolescents, adults, older adults, women during pregnancy and the postpartum period, and individuals with disabilities. The findings further provide guidance on the dose of physical activity needed across the lifecycle to realize these significant health benefits.

Future Physical Activity Guidelines Advisory Committees will be asked to carefully review the most recent evidence so that the Federal government can fully update the *2008 Physical Activity Guidelines for Americans*. Given the exceedingly low physical activity participation rates in this country, it will be critically important for the next Committee to identify proven strategies and approaches to increase population-level physical activity across the lifespan.

Integrating the Evidence

The research base reviewed by the 2015 DGAC provides clear evidence that persistent, prevalent, preventable health problems, notably overweight and obesity, cardiovascular disease, type 2 diabetes and certain cancers, have adversely affected the health of the U.S. public for decades and raise the urgency for immediate attention and bold action. Evidence points to specific areas of current food and nutrient concerns and it pinpoints the characteristics of healthy dietary and physical activity patterns that can reduce chronic disease risk, promote healthy weight status, and foster good health across the lifespan. In addition, research evidence is converging to show that healthy dietary patterns also are more sustainable and associated with more favorable health as well as environmental outcomes.

Effective models of "what works" to promote lifestyle behavior change exist. While they can be improved, especially in terms of our capacity for scaling-up in community and health care settings, the evidence to date can be used to guide programs and services for individuals and families. They also can be used to assist the public and private sectors and communities in facilitating innovative environmental change to promote the population's health.

It will take concerted, bold actions on the part of individuals, families, communities, industry, and government to achieve and maintain the healthy diet patterns and the levels of physical activity needed to promote the health of the U.S. population. These actions will require a paradigm shift to an environment in which population health is a national priority and where individuals and organizations, private business, and communities work together to achieve a population-wide "culture of health" in which healthy lifestyle choices are easy, accessible, affordable and normative—both at home and away from home. In such a culture, health care and public health professionals also would embrace a new leadership role in prevention, convey the importance of lifestyle behavior change to their patients/clients, set standards for prevention in their own facilities, and help patients/clients in accessing evidence-based and effective nutrition and comprehensive lifestyle services and programs.

The **2015 Dietary Guidelines Advisory Committee** was composed of 14 members.

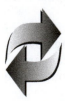

Adele Hite

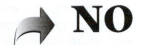

Healthy Nation Coalition's Letter to the Secretaries of Health and Human Services and the United States Department of Agriculture Regarding the *Scientific Report of the 2015 Dietary Guidelines Advisory Committee*

Secretary Sylvia Mathews Burwell and Secretary Tom Vilsack United States Department of Health and United States Department of Agriculture Human Services 1400 Independence Ave., SW 200 Independence Ave., SW Washington, D.C. 20250 Washington, D.C. 20201

Dear Secretary Burwell and Secretary Vilsack, As the Dietary Guidelines Advisory Committee (DGAC) submits its Report to your departments, we write to express concern about the state of federal nutrition policy and its long history of failure in preventing the increase of chronic disease in America. The tone, tenor, and content of the DGAC's public meetings to date suggest that the 2015 *Dietary Guidelines for Americans* (*DGA*) will perpetuate the same ineffective federal nutrition guidance that has persisted for nearly four decades, but has not achieved positive health outcomes for the American public.

We urge you to adhere to the initial Congressional mandate that the *DGA* act as "nutritional and dietary information and guidelines *for the general public*" and are "based on the *preponderance of the scientific and medical knowledge* which is current at the time the report is prepared" (emphasis added).[1]

Below we lay out specific objections to the *DGA*:

- they have contributed to the increase of chronic diseases;
- they have not provided guidance compatible with adequate essential nutrition;
- they represent a narrow approach to food and nutrition inconsistent with the nation's diverse cultures, ethnicities, and socioeconomic classes;

- they are based on weak and inconclusive scientific data;
- and they have expanded their purpose to issues outside their original mandate.

As you prepare to consider the 2015 DGAC's recommendations next year, we urge you to fulfill your duty to create the dietary foundation for good health for all Americans by focusing on adequate essential nutrition from whole, nourishing foods, rather than replicating guidance that is clearly failing.

The DGA have contributed to the rapid rise of chronic disease in America.

In 1977, dietary recommendations (called *Dietary Goals*) created by George McGovern's Senate Select Committee advised Americans to decrease intake of saturated fat and cholesterol from animal products and increase their consumption of grains, cereal products, and vegetable oils in order to reduce risk of chronic disease. These *Goals* were institutionalized as the *DGA* in 1980, and all *DGA* since then have asserted this same guidance. During this time period, the prevalence of heart failure and stroke has increased dramatically.[2] Rates of new cases of all cancers have risen. Most notably, rates of diabetes have tripled. In addition, although body weight is not itself a measure of health, rates of overweight and obesity have increased dramatically. In all cases, the health divide between black and white Americans has persisted or worsened.

While some argue that Americans have not followed the *DGA*, all available data show Americans have shifted their diets in the direction of the recommendations: consuming more grains, cereals, and vegetable oils, while consuming less saturated fat and cholesterol from whole foods such as meat, butter, eggs, and full-fat milk. Whether or not the public has followed all aspects of *DGA* guidance does not absolve the U.S. Departments of Agriculture (USDA) and Health and Human Services (DHHS) from ensuring that the dietary guidance provided to Americans first and foremost does no harm.

The DGA fail to provide guidance compatible with essential nutrition needs.

The 1977 *Dietary Goals* marked a radical shift in federal dietary guidance. Before then, federal dietary recommendations focused on foods Americans were encouraged to eat in order to acquire adequate nutrition; the *DGA* focus on specific food components to limit or avoid in order to prevent chronic disease. The *DGA* have not only failed to prevent chronic disease, in some cases, they have failed to provide basic guidance consistent with nutritionally adequate diets.

- . . . 2010 *DGA* for sodium were incompatible with potassium guidelines and with nutritionally adequate diets in general.
- Choline was recognized as an essential nutrient in 1998, after the *DGA* were first created. It is crucial for healthy prenatal brain development. Current choline intakes are far below adequate levels, and choline deficiency is thought to contribute to liver disease, atherosclerosis and neurological disorders. Eggs and meat, two foods restricted by current *DGA* recommendations, are important sources of choline. Guidance that limits their consumption thus restricts intake of adequate choline.
- In young children, the reduced fat diet recommended by the *DGA* has also been linked to lower intakes of important essential nutrients, including calcium, zinc, and iron.

Following USDA and DHHS guidance should not put the most vulnerable members of the population at risk for nutritional inadequacy. *DGA* recommendations should be emphasizing whole foods that provide essential nutrition, rather than employing a reductionist approach based on single food components to exclude these foods from the diet.

The DGA's narrow approach to food and health is inappropriate for a diverse population.

McGovern's 1977 recommendations were based on research and food patterns from middle class Caucasian American populations. Since then, diversity in America has increased, while the *DGA* have remained unchanged. *DGA* recommendations based on majority-white, high socioeconomic status datasets have been especially inappropriate for minority and low-income populations. When following *DGA* recommendations, African American adults gain *more* weight than their Caucasian counterparts, and low-income individuals have *increased* rates of diabetes, hypertension, and high cholesterol. Longstanding differences in environmental, genetic and metabolic characteristics may mean recommendations that are merely ineffective in preventing chronic disease in white, middle class Americans are downright detrimental to the long-term health of black and low-income Americans.

The *DGA* plant-based diet not only ignores human biological diversity, it ignores the diversity of American foodways. *DGA* guidance rejects foods that are part of the cultural heritage of many Americans and indicates that traditional foods long considered to be important to a nourishing diet should be modified, restricted, or eliminated altogether: ghee (clarified butter) for Indian Americans; chorizo and eggs for Latino Americans; greens with fatback for Southern and African Americans; liver pâtés for Jewish and Eastern European Americans.

Furthermore, recommendations to prevent chronic disease that focus solely on plant-based diets is a blatant misuse of public health authority that has stymied efforts of researchers, academics, healthcare professionals, and insurance companies to pursue other dietary approaches adapted to specific individuals and diverse populations, specifically, the treatment of diabetes with reduced-carbohydrate diets that do not restrict saturated fat. In contradiction of federal law, the *DGA* have had the effect of limiting the scope of medical nutrition research sponsored by the federal government to protocols in line with *DGA* guidance.

The DGA are not based on the preponderance of current scientific and medical knowledge.

The science behind the current *DGA* recommendations is untested and inconsistent. Scientific disagreements over the weakness of the evidence used to create the 1977 *Dietary Goals* have never been settled. Recent published accounts have raised questions about whether the scientific process has been undermined by politics, bias, institutional inertia, and the influence of interested industries.

Significant scientific controversy continues to surround specific recommendations that:

1) *Dietary saturated fat increases the risk of heart disease:* Two recent meta-analyses concluded there is no strong scientific support for dietary recommendations that restrict saturated fat. Studies cited by the 2010 *DGAC Report* demonstrate that in some populations, lowering dietary saturated fat actually worsens some biomarkers related to heart disease.

2) *Dietary cholesterol increases the risk of heart disease:* Due to a lack of evidence, nearly all other Western nations have dropped their limits on dietary cholesterol. In 2013, a joint panel of the American Heart Association and the American College of Cardiology did the same.

3) *Polyunsaturated vegetable oils reduce the risk of heart disease and should be consumed as the primary source of dietary fat:* Recent research renews concerns raised in response to the 1977 *Dietary Goals* that diets high in the omega-6 fatty acids present in vegetable oils may actually increase risk of chronic disease or death.

4) *A diet high in carbohydrate, including whole grains, reduces risk of chronic disease:* Clinical trials have demonstrated that diets with lower carbohydrate content improve risk factors related to heart disease and diabetes. Janet King, Chair of the 2005 DGAC, has stated that "evidence has begun to accumulate suggesting that a lower intake of carbohydrate may be better for cardiovascular health."

5) *A low-sodium diet reduces risk of chronic disease:* A 2013 Institute of Medicine report concludes there is insufficient evidence to recommend reducing sodium intake to the very low levels set by the *DGA* for African-Americans of any age and adults over 50.

In all of these cases, contradictory evidence has been ignored in favor of maintaining outdated recommendations that have failed to prevent chronic disease.

More generally, "intervention studies, where diets following the *Dietary Guidelines* are fed long-term to human volunteers, do not exist," and food patterns recommended by the *DGA* "have not been specifically tested for health benefits." The observational research being used for much of the current DGAC activities may suggest possible associations between diet and disease, but such hypotheses must then be evaluated through rigorous testing. Applying premature findings to public health policy without adequate testing may have resulted in unintended negative health consequences for many Americans.

The DGA have overstepped their original purpose.

The *DGA* were created to provide nutrition information to all Americans. However, the current 112-page *DGA*, with 29 recommendations, are considered too complex for the general public and are directed instead at policymakers and healthcare professionals, contradicting their Congressional mandate.

Federal dietary guidance now goes far beyond nutrition information. It tells Americans how much they should weigh and how to lose weight, even recommending that each American write down everything that is eaten on a daily basis. This focus on obesity and weight loss has contributed to extensive and unrecognized "collateral damage": fat-shaming, eating disorders, discrimination, and poor health from restrictive food habits. At the same time, researchers at the Centers for Disease Control have shown that overweight and obese people are often as healthy as their "normal" weight counterparts. Guidance related to body weight should meet individual health requirements and be given by a trained healthcare practitioner, not be dictated by federal policy.

The *DGA* began as an unmandated consumer information booklet. They are now a powerful political document that regulates a vast array of federal programs and services, dictates nationwide nutrition standards, influences agricultural policies and health-related research, and directs how food manufacturers target consumer demand. Despite their broad scope, the *DGA* are subject to no evaluation or accountability process based on health outcomes. Such an evaluation would demonstrate that they have failed to fulfill their original goal: to decrease rates of chronic disease in America.

Despite this failure, current DGAC proceedings point to an expansion of their mission into sustainable agriculture and environmental concerns. While these are important issues, they demonstrate continued "mission creep" of the *DGA*. The current narrow *DGA* focus on plant-based nutrition suggests a similarly biased approach will be taken to environmental issues, disregarding centuries of traditional farming practices in which livestock play a central role in maintaining soil quality and ecological balance. Instead of warning Americans not to eat eggs and meat due to concerns about saturated fat, cholesterol, and obesity, it is foreseeable that similar warnings will be given, but for "environmental" reasons. This calls for an immediate refocusing of the purpose of the *DGA* and a return to nutritional basics.

Solution: A return to essential nutrition guidance

As our nation confronts soaring medical costs and declining health, we can no longer afford to perpetuate guidelines that have failed to fulfill their purpose. Until and unless better scientific support is secured for recommendations regarding the prevention of chronic disease, the *DGA* should focus on food-based guidance that assists Americans in acquiring adequate essential nutrition.

Shifting the focus to food-based guidance for adequate essential nutrition will create *DGA* that:

- **are based on universally accepted and scientifically sound nutritional principles:** Although more knowledge is needed, the science of essential nutrient requirements is firmly grounded in clinical trials and healthcare practice, as well as observational studies.
- **apply to all Americans:** Essential nutrition requirements are appropriate for everyone. Lack of essential nutrients will lead without exception to diseases of deficiency.
- **include traditionally nourishing foods:** A wide variety of eating patterns can provide adequate essential nutrition; no nourishing dietary approaches or cultural food traditions would be excluded or discouraged.
- **expand opportunities for research:** With dietary guidance focused on adequate essential nutrition, researchers, healthcare providers, and insurance companies may pursue dietary programs and practices tailored to individual risk factors and diverse communities without running afoul of the *DGA* and while ensuring that basic nutrition needs are always met.
- **direct attention towards health and well-being:** Focus will be directed away from intermediate markers, such as weight, which may be beyond individual control, do not consistently predict health outcomes, and are best dealt with in a healthcare setting.

- **are clear, concise, and useful to the public:** Americans will be able to understand and apply such guidance to their own dietary patterns, minimizing the current widespread confusion and resentment resulting from federal dietary guidance that is poorly grounded in science.

It is the duty of USDA and DHHS leadership to end the use of controversial, unsuccessful and discriminatory dietary recommendations. USDA and DHHS leadership must refuse to accept any *DGA* that fail to establish federal nutrition policy based on the foundation of good health: adequate essential nutrition from wholesome, nourishing foods. It is time to create *DGA* that work for all Americans.

On behalf of the undersigned,
Adele Hite, MPH RD Director Healthy Nation Coalition Durham, NC adele.hite@gmail.com

Notes

1. **101st Congress,** *National Nutrition Monitoring and Related Research Act of* 1990, 1990.
2. **National Heart, Lung, and Blood Institute,** *Morbidity and Mortality: 2007 Chart Book on Cardiovascular, Lung, and Blood Diseases* (Bethesda, MD: U.S. Department of Health and Human Services, National Institutes of Health, 2007), http://www.nhlbi.nih.gov/resources/docs/07-chtbk.pdf.

ADELE HITE is a registered dietitian and director and co-founder of Healthy Nation Coalition. Her area of research focuses on a critical examination of the U.S. *Dietary Guidelines for Americans.*

EXPLORING THE ISSUE

Will the Government's Dietary Guidance Improve Health?

Critical Thinking and Reflection

1. Compare what is published in the actual *Dietary Guidelines for Americans (DGA) 2015* (*DGA 2015*) to the recommendations from the technical *Scientific Report of the 2015 Dietary Guidelines Advisory Committee*. Explain the similarities and differences in the two.
2. Review the actual *DGA 2015* available at http://health.gov/dietaryguidelines/. Explain how the *DGA 2015* include or ignore suggestions from the Healthy Nation Coalition's comment letter to the Secretaries of HHS and USDA.
3. The rates of cardiovascular disease, obesity, type 2 diabetes, and certain types of cancer have increased over the last 40 years and health care expenditures have increased since the introduction of the *Dietary Goals* in 1977. In 2015, the American government spent over a trillion dollars on health care, or 27 percent of total government expenditures, which is much higher than the health care expenditures of any other developed country in the world. Write a letter to your U.S. senator explaining how increases in appropriation to nutrition programs are needed to improve the health of Americans. In your letter, describe specific programs that you believe will improve the nation's health and nutrition status.
4. The Food and Agriculture Organization of the United Nations lists food guides from countries throughout the world, which is available at http://www.fao.org/nutrition/nutrition-education/food-dietary-guidelines/en/. Using the information from the website, prepare a table comparing the food guides of 8 to 10 countries.
5. List the negative things that the DGAC describes about the nutrition and health status of Americans. Select one item from your list and prepare a two-page educational brochure for the general public that describes the nutrition or health status you selected and strategies to ameliorate it.

Is There Common Ground?

Both the Dietary Guidelines Advisory Committee (DGAC) and Adele Hite, representing a coalition of over 600 health advocates from 45 states, acknowledge that chronic diseases such diabetes, cardiovascular disease, and obesity continue to be major problems among Americans. The DGAC and Hite both want to create policies that will improve the health of Americans and agree that changes are needed. So the goals of both groups are to improve the nation's health but they vary in their approaches.

Hite contends that the government's 35 years of nutrition guidance has contributed to the increase of chronic diseases and that the guidance is not based on scientific evidence. The DGAC uses the socio-ecological model and believes that it will require a paradigm shift and that the entire nation needs to work harder to make changes and the national priority needs to focus on improving health.

Additional Resources

Appel LJ, Lichtenstein AH, Callahan EA, Sinaiko A, Van horn L, Whitsel L. Reducing sodium intake in children: A public health investment. *J Clin Hypertens*. 2015;17(9):657–62.

Banfield EC, Liu Y, Davis JS, Chang S, Frazier-wood AC. Poor adherence to US dietary guidelines for children and adolescents in the National Health and Nutrition Examination Survey population. *J Acad Nutr Diet*. 2015. doi: http://dx.doi.org/10.1016/j.jand.2015.08.010.

Hawkes C, Haddad L, Udomkesmalee E. The Global Nutrition Report 2015: What we need to do to advance progress in addressing malnutrition in all its forms. *Public Health Nutr*. 2015;18(17):3067.

Hite AH, Feinman RD, Guzman GE, Satin M, Schoenfeld PA, Wood RJ. In the face of contradictory evidence:

Report of the Dietary Guidelines for Americans Committee. *Nutrition.* 2010;26(10):915–24.

Kim SA, Blanck HM, Cradock A, Gortmaker S. Networking to improve nutrition policy research. *Prev Chronic Dis.* 2015;12:E148.

Mcnamara DJ. The fifty year rehabilitation of the egg. *Nutrients.* 2015;7(10):8716–22.

Internet References . . .

Food and Agriculture Organization of the United Nations

www.fao.org/home/en/

Healthy Nation Coalition

forahealthynation.org

The U.S. Office of Disease Prevention and Health Promotion

health.gov

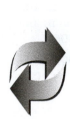

Selected, Edited, and with Issue Framing Material by:
Janet M. Colson, *Middle Tennessee State University*

ISSUE

Are the 2015 *Dietary Guidelines* Based on Sound Science?

YES: Barbara E. Millen, from "Part C: Methodology" and "Appendix E-4 NHANES Data Used in DGAC Data Analysis," *Scientific Report of the 2015 Dietary Guidelines Advisory Committee* (2015)

NO: Edward Archer, Gregory A. Hand, Steven N. Blair, from, "Validity of U.S. Nutritional Surveillance: National Health and Nutrition Examination Survey Caloric Energy Intake Data, 1971−2010" PLOS ONE | www.plosone.org (2013)

Learning Outcomes

After reading this issue, you will be able to:

- Outline the selection process and nutrition health expertise of the Dietary Guidelines Advisory Committee (DGAC) members.
- List three scientific approaches used by the DGAC to review the literature regarding links between dietary intake and health status.
- Explain why the DGAC used results from the National Health and Nutrition Examination Survey (NHANES) and What We Eat in America (WWEIA) to establish dietary intakes.
- Describe the steps Archer and colleagues used to validate the NHANES self-reported energy intakes and results of their study.

ISSUE SUMMARY

YES: The 2015 DGAC titled their report as being "Scientific" yet acknowledge that most food and nutrient intakes used to formulate the report are based on 24-hour recalls from the NHANES and WWEIA data. The DGAC also point out that the "strengths and shortcomings of these dietary assessment methods have been discussed over time and that no assessment method is perfect."

NO: Archer and colleagues criticize the methods used by NHANES to collect dietary data and question the validity of the data collected using the 24-hour recall method. They validated the self-reported energy intakes of over 60,000 NHANES participants and found that the majority of people underreport energy intake and consider the NHANES energy intake data physically implausible.

Methods used to describe the dietary intake of populations have been criticized by the scientific community for years and was pointed out by nutrition and health experts in 1977, when the original *Dietary Goals* were published. According to the preface of the *Dietary Goals for the United States—Second Edition*, dietary data used to describe the U.S. diet were derived from three sources:

1) Food disappearance: Food that disappears into civilian food consumption—sometimes referred to as the U.S. per capita food supply. . . . The nutritive value of these amounts of foods is estimated by the Agricultural Research Service of USDA.

2) Household food consumption: These food consumption data are collected every ten years or so from representative samples of households across the country by the Agricultural Research Service. These data are foods used by households over a seven-day period in terms of food brought into the kitchen—as purchased, or obtained from home gardens, or as gifts or pay. Nutritive values of these amounts of foods are estimated and compared to the RDA's for family members.

3) Food intake or food actually eaten by individuals: These data are usually collected by recall methods of a day or a period of a few days. They include amounts of foods eaten at home or away from home.

The percentages of energy from carbohydrate, protein, and fat described in the *Dietary Goals* were estimated based on the USDA's 1974 food disappearance data. The limitations of using this type of data to describe the nutritional status of the nation have been recognized for years. Senator Charles Percy, ranking minority member of the U.S. Senate Committee who introduced the *Dietary Goals for the United States*, and two colleagues were very critical of the methods used to gather dietary data. In the Forward of the second edition of the *Dietary Goals* they point out:

> Finally, [we] want to emphasize the limitations, acknowledged in this edition, in setting goals and food selection recommendations on the basis of food disappearance data, because of the difference between disappearance data, household food consumption data and intake data . . .
>
> These data were used because they are the best available at this time. However, in some cases they may not accurately reflect actual food intake. For example, the recommendations to reduce animal fat intake from the present level shown by food disappearance data must be viewed with some reservation because food disappearance data does not adjust for fat loss from retail preparation of meat, fat trimming before and after cooking, fat loss during cooking and table waste. The same case could be made for vegetable fat because many vegetable oils used in cooking are discarded and not consumed. Better food intake information, expected shortly, may produce more reliable and perhaps altered recommendations.

Dietary intake data from the NHANES I (1971–75) had not been analyzed by 1977, therefore was not available to be used in the report. Beginning with the 1980 *Dietary Guidelines for Americans*, nutritional information of the nation has used results of the most current NHANES, as did the Dietary Guidelines Advisory Committee (DGAC) in their *Scientific Report of the 2015 Dietary Guidelines Advisory (Scientific Report)* that they submitted to the Secretaries of HHS and USDA in January 2015. Additionally, the DGAC used data from What We Eat in America (WWEIA) to describe typical U.S. diet patterns. The WWEIA website describes WWEIA as the:

> integration of two nationwide surveys—USDA's Continuing Survey of Food Intakes by Individuals (CSFII) and HHS' NHANES. Under the integrated framework, DHHS is responsible for the sample design and data collection. USDA is responsible for the survey's dietary data collection methodology, development and maintenance of the food and nutrient databases used to code and process the data, and data review and processing. The two surveys were integrated in 2002.

Researcher Edward Asher and colleagues criticize the use of NHANES data in their article published in the June 2015 issue of *Mayo Clinic Proceedings*. The title of their critical review vividly describes their opinion: "The Inadmissibility of What We Eat in America [WWEIA] and NHANES Dietary Data in Nutrition and Obesity Research and the Scientific Formulation of National Dietary Guidelines." In their review, they argue that:

> the essence of science is the ability to discern fact from fiction, and we presented evidence from multiple fields to support the position that the data generated by nutrition epidemiologic surveys and questionnaires are not falsifiable. As such, these data are pseudoscientific and inadmissible in scientific research. Therefore, these protocols and the resultant data should not be used to inform national dietary guidelines or public health policy, and the continued funding of these methods constitutes an unscientific and major misuse of research resources.

The first selection (YES) for this issue describes the methods used by the Secretaries of HHS and USDA to select the DGAC and the steps the DGAC followed while writing the technical report to the Secretaries. These sections of the *Scientific Report* were selected to lay a foundation of the rigor associated with the DGAC member selection and the protocol the DGAC follow when preparing the technical report. The second (NO) is a study by Edward Asher and colleagues who question the validity of NHANES and WWEIA data; it is interesting to note that the article was published during the two-year period that the DGAC were reviewing the data. The DGAC even refer to Archer's article in their discussion of the strengths and shortcomings of using NHANES and WWEIA data.

(Refer to "Appendix E-4: NHANES Data Used in 1 DGAC Data Analyses" on the following pages.) In the sentence, "This has also been discussed for several years in the scientific literature . . . and in recent articles," one of the "recent articles" to which they refer is the NO article by Archer et al.

YES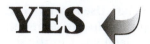

Barbara E. Millen

Part C: Methodology

Committee Appointment

Beginning with the 1985 edition, the U.S. Department of Agriculture (USDA) and U.S. Department of Health and Human Services (HHS) have appointed a Dietary Guidelines Advisory Committee (DGAC) of nationally recognized experts in the field of nutrition and health to review the scientific evidence and medical knowledge current at the time. This Committee has been an effective mechanism for obtaining a comprehensive and systematic review of the science which contributes to successful Federal implementation as well as broad public acceptance of the Dietary Guidelines. The 2015 DGAC was established for the single, time-limited task of reviewing the 2010 edition of *Dietary Guidelines for Americans* and developing nutrition and related health recommendations in this Advisory Report to the Secretaries of USDA and HHS.

. . .

Nominations were sought from the public through a Federal Register notice published on October 26, 2012. Criteria for nominating prospective members of the DGAC included knowledge about current scientific research in human nutrition and chronic disease, familiarity with the purpose, communication, and application of the Dietary Guidelines, and demonstrated interest in the public's health and well-being through their research and educational endeavors. They also were expected to be respected and published experts in their fields. Expertise was sought in several specialty areas, including, but not limited to, the prevention of chronic diseases (e.g., cancer, cardiovascular disease, type 2 diabetes, overweight and obesity, and osteoporosis); energy balance (including physical activity); epidemiology; food processing science, safety, and technology; general medicine; gerontology; nutrient bioavailability; nutrition biochemistry and physiology; nutrition education and behavior change; pediatrics; maternal/gestational nutrition; public health; and/or nutrition-related systematic review methodology.

The Secretaries of USDA and HHS jointly appointed individuals for membership to the 2015 DGAC. The chosen individuals are highly respected by their peers for their depth and breadth of scientific knowledge of the relationship between dietary intake and health in all relevant areas of the current Dietary Guidelines.

To ensure that recommendations of the Committee took into account the needs of the diverse groups served by USDA and HHS, membership included, to the extent practicable, a diverse group of individuals with representation from various geographic locations, racial and ethnic groups, women, and persons with disabilities.

. . .

Individuals were appointed to serve as members of the Committee to represent balanced viewpoints of the scientific evidence, and not to represent the viewpoints of any specific group.

. . .

Charge to the 2015 Dietary Guidelines Advisory Committee

The *Dietary Guidelines for Americans* provide science-based advice on how nutrition and physical activity can help promote health across the lifespan and reduce the risk for major chronic diseases in the U.S. population ages 2 years and older.

The *Dietary Guidelines* form the basis of Federal nutrition policy, standards, programs, and education for the general public and are published jointly by HHS and USDA every 5 years. The charge to the Dietary Guidelines Advisory Committee, whose duties were time-limited and solely advisory in nature, was described in the Committee's charter as follows:

- Examine the *Dietary Guidelines for Americans*, 2010 and determine topics for which new scientific evidence is likely to be available that may inform revisions to the current guidance or suggest new guidance.

Scientific Report of the 2015 Dietary Guidelines Advisory Committee: Part C: Methodology, February 2015.

- Place its primary focus on the systematic review and analysis of the evidence published since the last DGAC deliberations.
- Place its primary emphasis on the development of food-based recommendations that are of public health importance for Americans ages 2 years and older.
- Prepare and submit to the Secretaries of HHS and USDA a report of technical recommendations with rationales, to inform the development of the *2015 Dietary Guidelines for Americans*. DGAC responsibilities included providing authorship for this report; however, responsibilities did not include translating the recommendations into policy or into communication and outreach documents or programs.

· · ·

- Complete all work within the 2-year charter timeframe.

The Committee Process

Committee Membership

Fifteen members were appointed to the Committee, one of whom resigned within the first 3 months of appointment due to new professional obligations. The Committee served without pay and worked under the regulations of the Federal Advisory Committee Act (FACA). The Committee held seven public meetings over the course of 1½ years. Meetings were held in June 2013 and January, March, July, September, November, and December 2014. The members met in person on the campus of the National Institutes of Health in Bethesda, Maryland, for six of the seven meetings. The Committee met by webinar for the November 2014 meeting. All meetings were made publically available live by webcast. In addition, members of the general public were able to attend the Committee's first two meetings in person in the Washington DC area. For the remaining meetings, members of the public were able to observe by webcast. All meetings were announced in the *Federal Register*. Meeting summaries, presentations, archived recordings of all of the meetings, and other documents pertaining to Committee deliberations were made available at www.DietaryGuidelines.gov.

· · ·

Public Comments

Written public comments were received throughout the Committee's deliberations through an electronic database and provided to the Committee. This database allowed for the generation of public comment reports as a result of a query by key topic area(s).

· · ·

Approaches to Reviewing the Evidence

The Committee used a variety of scientifically rigorous approaches to address its science-based questions, and some questions were addressed using multiple approaches. The Committee used the state-of-the-art methodology, systematic reviews, to address 27 percent of its science-based research questions. These reviews are publically available in the Nutrition Evidence Library (NEL) at www.NEL.gov. The scientific community now regularly uses systematic review methodologies, so, unlike the 2010 DGAC, the 2015 Committee was able to use existing sources of evidence to answer an additional 45 percent of the questions it addressed. These sources included existing systematic reviews, meta-analyses, or reports. The remainder of the questions, 30 percent, were answered using data analyses and food pattern modeling analyses. These three approaches allowed the Committee to ask and answer its questions in a systematic, transparent, and evidence-based manner.

For all topics and questions, regardless of the path used to identify and evaluate the scientific evidence, the Committee developed conclusion statements and implications statements. Conclusion statements are a direct answer to the question asked, reflecting the strength of evidence reviewed (see additional details, below, in "Develop Conclusion Statements and Grade the Evidence"). Implications statements were developed to put the Conclusion in necessary context and varied in length depending on the topic or question. The primary purpose of these statements in this report is to describe what actions the Committee recommends that individuals, programs, or policies might take to promote health and prevent disease in light of the conclusion statement. However, some implications statements also provided important statements of fact or references to other processes or initiatives that the Committee felt were critical in providing a complete picture of how their advice should be applied to reach the desired outcomes.

Based on the existing body of evidence, research gaps, and limitations, the DGAC also formulated research recommendations that could advance knowledge related to its question and inform future Federal food and nutrition guidance as well as other policies and programs.

· · ·

Systematic Review of the Scientific Evidence

The USDA's Nutrition Evidence Library (NEL), was responsible for assisting the 2015 DGAC in reviewing the science and supporting development of the 2015 DGAC Report. The NEL used state-of-the-art methodology informed by the Agency for Healthcare Research and Quality (AHRQ), the Cochrane Collaboration, the Academy of Nutrition and Dietetics and the 2011 Institute of Medicine systematic review (SR) standards to review, evaluate, and synthesize published, peer-reviewed food and nutrition research. The NEL's rigorous, protocol-driven methodology is designed to maximize transparency, minimize bias, and ensure SRs are relevant, timely, and high-quality. Using the NEL evidence-based approach enables HHS and USDA to comply with the Data Quality Act, which states that Federal agencies must ensure the quality, objectivity, utility, and integrity of the information used to form Federal guidance.

. . .

The NEL employed a six-step SR process, which leveraged a broad range of expert inputs:

- Step 1: Develop systematic review questions and analytic frameworks
- Step 2: Search, screen, and select studies to review
- Step 3: Extract data and assess the risk of bias of the research
- Step 4: Describe and synthesize the evidence
- Step 5: Develop conclusion statements and grade the evidence
- Step 6: Identify research recommendations

Develop Systematic Review Questions and Analytic Frameworks

The DGAC identified, refined, and prioritized the most relevant topics and then developed clearly focused SR questions that were appropriate in scope, reflected the state of the science, and targeted important policy relevant to public health issue(s). Once topics and systematic review questions were generated, the DGAC developed an analytical framework for each topic in accordance with NEL methodology.

. . .

The core elements of a SR question include Population, Intervention or Exposure, Comparator, and Outcomes (PICO). These elements represent key aspects of the topic that need to be considered in developing a SR framework. An analytic framework is a type of evidence model that defines and links the PICO elements and key confounders. The analytical framework serves as a visual representation of the overall scope of the project, provides definitions for key SR terms, helps to ensure that all contributing elements in the causal chain will be examined and evaluated, and aids in determining inclusion and exclusion criteria and the literature search strategy.

. . .

The NEL established and the DGAC approved standard inclusion and exclusion criteria to promote consistency across reviews and ensure that the evidence being considered in NEL SRs was most relevant to the U.S. population. The DGAC used these standard criteria and revised them a priori as needed to ensure that they were appropriate for the specific SR being conducted. In general, criteria were established based on the analytical framework to ensure that each study included the appropriate population, intervention/exposure, comparator(s), and outcomes. They were typically established for the following study characteristics:

- Study design
- Date of publication
- Publication language
- Study setting
- Study duration
- Publication status (i.e., peer reviewed)
- Type, age, and health status of study subjects
- Size of study groups
- Study dropout rate

. . .

Existing Sources of Evidence: Reports, Systematic Reviews, and Meta-analyses

For a number of topics, the DGAC chose to consider existing high-quality sources of evidence such as existing reports from leading scientific organizations or

Federal agencies, SRs, and/or MA to fully or partially address questions. (These three categories of existing sources of evidence are collectively referred to in this report as "existing reports.") This was done to prevent duplication of effort and promote time and resource management.

. . .

First, an analytical framework was developed that clearly described the population, intervention/exposure, comparator, and outcomes (intermediate and clinical) of interest for the question being addressed. When Committee members were aware of high-quality existing reports that addressed their question(s), they decided a priori to use existing report(s), rather than to conduct a de novo NEL SR. A literature search was then conducted to identify other existing reports to augment the existing report(s) identified by the Committee. The literature was searched by a NEL librarian to identify relevant studies. The process used to create and execute the literature search is described in detail above (see "Search, Screen, and Select Studies to Review"). In other cases, the Committee was not aware of any existing reports and intended to conduct a de novo NEL SR. However, as part of the duplication assessment step of the NEL process, one or more existing SRs or MA were identified that addressed the question that led to the Committee deciding to proceed using existing SRs/MA rather than complete an independent review of the primary literature. This process is also described above. Finally, for some questions, the Committee used existing reports as the primary source of evidence to answer a question, but chose to update one or more of those existing reports using the NEL process to identify and review studies that had been published after the completion of the literature search for the existing report(s).

. . .

Next, the Committee graded their conclusion statement using a table of strength of evidence grades adapted specifically to use with existing reports. In cases where the DGAC used an existing report with its own formally graded conclusions, the Committee acknowledged the grade assigned within that existing report, and then assigned a DGAC grade that was the closest equivalent to the grade assigned in the existing report.

Data Analyses

Federal Data Acquisition

Earlier Committees used selected national, Federal data about the dietary, nutritional, and health status of the U.S. population. In the 2015 DGAC, a Data Analysis Team (DAT) was established to streamline the data acquisition process and efficiently support the data requests of the Committee. During the Committee's work, the data used by the DGAC were publically available through www.DietaryGuidelines.gov. Upon publication, the data became available through the report's references and appendices.

Upon request from the DGAC, the DAT either conducted data analyses or compiled data from their agencies' publications for the DGAC to use to answer specific research questions. The DGAC took the strengths and limitations of data analyses into account in drawing conclusions. The grading rubric used for questions answered using NEL systematic reviews do not apply to questions answered using data analyses; therefore, these conclusions were not graded.

Most of the analyses used the National Health and Nutrition Examination (NHANES) data and its dietary component, What We Eat in America (WWEIA), NHANES. These data were used to answer questions about food and nutrient intakes because they provide national and group level estimates of dietary intakes of the U.S. population, on a given day as well as usual intake distributions. These data contributed substantially to questions answered using data analyses (see Appendix E-4: *NHANES Data Used in DGAC Data Analyses* for additional discussion of the NHANES data used by the 2015 DGAC).

Other Data Sources
The DGAC also used data from the National Health Interview Survey, the National Cancer Institute's Surveillance, Epidemiology, and End Results (SEER) statistics, and heart disease and stroke statistics from the 2014 report of the American Heart Association. In addition, the Committee used USDA National Nutrient Database for Standard Reference, Release 27, 2014 to list food sources ranked by amounts of selected nutrients (calcium, fiber, iron, potassium, and Vitamin D) and energy per standard food portions and per 100 grams of foods.

Appendix E-4: NHANES Data Used in DGAC Data Analyses

Most of the DGAC data analyses used the National Health and Nutrition Examination (NHANES) data and its dietary component, What We Eat in America (WWEIA), NHANES (Zipf et al., 2013). These data were used to answer questions about food and nutrient intakes because they provide national and group level estimates of dietary intakes of the U.S. population on a given day as well as usual intake distributions. These data contributed substantially to questions answered using data analyses.

. . .

NHANES

NHANES consists of ongoing, comprehensive, cross-sectional, population-based surveys designed to collect data on health, nutritional status, and health behaviors of the non-institutionalized civilian population living in households in the United States. It is conducted by the National Center for Health Statistics (NCHS) of the Centers for Disease Control and Prevention (CDC). NHANES has had a long history starting in the early 1960s; it has been monitoring food and nutrient intake and nutritional status of the U.S. population since 1971, starting with NHANES I. Since then, several cycles of NHANES have been conducted as a series of cross-sectional surveys focusing on different population groups in terms of age and race/ethnicity, or health topics. In 1999, NHANES became a continuous survey, sampling U.S. residents of all ages, with a changing focus on a variety of health and nutrition measurements to meet emerging needs. The goals of the continuous NHANES are to provide prevalence data on selected diseases and risk factors for the U.S. population; to monitor trends in selected diseases, behaviors, and environmental exposures; to explore emerging public health needs; and to maintain a national probability sample of baseline information on health and nutritional status of the U.S. household population.

NHANES has a complex, multi-stage, probability sampling design and examines a nationally representative sample of about 5,000 persons each year. In NHANES, certain subgroups have been periodically oversampled. These include low income, older Americans, infants and children, pregnant women and certain race/ethnic groups (e.g., Hispanics, including Mexican Americans, African Americans, and more recently, Asian Americans). The NHANES survey is unique because it combines personal interviews with standardized physical examinations and laboratory tests administered by a specially trained staff that travels with the Mobile Examination Center (MEC) to survey sites selected to represent the U.S. population. In the continuous NHANES, dietary intake is assessed through two 24-hr recalls, administered by trained dietary interviewers using the USDA's Automated Multiple Pass Method (AMPM) through What We Eat in America (WWEIA). The first 24-hr recall (day 1) is collected in-person at the MEC and a subsequent 24-hr recall (day 2) is obtained 7 to 10 days later over the telephone. Information on dietary supplements consumed during the 24-hour recall period is also collected. The strengths of the WWEIA, NHANES dietary data include that because two 24-hour recalls are available in WWEIA, NHANES (from 2003 onwards), usual intake distributions can be estimated based on statistical techniques that reduce the effect of intra-individual variation in food and nutrient intakes in 24-hour recalls.

The WWEIA, NHANES dietary data are one of the few sources that can provide national estimates of total nutrient intake from diet and dietary supplements for the U.S. population. Moreover, dietary intakes can be described by specific socio-demographic groups including race/ethnic groups, income status, and participation in Federal nutrition assistance programs (e.g., Supplemental Nutrition Assistance Program). Dietary data from WWEIA, NHANES can be linked to thorough anthropometric, laboratory, and clinical evaluation data as well health outcomes to examine cross-sectional associations at the national and large subgroup levels. It must be recognized that WWEIA, NHANES dietary data are not designed for individual-level assessment. These data can be useful to inform nutrition policy, but not sufficient by themselves to form policy recommendations.

No single perfect method for assessing dietary intake information is available in surveys and different methods may be indicated for specific purposes. NCHS has been actively involved in researching and reviewing its data collection methods, including dietary data, over the years internally and in consultation with expert groups. The methods used in NHANES are adapted in light of its large sample size and complex design, cost and feasibility, and respondent burden to ensure a high response rate to derive nationally representative estimates. Some examples of adaptations in methods include the transition to USDA's standardized automated multi-pass method for collection of dietary

Table C.1

Nutrition Evidence Library Bias Assessment Tool (BAT) The NEL Bias Assessment Tool (NEL BAT) is used to assess the risk of bias of each individual study included in a SR. The types of bias that are addressed in the NEL BAT include:	
Selection Bias	Systematic differences between baseline characteristics of the groups that are compared; error in choosing the individuals or groups taking part in a study
Performance Bias	Systematic differences between groups in the intervention/exposure received, or in experience with factors other than the interventions/exposures of interest
Detection Bias	Systematic differences between groups in how outcomes are determined; outcomes are more likely to be observed or reported in certain subjects
Attrition Bias	Systematic differences between groups in withdrawals from a study, particularly if those who drop out of the study are systematically different from those who remain in the study
Adapted from: Cochrane Bias Methods Group: http://bmg.cochrane.org/assessing-risk-bias-included-studies	

recalls by trained interviewers that has been evaluated and associated with reduced measurement error. Other examples include collection of an additional 24-hour dietary recall in NHANES since 2003 (for a total of two 24-hour recalls), coupled with targeted food frequency questionnaires over various NHANES cycles.

The strengths and shortcomings of these dietary assessment methods have been discussed over time in various meetings (e.g., International Conference on Diet and Activity Methods and American Society for Nutrition/ Experimental Biology), workshops, and expert groups. This has also been discussed for several years in the scientific literature and in recent articles. No assessment method is perfect and the choice of dietary method is based on the purpose for which it is intended. For NHANES, repeated 24-hour recalls remain the backbone of dietary assessment and monitoring. These data are useful in providing national-and group-level estimates of dietary intakes of the U.S. population, on a given day as well as in describing usual intake distributions using appropriate statistical approaches, to inform nutrition policy.

The NEL BAT is tailored by study design, with different sets of questions applying to randomized controlled trials (14 questions), non-randomized controlled trials (14 questions), and observational studies (12 questions). Abstractors complete the NEL BAT after data extraction for each article. There are four response options:

- **Yes:** Information provided in the article is adequate to answer "yes".
- **No:** Information provided in the article clearly indicates an answer of "no".
- **Cannot Determine:** No information or insufficient information is provided in the article, so an answer of "yes" or "no" is not possible.
- **N/A:** The question is not applicable to the article.

The NEL Bias Assessment Tool (NEL BAT)		
Risk of Bias Questions	**Study Designs**	**Type of Bias**
Were the inclusion/exclusion criteria similar across study groups?	Controlled trials Observational studies	Selection Bias
Was the strategy for recruiting or allocating participants similar across study groups?	Controlled trials Observational studies	Selection Bias
Was the allocation sequence randomly generated?	RCTs	Selection Bias
Was the group allocation concealed (so that assignments could not be predicted)?	RCTs	Selection Bias Performance Bias

(Continued)

Risk of Bias Questions	Study Designs	Type of Bias
Was distribution of health status, demographics, and other critical confounding factors similar across study groups at baseline? If not, does the analysis control for baseline differences between groups?	RCTs Controlled trials Observational studies	Selection Bias
Did the investigators account for important variations in the execution of the study from the proposed protocol or research plan?	RCTs Controlled trials Observational studies	Performance Bias
Was adherence to the study protocols similar across study groups?	RCTs Controlled trials Observational studies	Performance Bias
Did the investigators account for the impact of unintended/unplanned concurrent interventions or exposures that were differentially experienced by study groups and might bias results?	RCTs Controlled trials Observational studies	Performance Bias
Were participants blinded to their intervention or exposure status?	RCTs Controlled trials	Performance Bias
Were investigators blinded to the intervention or exposure status of participants?	RCTs Controlled trials	Performance Bias
Were outcome assessors blinded to the intervention or exposure status of participants?	RCTs Controlled trials Observational studies	Detection Bias
Were valid and reliable measures used consistently across all study groups to assess inclusion/exclusion criteria, interventions/exposures, outcomes, participant health benefits and harms, and confounding?	RCTs Controlled trials Observational studies	Detection Bias
Was the length of follow-up similar across study groups?	RCTs Controlled trials Observational studies	Attrition Bias
In cases of high or differential loss to follow-up, was the impact assessed (e.g., through sensitivity analysis or other adjustment method)?	RCTs Controlled trials Observational studies	Attrition Bias
Were other sources of bias taken into account in the design and/or analysis of the study (e.g., through matching, stratification, interaction terms, multivariate analysis, or other statistical adjustment such as instrumental variables)?	RCTs Controlled trials Observational studies	Attrition, Detection, Performance, and Selection Bias
Were the statistical methods used to assess the primary outcomes adequate?	RCTs Controlled trials Observational studies	Detection Bias

Table C.2

NEL Grading Rubric USDA Nutrition Evidence Library Conclusion Statement Evaluation Criteria for judging the strength of the body of evidence supporting the Conclusion Statement				
Elements	Grade I: Strong	Grade II: Moderate	Grade III: Limited	Grade IV: Grade Not Assignable*
Risk of bias (as determined using the NEL Bias Assessment Tool)	Studies of strong design free from design flaws, bias and execution problems	Studies of strong design with minor methodological concerns OR only studies of weaker study design for question	Studies of weak design for answering the question OR inconclusive findings due to design flaws, bias or execution problems	Serious design flaws, bias, or execution problems across the body of evidence
Quantity • Number of studies • Number of subjects in studies	Several good quality studies; large number of subjects studied; studies have sufficiently large sample size for adequate statistical power	Several studies by independent investigators; doubts about adequacy of sample size to avoid Type I and Type II error	Limited number of studies; low number of subjects studied and/or inadequate sample size within studies	Available studies do not directly answer the question OR no studies available

(Continued)

Elements	Grade I: Strong	Grade II: Moderate	Grade III: Limited	Grade IV: Grade Not Assignable*
Consistency of findings across studies	Findings generally consistent in direction and size of effect or degree of association and statistical significance with very minor exceptions	Some inconsistency in results across studies in direction and size of effect, degree of association or statistical significance	Unexplained inconsistency among results from different studies	Independent variables and/or outcomes are too disparate to synthesize OR single small study unconfirmed by other studies
Impact • Directness of studied outcomes • Magnitude of effect	Studied outcome relates directly to the question; size of effect is clinically meaningful	Some study outcomes relate to the question indirectly; some doubt about the clinical significance of the effect	Most studied outcomes relate to the question indirectly; size of effect is small or lacks clinical significance	Studied outcomes relate to the question indirectly; size of effect cannot be determined
Generalizability to the U.S. population of interest	Studied population, intervention and outcomes are free from serious doubts about generalizability	Minor doubts about generalizability	Serious doubts about generalizability due to narrow or different study population, intervention or outcomes studied	Highly unlikely that the studied population, intervention AND/OR outcomes are generalizable to the population of interest

Table C.3

	AMSTAR (Assessment of Multiple Systematic Reviews) Tool	YES	NO	Can't Answer	N/A
1	**Was an 'a priori' design provided?** *The research question and inclusion criteria should be established before the conduct of the review.*				
2	**Was there duplicate study selection and data extraction?** *There should be at least two independent data extractors and a consensus procedure for disagreements should be in place.*				
3	**Was a comprehensive literature search performed?** *At least two electronic sources should be searched. The report must include years and databases used (e.g. Central, EMBASE, and MEDLINE). Key words and/or MESH terms must be stated and where feasible the search strategy should be provided. All searches should be supplemented by consulting current contents, reviews, textbooks, specialized registers, or experts in the particular field of study, and by reviewing the references in the studies found.*				
4	**Was the status of publication (i.e., grey literature) used as an inclusion criterion?** **The authors should state that they searched for reports regardless of their publication type. The authors should state whether or not they excluded any reports (from the systematic review), based on their publication status, language, etc.*				
5	**Was a list of studies (included and excluded) provided?** *A list of included and excluded studies should be provided.*				
6	**Were the characteristics of the included studies provided?** *In an aggregated form such as a table, data from the original studies should be provided on the participants, interventions and outcomes. The ranges of characteristics in all the studies analyzed e.g. age, race, sex, relevant socioeconomic data, disease status, duration, severity, or other diseases should be reported.*				
7	**Was the scientific quality of the included studies assessed and documented?** *'A priori' methods of assessment should be provided (e.g., for effectiveness studies if the author(s) chose to include only randomized, double-blind, placebo controlled studies, or allocation concealment as inclusion criteria); for other types of studies alternative items will be relevant.*				
8	**Was the scientific quality of the included studies used appropriately in formulating conclusions?** *The results of the methodological rigor and scientific quality should be considered in the analysis and the conclusions of the review, and explicitly stated in formulating recommendations.*				

(Continued)

		YES	NO	Can't Answer	N/A
9	**Were the methods used to combine the findings of studies appropriate?** *For the pooled results, a test should be done to ensure the studies were combinable, to assess their homogeneity (i.e. Chisquared test for homogeneity, I2). If heterogeneity exists a random effects model should be used and/or the clinical appropriateness of combining should be taken into consideration (i.e. is it sensible to combine?).*				
10	**Was the likelihood of publication bias assessed?** *An assessment of publication bias should include a combination of graphical aids (e.g., funnel plot, other available tests) and/or statistical tests (e.g., Egger regression test).*				
11	**Was the conflict of interest stated?** *Potential sources of support should be clearly acknowledged in both the systematic review and the included studies.*				

* The guidance for answering this question was adapted for the 2015 Dietary Guidelines Advisory Committee.

Table C.4

Strength of evidence terminology to support a conclusion statement when a question is answered with existing reports	
Strong	The conclusion statement is substantiated by a large, high quality, and/or consistent body of evidence that directly addresses the question. There is a high level of certainty that the conclusion is generalizable to the population of interest, and it is unlikely to change if new evidence emerges.
Moderate	The conclusion statement is substantiated by sufficient evidence, but the level of certainty is restricted by limitations in the evidence, such as the amount of evidence available, inconsistencies in findings, or methodological or generalizability concerns. If new evidence emerges, there could be modifications to the conclusion statement.
Limited	The conclusion statement is substantiated by insufficient evidence, and the level of certainty is seriously restricted by limitations in the evidence, such as the amount of evidence available, inconsistencies in findings, or methodological or generalizabilty concerns. If new evidence emerges, there could likely be modifications to the conclusion statement.
Grade not assignable	A conclusion statement cannot be drawn due to a lack of evidence, or the availability of evidence that has serious methodological concerns.

The completed NEL BAT is used to rate the overall risk of bias for the article by tallying the responses to each question. Each "Yes" response receives 0 points, each "Cannot Determine" response receives 1 point, each "No" response receives 2 points, and each "N/A" response receives 0 points. Since 14 questions are answered for randomized controlled trials and non-randomized controlled trials, they will be assigned a risk of bias rating out of a maximum of 28 points; while observational studies will be out of 24 points. The lower the number of points received, the lower the risk of bias.

BARBARA MILLEN, founder and president of Millennium Prevention, Inc., was chair of the 14-member 2015 Dietary Guidelines Advisory Committee.

Edward Archer, Gregory A. Hand, and Steven N. Blair

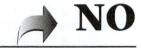

Validity of U.S. Nutritional Surveillance: National Health and Nutrition Examination Survey Caloric Energy Intake Data, 1971–2010

Introduction

The rise in the population prevalence of obesity has focused attention on U.S. nutritional surveillance research and the analysis of trends in caloric energy intake (EI). Because these efforts provide the scientific foundation for many public health policies and food-based guidelines, poor validity in dietary measurement protocols can have significant long-term implications for our nation's health.

In the U.S., population-level estimates of EI are derived from data collected as part of the National Health and Nutrition Examination Survey (NHANES), a complex, cross-sectional sample of the U.S. population. The primary method used in NHANES to approximate EI is the 24-hour dietary recall interview (24HR). The data collected are based on the subject's self-reported, retrospective perceptions of food and beverage consumption in the recent past. To calculate EI estimates, these subjective data are translated into nutrient food codes and then assigned numeric energy (i.e., caloric) values from food and nutrient databases. Prior to 2001–2002, the NHANES relied upon databases of varying quality and composition for the *post-hoc* conversion of food and beverage consumption (24HR) data into energy values. After 2001–2002, the NHANES and the U.S. Department of Agriculture's (USDA) Continuing Survey of Food Intakes by Individuals were integrated into the "What We Eat in America" program, and the translation process was standardized via use of successive versions of the USDA's National Nutrient Database for Standard Reference (NNBS).

Misreporting

Given the indirect, pseudo-quantitative nature of the method (i.e., assigning numeric values to subjective data without objective corroboration), nutrition surveys frequently report a range of energy intakes that are not representative of the respondents' habitual intakes, and estimates of EI that are physiologically implausible (i.e., incompatible with survival) have been demonstrated to be widespread. For example, in a group of "highly educated" participants, Subar et al. (2003) demonstrated that when total energy expenditure (TEE) via doubly labeled water (DLW) was compared to reported energy intake (rEI), the raw correlations between TEE and rEI were 0.39 for men and 0.24 for women. Men and women underreported energy intake by 12–14% and 16–20%, respectively. The level of underreporting increased significantly after correcting for the weight gain of the sample over the study period, and underreporting was greater for fat than for protein, thereby providing additional support for the well-documented occurrence of the selective misreporting of specific macronutrients (e.g., fat and sugars). These results are consistent with earlier work, in which the correlations between DLW-derived TEE and seven 24HR and the average of two seven-day dietary recalls were 0.33 and 0.30, respectively.

Because the NHANES collected dietary data over the period in which the population prevalence of obesity was increasing, these data have been used (despite the widely acknowledged issues) to examine the association of trends in EI with increments in mean population body mass index (BMI) and rates of obesity. Given that implausible rEI values and the misreporting of total dietary intake render the relationships between dietary factors, BMI and other indices of health ambiguous, and diminish the usefulness of nutrition data as a tool to inform public health policy, this report examines the validity of U.S. nutrition surveillance EI data

Archer E, Hand GA, Blair SN (2013). Validity of U.S. Nutritional Surveillance: National Health and Nutrition Examination Survey Caloric Energy Intake Data, 1971–2010. *PLoS ONE* 8(10): e76632. doi:10.1371/journal.pone.0076632 from NHANES I (1971–1974) through NHANES 2010 (nine survey periods) using two protocols: the ratio of reported energy intake (rEI) to basal metabolic rate (rEI/BMR) and the disparity between rEI and estimated total energy expenditure (TEE) from the Institute of Medicine's (IOM) predictive equations.

Methods

Population

Data were obtained from the National Health and Nutrition Examination Surveys for the years 1971–2010. The NHANES is a complex multi-stage, cluster sample of the civilian, noninstitutionalized U.S. population conducted by the Centers for Disease Control and Prevention (CDC).

The National Center for Health Statistics ethics review board approved protocols and written informed consent was obtained from all NHANES participants.

Inclusion Criteria

The study sample was limited to adults aged ≥20 and, ≥74 years at the time of the NHANES in which they participated, and had a body mass index (BMI) ≥18 kg/m^2, and with complete data on age, sex, height, weight, and dietary energy intake.

Dietary Data

Estimates of EI were obtained from a single 24HR from each of the nine NHANES study periods. Energy content

Table 1

rEI/BMR values for all men and women from NHANES I through NHANES 2009–2010.
Reported Energy Intake (rEI)/Basal Metabolic Rate (BMR) rEI/BMR >1.35 = plausible U.S.
Men & Women (20–74 years); NHANES I–NHANES 2009–2010

NHANES Survey Year	Sex	Estimate rEI/RMR (mean)	Standard Error	95% Confidence Interval Lower	Upper	rEI Value Plausible Y = Yes N = No
NHANES I	Men (n = 4652)	1.30	0.012	1.28	1.32	N
	Women (n = 7709)	1.10	0.010	1.08	1.12	N
NHANES II	Men (n = 5236)	1.28	0.010	1.26	1.30	N
	Women (n = 6006)	1.08	0.008	1.06	1.09	N
NHANES III	Men (n = 6122)	1.36	0.011	1.34	1.39	Y
	Women (n = 7127)	1.22	0.009	1.20	1.24	N
NHANES 1999–00	Men (n = 1600)	1.31	0.018	1.27	1.34	N
	Women (n = 1886)	1.23	0.016	1.19	1.26	N
NHANES 2001–2002	Men (n = 1782)	1.31	0.015	1.28	1.34	N
	Women (n = 2029)	1.24	0.011	1.22	1.26	N
NHANES 2003–2004	Men (n = 1671)	1.32	0.013	1.30	1.35	Y
	Women (n = 1838)	1.23	0.018	1.20	1.27	N
NHANES 2005–2006	Men (n = 1749)	1.34	0.013	1.31	1.36	Y
	Women (n = 1998)	1.21	0.014	1.18	1.24	N
NHANES 2007–08	Men (n = 2154)	1.27	0.017	1.24	1.30	N
	Women (n = 2306)	1.19	0.020	1.15	1.23	N
NHANES 2009–2010	Men (n = 2319)	1.29	0.013	1.26	1.31	N
	Women (n = 2532)	1.20	0.007	1.18	1.21	N
All Surveys	**Men (n = 27285)**	**1.31**	**0.005**	**1.30**	**1.32**	**N**
	Women (n = 33431)	**1.19**	**0.005**	**1.18**	**1.20**	**N**

of the self-reported food consumption was determined by NHANES using nutrient databases based on previous versions of the USDA National Nutrient Database for Standard Reference (NNDS).

Determination of Physiologically Credible rEI Values

The ratio of rEI to BMR (rEI/BMR) <1.35 was used to determine EI values that were implausible. BMR was estimated via the Schofield predictive equations. The <1.35 cut-off for implausible EI values was used because *"it is highly unlikely that any normal, healthy free-living person could habitually exist at a PAL [i.e., TEE/BMR] of less than 1.35"*.

It is important to note that the <1.35 cut-off does not assess all forms of misreporting (e.g., over-reporting). To avoid the confounding effects of potential over-reporting, all rEI/BMR values >2.40 were excluded from analyses of underreporting. One form of misreporting that neither cut-off addresses is the underreporting of EI from a high caloric intake associated with elevated levels of physical activity.

Disparity of the rEI and Estimated Total Energy Expenditure (TEE)

In 2002, the IOM used datasets derived from studies using DLW to create factorial equations to estimate energy requirements for the US population. IOM TEE values were

Table 2

rEI/BMR index for all women by BMI categories from NHANES I through NHANES 2009–2010. Reported Energy Intake (rEI)/Basal Metabolic Rate (BMR) rEI/BMR >1.35 = plausible U.S. Women (20–74 years); NHANES I–NHANES 2009–2010

NHANES Survey Year	BMI Category	Estimate rEI/BMR (Mean)	Standard Error	95% Confidence Interval Lower	95% Confidence Interval Upper	rEI Value Plausible Y = Yes N = No
NHANES I	Normal (n = 4222)	1.20	0.013	1.18	1.23	N
	Overweight (n = 2028)	1.00	0.012	0.98	1.02	N
	Obese (n = 1459)	0.88	0.014	0.86	0.91	N
NHANES II	Normal (n = 3171)	1.18	0.010	1.16	1.20	N
	Overweight (n = 1671)	0.98	0.012	0.96	1.01	N
	Obese (n = 1164)	0.89	0.012	0.87	0.91	N
NHANES III	Normal (n = 2661)	1.32	0.014	1.30	1.35	Y
	Overweight (n = 2150)	1.18	0.019	1.14	1.22	N
	Obese (n = 2316)	1.07	0.015	1.04	1.10	N
NHANES 2003–2004	Normal (n = 550)	1.35	0.031	1.29	1.41	Y
	Overweight (n = 546)	1.19	0.027	1.14	1.25	N
	Obese (n = 742)	1.15	0.026	1.10	1.20	N
NHANES 2005–2006	Normal (n = 615)	1.34	0.026	1.29	1.39	Y
	Overweight (n = 558)	1.19	0.028	1.13	1.24	N
	Obese (n = 825)	1.10	0.024	1.05	1.15	N
NHANES 2007–2008	Normal (n = 634)	1.30	0.038	1.23	1.38	Y
	Overweight (n = 694)	1.17	0.026	1.12	1.22	N
	Obese (n = 978)	1.10	0.020	1.06	1.14	N
NHANES 2009–2010	Normal (n = 690)	1.31	0.022	1.26	1.35	Y
	Overweight (n = 745)	1.23	0.024	1.18	1.28	N
	Obese (n = 1097)	1.08	0.006	1.06	1.09	N

Table 3

rEI/BMR index for all men by BMI categories from NHANES I through NHANES 2009–2010. Reported Energy Intake (rEI)/Basal Metabolic Rate (BMR) rEI/BMR >1.35 = plausible U.S. Men (20–74 years); NHANES I–NHANES 2009–2010

NHANES Survey Year	BMI Category	Estimate rEI/BMR (Mean)	Standard Error	95% Confidence Interval		rEI Value Plausible Y = Yes N = No
				Lower	Upper	
NHANES I	Normal (n = 2115)	1.41	0.016	1.38	1.44	Y
	Overweight (n = 1945)	1.24	0.017	1.21	1.28	N
	Obese (n = 592)	1.08	0.025	1.04	1.13	N
NHANES II	Normal (n = 2431)	1.37	0.009	1.35	1.39	Y
	Overweight (n = 2111)	1.25	0.015	1.22	1.28	N
	Obese (n = 694)	1.08	0.018	1.05	1.12	N
NHANES III	Normal (n = 2275)	1.47	0.018	1.43	1.50	Y
	Overweight (n = 2482)	1.35	0.015	1.32	1.38	Y
	Obese (n = 1365)	1.20	0.018	1.17	1.24	N
NHANES 2003–2004	Normal (n = 465)	1.46	0.029	1.41	1.52	Y
	Overweight (n = 659)	1.35	0.025	1.30	1.40	Y
	Obese (n = 547)	1.18	0.035	1.11	1.24	N
NHANES 2005–2006	Normal (n = 413)	1.51	0.030	1.45	1.57	Y
	Overweight (n = 735)	1.33	0.023	1.29	1.38	Y
	Obese (n = 601)	1.22	0.014	1.19	1.25	N
NHANES 2007–2008	Normal (n = 539)	1.40	0.038	1.32	1.47	Y
	Overweight (n = 835)	1.29	0.017	1.26	1.32	N
	Obese (n = 790)	1.15	0.019	1.12	1.19	N
NHANES 2009–2010	Normal (n = 563)	1.38	0.027	1.33	1.44	Y
	Overweight (n = 872)	1.35	0.021	1.31	1.39	Y
	Obese (n = 884)	1.16	0.016	1.13	1.19	N

subtracted from the NHANES rEI to calculate disparity values. Negative values indicate underreporting.

assumes a physical activity level (PAL) of ≥1.4 and <1.6, which is indicative of a "low active" population.

IOM Equations for Predicting TEE Normal Weight (NW) Adults only (≥19years)

Equation 1 Men: TEE = 864 − (9.72 × age [y]) + PA* × (14.2 × weight [kg] + 503 × height[m]) (±202).

Equation 2 Women: TEE = 387 − (7.31 ± age [y] + PA* × (10.8 ± weight [kg] + 660.7 × height[m]) (±156).

* Physical activity (PA) values were 1.12 and 1.14 for NW men and women, respectively. The use of these values

IOM Equations for Predicting TEE Overweight (OW)/ Obese (OB) Adults Only (≥19 years)

Equation 3 Men: TEE = 1086 − (10.1 × age [y]) + PA* × (13.7 × weight [kg] + 416 × height [m]).

Equation 4 Women: TEE = 448 − (7.95 × age [y]) + PA* × (11.4 × weight [kg] + 619 × height [m]).

*PA values were 1.12 and 1.16 for OW/OB men and women, respectively. The use of these values assumes a

Figure 1

Percent of plausible reporters (i.e., rEI/BMR >1.35) by sex from NHANES I to NHANES 2009−2010; U.S. men and women (20−74 years).

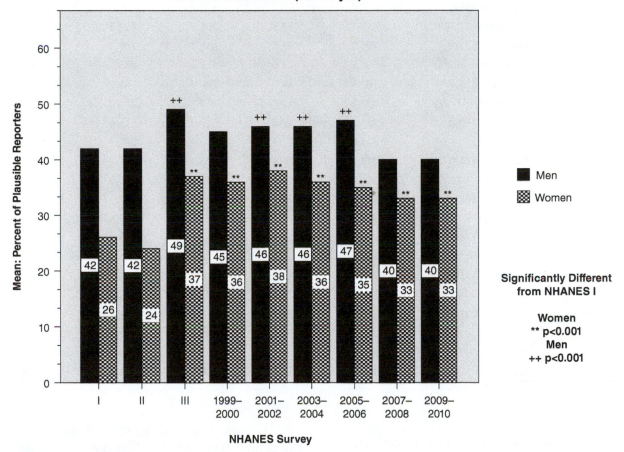

Percent of Plausible Reporters (rEI/BMR >1.35) US Men & Women (20–74 yrs)

physical activity level (PAL) of ≥1.4 and <1.6, which is indicative of a "low active" population.

Note: age (years); weight (kg); height (m; meters); BMI = body mass index, (kg/m²), IOM = Institute of Medicine; TEE = total energy expenditure.

Anthropometry

Body mass was measured to ±0.1 kg. Height was measured to ±0.1 cm. BMI was calculated as weight (kg)/height (m)². The sample was divided into three standard BMI categories: BMI ≥18 kg/m² and <25 kg/m² were normal weight

(NW), BMI between 25 kg/m² and 29.9 kg/m² were overweight (OW), and ≥30 kg/m² were obese (OB).

Statistical Analyses

Data processing and statistical analyses were performed using SASR, V 9.2 and SPSSR V.19 in 2012−2013. Analyses accounted for the NHANES' complex survey design via the incorporation of stratification, clustering and post-stratification weighting to maintain a nationally representative sample for each survey period. All analyses included adjusted means, and α <0.05 (2-tailed) was used to identify statistical significance.

Table 4

Disparity of rEI and TEE for men and women (20−74 years).
Disparity between rEI and IOM TEE U.S. Men & Women (20−74 years)
NHANES I–NHANES 2009−2010

NHANES Survey Year	Sex	EstimaterEI minus TEE (mean)*	Standard Error	95% Confidence Interval (CI)		Validity: 95% CI includes zero (Y = Yes, N = No)
				Lower	Upper	
NHANES I	Men (n = 4652)	−290.8	20.3	−330.7	−250.9	N
	Women (n = 7709)	−479.7	14.5	−508.1	−451.3	N
NHANES II	Men (n = 5236)	−323.2	17.8	−358.1	−288.3	N
	Women (n = 6006)	−505.8	11.6	−528.4	−483.1	N
NHANES III	Men (n = 6122)	−183.3	19.1	−220.8	−145.7	N
	Women (n = 7127)	−325.3	13.5	−351.7	−298.8	N
NHANES 1999−2000	Men (n = 1600)	−285.3	37.7	−359.3	−211.4	N
	Women (n = 1886)	−328.7	27.3	−382.3	−275.1	N
NHANES 2001−2002	Men (n = 1782)	−270.3	26.8	−322.9	−217.7	N
	Women (n = 2029)	−306.0	15.5	−336.3	−275.6	N
NHANES 2003−2004	Men (n = 1671)	−255.6	24.7	−304.0	−207.3	N
	Women (n = 1838)	−308.2	27.2	−361.5	−254.8	N
NHANES 2005−2006	Men (n = 1749)	−232.2	25.3	−281.8	−182.6	N
	Women (n = 1998)	−347.5	20.8	−388.4	−306.6	N
NHANES 2007−08	Men (n = 2154)	−355.0	32.1	−417.9	−292.0	N
	Women (n = 2306)	−379.4	28.5	−435.3	−323.5	N
NHANES 2009−2010	Men (n = 2319)	−330.9	22.7	−375.4	−286.4	N
	Women (n = 2532)	−366.9	9.8	−386.1	−347.7	N
All Surveys	**Men (n = 27285)**	**−281.4**	**9.1**	**−299.3**	**−263.5**	**N**
	Women (n = 33431)	**−364.6**	**7.0**	**−378.3**	**−351.0**	**N**

Results

Examination of Underreporting via rEI/BMR

Table 1 depicts the rEI/BMR values for men and women from NHANES I through NHANES 2009−2010. rEI was from NHANES 24HR data and BMR was calculated using the Schofield predictive equations. Values <1.35 are considered implausible and indicative of underreporting.

As Table 1 depicts, the 95% confidence intervals (CI) suggest that all mean rEI values for women and six of nine mean rEI values for men were apparently implausible.

Table 2 depicts the rEI/BMR index for all women by BMI categories from NHANES I through NHANES 2009−2010.

As Table 2 depicts, the 95% CI suggest that in 20 of the 27 measurement categories (i.e., three BMI categories and nine surveys) the rEI values were not in the physiologically plausible range. The overall mean for rEI/BMR values for the total sample of women (n = 33,431) across all NHANES was 1.19 (95% CI: 1.18, 1.20) and therefore not physiologically plausible.

Table 3 depicts the rEI/BMR index for all men by BMI categories from NHANES I through NHANES 2009−2010.

As shown in Table 3, the 95% CI suggest that in 12 of 27 measurement categories (i.e., three BMI categories and nine surveys), the rEI values were not in the physiologically plausible range. The overall mean value for rEI/BMR for the total sample of men (n = 27,285) across all NHANES was 1.31 (95% CI: 1.30, 1.32), and therefore not in the physiologically plausible range.

Table 5

Disparity between rEI and the TEE for women (20−74 years) by BMI categories.
Disparity between rEI and IOM TEE; U.S. Women by BMI categories (20−74 years)
NHANES I−NHANES 2009−2010

NHANES Survey Year	BMI Category	Estimate rEI minus TEE (mean)	Standard Error	95% Confidence Interval (CI)		Validity: 95% CI includes zero (Y = Yes, N = No)
				Lower	Upper	
NHANES I	Normal n = 4222)	−316.0	17.7	−350.8	−281.2	N
	Overweight (n = 2028)	−595.3	17.7	−629.9	−560.6	N
	Obese (n = 1459)	−856.0	23.5	−902.0	−809.9	N
NHANES II	Normal (n = 3171)	−351.6	13.7	−378.5	−324.8	N
	Overweight (n = 1671)	−617.6	17.1	−651.1	−584.1	N
	Obese (n = 1164)	−850.6	19.5	−888.9	−812.3	N
NHANES III	Normal (n = 2661)	−158.6	17.7	−193.3	−123.9	N
	Overweight (n = 2150)	−357.1	26.5	−409.1	−305.2	N
	Obese (n = 2316)	−594.2	22.6	−638.5	−549.9	N
NHANES 2003−2004	Normal (n = 550)	−116.3	39.2	−193.2	−39.4	N
	Overweight (n = 546)	−339.0	37.7	−413.0	−265.0	N
	Obese (n = 742)	−477.1	42.2	−560.0	−394.2	N
NHANES 2005−2006	Normal (n = 615)	−131.1	34.1	−198.0	−64.3	N
	Overweight (n = 558)	−342.8	38.0	−417.4	−268.3	N
	Obese (n = 825)	−567.3	38.7	−643.2	−491.3	N
NHANES 2007−2008	Normal (n = 634)	−173.2	52.1	−275.4	−71.0	N
	Overweight (n = 694)	−374.1	35.8	−444.4	−303.7	N
	Obese (n = 978)	−567.3	33.2	−632.5	−502.1	N
NHANES 2009−2010	Normal (n = 690)	−173.0	27.8	−227.5	−118.4	N
	Overweight (n = 745)	−288.9	34.0	−355.7	−222.2	N
	Obese (n = 1097)	−590.5	14.0	−617.8	−563.1	N

Percent of Plausible Reporters

Figure 1 depicts the percent of plausible reporters (i.e., rEI/ BMR >1.35) by sex from NHANES I to NHANES 2009−2010.

As Figure 1 depicts, across the entire study period (i.e., 1971−2010) the majority of respondents did not report plausible rEI values in any survey. When stratified by sex and BMI categories, plausible reporting in OB women ranged from a low of 12% in NHANES I and II to a high of 31% in NHANES 2003−2004. At no point in the history of the NHANES did more than 43% of OW and OB women report plausible values. Plausible reporting in NW women ranged from a low of 32% in NHANES II to 52% in NHANES

2001−2002. Plausible rEI values in OB men ranged from a low of 23% in NHANES II to a high of 35% in NHANES 2005−2006. At no point in the history of NHANES did more than 49% of OW and OB men report plausible rEI values.

Disparity between NHANES rEI and IOM TEE

Table 4 depicts the disparity of rEI and TEE for men and women (20−74 years). These values were calculated by subtracting the IOM TEE from the NHANES rEI. Negative values indicate the kilocalorie-per-day (kcal/day) value of underreporting.

Table 6

**Disparity between rEI and the TEE for all men (20−74 years) by BMI categories.
Disparity between rEI and IOM TEE; U.S. Men by BMI categories (20−74 years)
NHANES I−NHANES 2009−2010**

NHANES Survey Year	BMI Category	Estimate rEI minus TEE (mean)	Standard Error	95% Confidence Interval (CI)		Validity: 95% CI includes zero (Y = Yes, N = No)
				Lower	Upper	
NHANES I	Normal (n = 2115)	−96.3	26.8	−149.0	−43.6	N
	Overweight (n = 1945)	−374.7	30.8	−435.1	−314.2	N
	Obese (n = 592)	−702.1	49.7	−799.7	−604.5	N
NHANES II	Normal (n = 2431)	−178.7	15.9	−209.9	−147.6	N
	Overweight (n = 2111)	−367.6	27.0	−420.5	−314.6	N
	Obese (n = 694)	−716.5	37.3	−789.8	−643.3	N
NHANES III	Normal (n = 2275)	−8.8	31.1	−69.8	52.2	Y
	Overweight (n = 2482)	−191.5	27.9	−246.3	−136.7	N
	Obese (n = 1365)	−494.4	38.0	−569.0	−419.9	N
NHANES 2003−2004	Normal (n = 465)	−6.8	47.3	−99.6	86.0	Y
	Overweight (n = 659)	−175.4	46.9	−267.4	−83.4	N
	Obese (n = 547)	−549.8	72.0	−691.1	−408.5	N
NHANES 2005−2006	Normal (n = 413)	70.4	53.0	−33.7	174.5	Y
	Overweight (n = 735)	−222.4	39.7	−300.3	−144.4	N
	Obese (n = 601)	−464.2	32.1	−527.2	−401.2	N
NHANES 2007−2008	Normal (n = 539)	−117.9	64.8	−245.2	9.3	Y
	Overweight (n = 835)	−286.7	31.3	−348.1	−225.2	N
	Obese (n = 790)	−608.0	42.2	−690.8	−525.2	N
NHANES 2009−2010	Normal (n = 563)	−154.4	43.5	−239.8	−69.1	N
	Overweight (n = 872)	−178.9	42.1	−261.5	−96.4	N
	Obese (n = 884)	−590.9	32.9	−655.4	−526.4	N

As Table 4 depicts, in no survey group (i.e., men & women in 9 surveys) does the 95% CI for the disparity between rEI and TEE include zero. This suggests that underreporting of EI occurred in both men and women, and across all surveys. The overall mean value for the disparity of rEI and IOM TEE for the total sample of women (n = 33,431) across all NHANES was −365 kcal/day (95% CI: −378, −351), or ,18% of TEE, and for the total sample of men (n = 27,285) was −281 kcal/day (95% CI: −299,−264), or ~10% of TEE.

When stratified by sex and BMI categories (see Tables 5 & 6), the disparities between rEI and TEE in OB women ranged from −856 kcal/day (95% CI: −902, −810), an underreporting of 41% of TEE, to −477 kcal/day (95% CI: −560, −394), an underreporting of 20% of TEE.

The disparities between rEI and TEE in OB men ranged from −717 kcal/day (95% CI: −790, −643) in NHANES II to −464 kcal/day (95% CI: −527, −401) underreporting of 25% and 15%, respectively.

Trends in Underreporting

After the removal of over-reporters, both protocols, that is rEI/ BMR (*Figure* 1) and the disparity between rEI and IOM TEE (*Table* 4) exhibited significant decreases in underreporting from NHANES II and NHANES III (p<0.001). There were significant negative linear trends for both men and women in changes in underreporting total caloric intake from NHANES I to NHANES 2009−2010 (rEI/BMR: p<0.001, and disparity: p = 0.028).

Trends in Over-reporting

Across the study period, approximately 4.9% of men and 2.9% of women reported rEI/BMR values suggestive of over-reporting (i.e., rEI/BMR >2.4) with no significant trends. The greatest increase in the percentage of over-reporters between survey periods occurred from NHANES II to NHANES III, with men increasing from 4.1% to 6.4%, and women from 1.7% to 3.4% (both p<0.001). The greatest absolute percentage of over-reporters was in NHANES III, with 6.4% of men over-reporting and NHANES 2003–2004, with 3.9% of women over-reporting.

Discussion

Validity of NHANES EI Data

Our results suggest that across the 39-year history of U.S. nutrition surveillance research, rEI data on the majority of respondents (67.3% of women and 58.7% of men) were not physiologically plausible. The historical average rEI/BMR values for all men and women were 1.31 and 1.19 respectively (*Table* 1). These values are indicative of substantial underreporting. The expected average values for healthy, free living men and women are ~1.55, with a range of >1.35 to <2.40. In no survey did at least 50% of the respondents report plausible EI values (Figure 1). These data are consistent with previous research demonstrating that the misreporting of EI in nutrition surveys is widespread. Goldberg et al. (1991) demonstrated that in 37 studies across 10 countries, >65% of the mean rEI/ BMR values were below the study-specific plausibility cut-off. In addition to the extensive underreporting in our sample, 4.9% of men and 2.9% of women reported rEI/BMR values suggestive of over-reporting (i.e., rEI/BMR >2.40).

Disparity between NHANES rEI and IOM Derived TEE

Throughout the study period (i.e., 1971–2010) the disparity between rEI and TEE values were large and variable across BMI and sex categories suggesting substantial systematic biases in underreporting (*Tables* 4, 5, 6). The overall mean disparity values for men and women were −281 kcal/day and −365 kcal/day, respectively. The greatest mean disparity values were −717 kcal/ day (25% of TDEE) and −856 kcal/day (41% of TEE) in OB men and women, respectively.

Trends in the Validity and Inferences from NHANES rEI Data

As depicted in Tables 1 and 2, and Figure 1, there were large decreases in underreporting between NHANES II and

NHANES III. This is clearly evidenced by the increase in rEI/BMR index (Table 1), the large and significant increase in the percent of plausible reporters (*Figure* 1), and the reduction in the disparity between NHANES rEI and NAS/IOM EER (*Table* 4). This decrement in underreporting between NHANES II and subsequent surveys across all sex and BMI categories is likely the result of improvements in survey protocols for NHANES III, such as the inclusion of more days of dietary recall (i.e., weekends), automated multi-pass methodology, and increased staff training and quality control. The extent of these improvements is notable; for example, the percentage of OB women reporting implausible values decreased from ~88% in NHANES II to 74% in NHANES III.

These changes in measurement protocols led to an apparent increase in mean rEI values that has been reported as an actual increase in population-level EI despite caveats that the *"Interpretation of trends in energy and nutrient intakes is difficult when methodologic changes occur between surveys."* Nevertheless, Briefel and Johnson state (without caveat) in their abstract, *"During the 30-year period, mean energy intake increased among adults . . . ."* The data presented in the present report refute this inference. When the NHANES dietary measurement protocols were altered after NHANES II, the improved method captured a higher percentage of actual intakes. The apparent increase in mean rEI was merely an artifact of improved measurement protocols and not indicative of a true increase in caloric consumption. Despite this fact, the apparent increase has been regularly published and uncritically accepted as a true upward trend in caloric consumption and the cause of the obesity epidemic.

Changes in Underreporting and Public Policy Recommendations

In addition to the ubiquity of misreporting, there is strong evidence that the reporting of 'socially undesirable' (e.g., high fat and/or high sugar) foods has changed as the prevalence of obesity has increased. Additionally, research has demonstrated that interventions emphasizing the importance of "healthy" behaviors may lead to increased misreporting as participants alter their reports to reflect the adoption of the "healthier" behaviors independent of actual behavior change. It appears that lifestyle interventions "teach" participants the socially desirable or acceptable responses. As such, the ubiquity of public health messages to "eat less and exercise more" may induce greater levels of misreporting and may explain the recent downward bias in both self-reported

EI and body weight, especially given that social desirability bias is often expressed in the underreporting of calorically dense foods.

Selective misreporting of specific macronutrients has important ramifications for epidemiological research and nutrition surveillance. Heitmann and Lissner (2005) demonstrated that the selective misreporting of dietary fat by groups at an increased risk of chronic non-communicable diseases may result in an overestimated association between fat consumption and disease. If the potentially negative effects of high-fat diets are overestimated due to selective misreporting, current recommendations for fat intake may be overly conservative.

Additional Systematic Biases of Nutrition Surveillance Data

In addition to known sources of systematic reporting error, there are numerous sources of systematic bias in nutrition surveillance research protocols that are not addressed via our data. Another potentially large source of error is the translation of food and beverage consumption data (e.g., 24HR) into nutrient energy values via nutrient composition databases. The accuracy of this translation relies on a number of assumptions that are rarely justified. As cited earlier, research on misreporting shows that reports do not accurately reflect the quantity or number of foods consumed, and are not representative of usual intakes. Given that the basic methodological assumptions are violated, it is not surprising that research has demonstrated that food data to nutrient energy conversions are *"riddled with potential pitfalls at all stages"* that *"hamper the interpretability of the results,"* and represent a major source of systematic error in national nutrition surveillance efforts.

Throughout its history, the NHANES has relied upon databases of varying quality and composition for the post-hoc conversion of food and beverage consumption (i.e., 24HR) data into energy values. This makes the analysis of trends extremely complex because the nutrient energy (i.e., caloric) values in the databases varied considerably over time. Additionally, research has demonstrated that the energy content of restaurant food (and especially fast-food outlets) vary significantly when compared to the industry values used in the NNDS, and an internal quality review of NHANES 2003–2004 data led to ~400 substantive changes in nutrient and energy values. The result of these limitations are discussed in detail elsewhere.

As with the improvements in the NHANES survey protocols, the progressive alterations to the nutrient database

combined with changes in the types of foods that are available for consumption led to artifactual differences in nutrient and energy consumption estimates that frustrate efforts to examine trends in caloric consumption. To account for these changes, researchers must maintain the real differences in the composition of foods while correcting for artifactual differences attributable to improvements in the quality of nutrient data. Given the lack of comprehensive crossover studies and metrics for adjustment as the food and nutrient databases evolved, papers examining trends in caloric consumption must be treated with skepticism.

Commercially Prepared Foods and Meals Away From Home

One of the most prominent systematic errors from 24HR data-to-nutrient energy conversions is due to the increased reliance on the food service industry and the substantial rise in meals eaten "away from home." As stated previously, the vast majority of foods and beverages in the NNDS have not been evaluated empirically and research has demonstrated that the energy and macro/micro nutrient content of commercially prepared foods varies significantly compared to the industry values used in the NNDS. When foods or commodities are not in the database, substitutions are necessitated. For these interpolations to be accurate, the analogues must be similar in composition to the consumed food or beverage. This is extremely difficult to perform in practice because no two foods or commodities are identical, and local vs. imported foods/commodities differ significantly. For example, in survey data collection, knowledge of the specific preparation and cut of beef are essential since the energy content of generic beef substitutions may differ dramatically (e.g., 166 kcals per 100 grams in round steak to 257 kcals in top sirloin) Given these realities, USDA estimates of caloric consumption may be increasingly inaccurate as the number of food and beverages supplied by the commercial sector expands rapidly.

Recent research has attempted to quantify the changes in consumer packaged foods and beverages, and their impact on the American diet. Nevertheless, these efforts suffer from the same limitations as all food data-to-nutrient energy value conversions via nutrient composition databases. Additionally, the translation of "as-purchased" foods and beverages (using information from the commercial sector) to "as-consumed" energy and macro/micronutrient content for national surveillance relies on the accurate quantification of food preparation and waste. Unfortunately, these data are limited and highly variable. In a report from the USDA's Economic Research Service, Muth et al. (2011) state that the current data are incomplete and overstate actual consumption because the level of *"documentation of food losses . . . ranged from little to none for estimates at the retail and customer levels."* These results clearly demonstrate the conceptual and methodological complexity of translating food and beverage purchases into nutrient energy and macro/micronutrient intake in the context of a rapidly evolving food supply.

Methods of Adjustment for Systematic Biases

There are various methods that attempt to improve estimates of caloric consumption derived from self-reported dietary intake. While these methods may improve the shape of the distribution of the estimates, none can address the significant systematic biases described in this report. For example, the National Research Council and the Iowa State University methods provide significantly improved estimates of the shape of the distribution, but do not substantially improve estimates of mean energy intake (10−15% underestimation) or protein consumption (6−7% underestimation).

Strengths and Limitations

A strength of the present study was the use of the established rEI/BMR method for the determination of physiologically implausible EI values. We used a liberal cutoff (i.e., ,1.35) that is below the study-specific theoretical cutoff for our smallest subgroup (i.e., *n* >400). The use of the more conservative cutoff of rEI/BMR <1.50 recommended by Goldberg et al. (1991) increased underreporting by 10% in women and 7% in men across all surveys. A second strength was the use of a rEI/BMR >2.4 for the elimination of potential over-reporters to correct the limitations of previous research.

Finally, the use of the IOM factorial equations for estimating TEE for specific subgroups (i.e., OW & OB respondents) in the calculation of disparity values is a significant strength. The results of this additional protocol demonstrated significant underreporting in all surveys, and that the disparity values closely paralleled the implausible values in 15 of the 18 sub-groups (i.e., men & women in 9 surveys). The close agreement between these two dissimilar protocols increases confidence in our results and conclusions.

A potential limitation to our analysis was the use of the Schofield predictive equation for estimating BMR.

The Schofield predictive equations may overestimate BMR in some populations. If the Schofield equation overestimated BMR, a greater percentage of survey respondents would be classified as underreporters. To address this potential limitation, we performed the analyses using the Mifflin equation, which has been validated in OW and OB populations such as the U.S. The results of those analyses were similar to those obtained using the Schofield equation, with substantial underreporting (>50%) in all surveys, significant trends in changes in underreporting, and a small increase in over-reporting. To remain consistent with past research on implausible rEI and underreporting, we chose to present the results from the Schofield predictive equations.

Conclusions

Throughout its history, NHANES dietary measurement protocols have failed to provide accurate estimates of the habitual caloric consumption of the U.S. population. Furthermore, successive changes to the nutrient databases used for the 24HR data-to-energy conversations and improvements in measurement protocols make it exceedingly difficult to discern temporal patterns in caloric intake that can be related to changes in population rates of obesity. As such, there are no valid population-level data to support speculations regarding trends in caloric consumption and the etiology of the obesity epidemic. Because underreporting and physiologically implausible rEI values are a predominant feature of U.S. nutritional surveillance, the ability to generate empirically supported public policy and dietary guidelines relevant to the obesity epidemic based on these data is extremely limited.

EDWARD ARCHER is an obesity theorist and computational physiologist at the Nutritional Obesity Research Center at the University of Alabama, Birmingham.

GREGORY HAND is Professor of Epidemiology and Founding Dean of the Robert C. Byrd Health Sciences Center School of Public Health at West Virginia University. He previously served as Professor of Exercise Science and Associate Dean for Research and Practice at the University of South Carolina, USA.

STEVEN BLAIR is Professor, Arnold School of Public Health, Departments of Exercise Science and Epidemiology and Biostatistics, University of South Carolina.

EXPLORING THE ISSUE

Are the 2015 *Dietary Guidelines* Based on Sound Science?

Critical Thinking and Reflection

1. Outline the steps in the systematic review process used by the DGAC to formulate their report to the Secretaries of HHS and USDA.
2. Summarize the research protocol used by NHANES. Include recruitment of subjects; data collected and methods used; and the location where data is collected.
3. Locate and summarize one primary research article that uses recent NHANES data to describe the food or nutritional quality of Americans' eating patterns.
4. Complete 24-hour diet recalls for five of your friends. Using a diet analysis program such as SuperTracker, determine the calories consumed in the 24-hour period. Compare your friends' average caloric intake to the average reported for adults in WWEIA data.
5. Using data from WWEIA, describe the sample of people used in the most recent data collection period. Include the number and percentage by age, sex, income, and racial background. Explain if you think this is a logical representative group of Americans to use when describing typical dietary patterns of Americans. List strengths and weaknesses of using this data to formulate U.S. dietary guidance.

Is There Common Ground?

The 14 members of the DGAC and the three authors (Archer, Hand, and Blair) of the NO article recognize that a strong science base is needed to develop nutrition guidance for the nation. All 17 of the individuals are very knowledgeable in current nutrition and health research and considered experts in a field related to nutrition, food, or health.

All recognize weaknesses of using 24-hour recalls from the NHANES and WWEIA data to describe the general nutrient and food intake patterns. In fact, the DGAC point out that the "strengths and shortcomings of these dietary assessment methods have been discussed over time and that no assessment method is perfect" and they even cite the article by Archer, Hand, and Blair. Therefore, common ground does exist. Why, however, do HHS and USDA allow this weak data to be used to formulate the official nutrition guidance for the nation?

Additional Resources

Archer E, Pavela G, Lavie CJ. The inadmissibility of What We Eat in America and NHANES dietary data in nutrition and obesity research and the scientific formulation of national dietary guidelines. *Mayo Clin Proc.* 2015;90(7):911–26.

Davy BM, Estabrooks PA. The validity of self-reported dietary intake data: Focus on the "What We Eat In America" component of the National Health and Nutrition Examination Survey research initiative. *Mayo Clin Proc.* 2015;90(7):845–7.

Hébert JR, Hurley TG, Steck SE, et al. Considering the value of dietary assessment data in informing nutrition-related health policy. *Adv Nutr.* 2014;5(4):447–55.

Slavin, J., U nutritionist: Keep dietary guidance evidence-based. *Star Tribune.* July 28, 2015.

Teicholz, N. The scientific report guiding the US dietary guidelines: Is it scientific? *BMJ.* 2015;351:h4962.

Internet References . . .

Food Politics

> Food.politics.com

Health.gov

> health.gov

National Health and Nutrition Examination Survey (NHANES)

> www.cdc.gov/nchs/nhanes.htm

SuperTracker

> supertracker.usda.gov

Selected, Edited, and with Issue Framing Material by:
Janet M. Colson, *Middle Tennessee State University*

ISSUE

Should We Eat Less Saturated Fat?

YES: Barbara E. Millen, from "Part D. Chapter 6: Cross-Cutting Topics of Public Health Importance: Saturated Fat," *Scientific Report of the 2015 Dietary Guidelines Advisory Committee* (2015)

NO: Richard A. Passwater, from "An Interview with Professor Fred A. Kummerow, Ph.D., Cholesterol and Saturated Fats Won't Kill You, but *Trans* Fat May (Parts 1 and 2)," *WholeFoods Magazine* (2014)

Learning Outcomes
After reading this issue, you will be able to:
• Discuss the two conclusions that the DGAC makes about saturated fats related to health and the studies on which their conclusions are based.
• Describe the early research conducted by biochemist Fred A. Kummerow related to lipid metabolism and why he contends that saturated fat is heart neutral.
• Differentiate between the results of studies reviewed by the DGAC and those described in the interview of Kummerow by Richard Passwater.

ISSUE SUMMARY

YES: The DGAC, led by Barbara E. Millen, followed the lead of the American Heart Association and the American College of Cardiology and recommend eating less saturated fat. It concludes there is "strong and consistent" evidence that replacing saturated fat with polyunsaturated fat reduces risk of cardiovascular disease and coronary mortality and only "limited evidence" that replacing saturated with monounsaturated fats is beneficial.

NO: Richard A. Passwater interviews biochemist Fred Kummerow, who at 100 years of age reports that he eats one egg, uses real butter, and drinks three glasses of whole milk each day. He says that "saturated fats are heart neutral and have no effect on cholesterol/HDL ratio or heart disease. They do provide calories, though, and should not be overdone in terms of daily calories."

In the 1950s, scientist Ancel Keys became famous in the health and nutrition community for his theory that eating too much saturated fat causes heart disease and proposed the idea that replacing saturated fat with polyunsaturated is cardio-protective. The American Heart Association agreed with his hypothesis and began to promote low-fat diets, especially those low in the "evil" saturated fats. Throughout the 1960s, health writers for popular publications such as *The New York Times*, *Time* magazine, and *Reader's Digest* promoted the "fat is evil, saturated fat is worse" message.

Finally, the federal government began to pay attention to the idea and introduced the *Dietary Goals for the United States* in 1977. The goals called for a limit on total fat intake to 30 percent of energy and recommended to limit saturated fat (SFA) to 10 percent of energy with polyunsaturated fat (PUFA) and monounsaturated fat (MUFA) each contributing 10 percent of energy, and daily cholesterol intake be limited to 300 mg.

Based on its 1974 report, the USDA estimated that Americans had been consuming about 42 percent of energy from fats, with 16 percent from SFA, 19 percent from MUFA, and only 7 percent from PUFA. To achieve the new dietary goals would require that Americans make some pretty drastic dietary changes to be able to decrease both SFA and MUFA, while increasing PUFA. This message continued when the first *Dietary Guidelines for Americans* (*DGA*) was published in 1980 and for the six editions that followed. The message that "fat is evil" resulted in a fat phobia in most Americans. One group that benefited from the low-fat craze was the food industry; thousands of "low-fat" or "cholesterol-free" products were developed netting billions in profit to food processors.

The recommendation to limit fat to 30 percent of calories continued until 2005 when the *DGA* introduced a desirable fat intake range from 20 to 35 percent of energy for adults with slightly higher levels for children. Additionally, the emphasis to consume 10 percent of energy from MUFA and another 10 percent from PUFA was changed to simply replace SFA calories with MUFA and/or PUFA.

America has followed the instructions and has cut back on fat, saturated fat, and cholesterol. But were these changes necessary and even beneficial?

As far back as 1977, Senator Percy and fellow senators, who were on the original *Dietary Goals* committee, stated that they had "serious reservations about certain aspects" of the *Dietary Goals* and had "become increasingly aware of the lack of consensus among nutrition scientists and other health professionals." This skepticism and lack of consensus continues today.

Numerous popular books, articles, and documentaries have bashed the "cut back on fat and cholesterol recommendation." Perhaps one of the earliest was cardiologist Dr. Robert Atkins. Beginning in 1972, Atkins promoted his low-carb diet claiming that eating steak, eggs, butter, pork rinds, and other fatty foods while restricting carbohydrate intake not only results in rapid weight loss, but also improves blood cholesterol and glucose levels. After three decades of criticism by the mainstream medical community, *New York Times* journalist Gary Taubes questions the criticism in his 2002 article "What If It's Been a Big Fat Lie." Part of his defense for Atkins includes:

> They spend 30 years ridiculing Robert Atkins, author of the phenomenally-best-selling 'Dr. Atkins' Diet Revolution' . . . accusing the Manhattan doctor of quackery and fraud, only to discover that the unrepentant Atkins was right all along. Or maybe it's this: they find that their very own dietary recommendations—eat less fat and more carbohydrates—are the cause of the rampaging epidemic of obesity in America. Or, just possibly this: they find out both of the above are true.

When Atkins first published his "Diet Revolution" in 1972, Americans were just coming to terms with the proposition that fat—particularly the saturated fat of meat and dairy products—was the primary nutritional evil in the American diet. Atkins managed to sell millions of copies of a book promising that we would lose weight eating steak, eggs and butter to our heart's desire, because it was the carbohydrates, the pasta, rice, bagels and sugar that caused obesity and even heart disease. Fat, he said, was harmless.

More recently, Nina Teicholz's best-selling book *The Big Fat Surprise: Why Butter, Meat and Cheese Belong in a Healthy Diet* sheds even more light on the possibility that "nutrition experts" have made a mistake on low-fat recommendations. She questions the nutrition advice that the government, the American Heart and Medical Associations, plus most nutrition professionals have preached over the last 50 years and agrees with Taubes that the diet-heart hypothesis is at the root of health problems.

The 2015 Dietary Guidelines Advisory Committee (DGAC) recommendations do not include any limitations on cholesterol and specify no upper limit on total fat but continue to set limits on SFA. They also stress to replace SFA with PUFA but question the benefits of increasing MUFA intake.

Many of the 29,000 comment letters about the DGAC report focused on the fat recommendations—some supported the report whereas others were critical. For example, the American Heart Association's letter (Comment ID #24235) "strongly supports" the DGAC's fat recommendations and concludes that lowering the SFA intake will also reduce cholesterol intake because SFA and cholesterol are often found in the same animal-derived foods such as eggs, cheese, and beef. They also recommend a limit of only 5 to 6 percent of energy from saturated fat instead of 10 percent.

The Center for Science in the Public Interest (CSPI) submitted a 59-page letter (Comment ID #27350) and agrees that SFA should be replaced with foods high in MUFA or PUFA but that SFA should be limited to 7 percent of energy instead of 10 percent: CSPI also disagrees with the DGAC's lift on the cholesterol limit and recommends that the "final Dietary Guidelines should advise Americans to limit cholesterol-rich foods (primarily whole eggs and egg yolks) to lower their risk of heart disease and type 2 diabetes."

In contrast to both AHA and CSPI, the Academy of Nutrition and Dietetics' letter (Comment ID #27125) disagrees with the recommendations to reduce SFA. It cites its 2014 position paper on dietary fats in which it concludes, "despite documented influence of saturated fat on surrogate disease markers, the effect of saturated fat intake on disease end points is not clear." The Academy also expresses its concern that "the evidence does not lead to the conclusion that saturated fats should be replaced with polyunsaturated fats for the greatest health benefit." Instead it proposes to replace carbohydrate with PUFA "because carbohydrate contributes a greater amount to the risk for cardiovascular disease than saturated fat."

So what are your thoughts? The first selection, by the DGAC, stresses the need to reduce SFA to improve health. Biochemists Richard A. Passwater and Fred A. Kummerow explain the historical background on lipid recommendations and provide the chemical basis about why SFA is not the culprit.

YES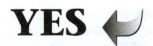

Barbara E. Millen

Part D. Chapter 6: Cross-Cutting Topics of Public Health Importance: Saturated Fat

Saturated Fat

Introduction

The relationship between different types of dietary fats and risk of CVD has been extensively studied in RCTs and epidemiologic studies. It is now well-established that higher intake of *trans* fat from partially hydrogenated vegetable oils is associated with increased risk of CVD and thus, should be minimized in the diet. Numerous RCTs have demonstrated that saturated fat (SFA) as compared to mono- (MUFA) or polyunsaturated fats (PUFA) or carbohydrates increases total and LDL cholesterol. Thus, limiting saturated fat consumption has been a longstanding dietary recommendation to reduce risk of CVD. In particular, previous DGACs have recommended consuming no more than 10 percent of daily calories from saturated fat.

However, recent meta-analyses of prospective observational studies did not find a significant association between higher saturated fat intake and risk of CVD in large populations. These data have re-ignited the debate regarding the current recommendation to limit saturated fat intake. Therefore, the DGAC chose to conduct a focused review of published systematic reviews and meta-analyses on saturated fat intake and CVD. A central issue in the relationship between saturated fat and CVD is the specific macronutrients that are used to replace it because consuming unsaturated fats versus carbohydrates in place of saturated fat can have different effects on blood lipids and risk of CVD. Thus, the Committee's assessment of the available evidence puts greater emphasis on the replacement macronutrient for saturated fat.

In the United States, the top sources of foods contributing to saturated fat intake are mixed dishes, particularly burgers and sandwiches, and snacks and sweets. Although saturated fat intake has declined in the past decades, current intake is still high at a median of 11.1 percent of daily calories. Therefore, saturated fat continues to be an area of public health concern and the DGAC deemed it important to re-evaluate and update the knowledge base on saturated fat intake and CVD risk.

Question: What is the relationship between intake of saturated fat and risk of cardiovascular disease?

Conclusions

Strong and consistent evidence from RCTs shows that replacing SFA with unsaturated fats, especially PUFA, significantly reduces total and LDL cholesterol. Replacing SFA with carbohydrates (sources not defined) also reduces total and LDL cholesterol, but significantly increases triglycerides and reduces HDL cholesterol.

Strong and consistent evidence from RCTs and statistical modeling in prospective cohort studies shows that replacing SFA with PUFA reduces the risk of CVD events and coronary mortality. For every 1 percent of energy intake from SFA replaced with PUFA, incidence of CHD is reduced by 2 to 3 percent. However, reducing total fat (replacing total fat with overall carbohydrates) does not lower CVD risk. Consistent evidence from prospective cohort studies shows that higher SFA intake as compared to total carbohydrates is not associated with CVD risk. **DGAC Grade: Strong**

Evidence is limited regarding whether replacing SFA with MUFA confers overall CVD (or CVD endpoint) benefits. One reason is that the main sources of MUFA in a typical American diet are animal fat, and because of the co-occurrence of SFA and MUFA in foods makes it difficult to tease out the independent association of MUFA with CVD. However, evidence from RCTs and prospective studies has demonstrated benefits of plant sources of monounsaturated fats, such as olive oil and nuts on CVD risk. **DGAC Grade: Limited**

Scientific Report of the 2015 Dietary Guidelines Advisory Committee: Part D: Science Base, Chapter 6: Cross-Cutting Topics of Public Health Importance: Saturated Fat, February 2015.

Implications

Recommendations on saturated fat intake should specify replacement macronutrients and emphasize replacing saturated fat with unsaturated fats, especially polyunsaturated fats. The Committee recommends retaining the 10 percent upper limit for saturated fat intake. In practice, non-hydrogenated vegetable oils that are high in unsaturated fats and relatively low in SFA (e.g., soybean, corn, olive, and canola oils) instead of animal fats (e.g., butter, cream, beef tallow, and lard) or tropical oils (e.g., palm, palm kernel, and coconut oils) should be recommended as the primary source of dietary fat. Partially hydrogenated oils containing *trans* fat should be avoided.

In low-fat diets, fats are often replaced with refined carbohydrates and this is of particular concern because such diets are generally associated with dyslipidemia (hypertriglyceridemia and low HDL-C concentrations). Therefore, dietary advice should put the emphasis on optimizing types of dietary fat and not reducing total fat.

When individuals reduce consumption of refined carbohydrates and added sugars, they should not replace them with foods high in saturated fat. Instead, refined carbohydrates and added sugars should be replaced by healthy sources of carbohydrates (e.g., whole grains, legumes, vegetables, and fruits), and healthy sources of fats (e.g., non-hydrogenated vegetable oils that are high unsaturated fats, and nuts/seeds). The consumption of "low-fat" or "nonfat" products with high amounts of refined grains and added sugars should be discouraged.

Dietary recommendations on macronutrient composition for reducing CVD risk should be dietary pattern-based emphasizing foods that characterize healthy dietary patterns. Individuals are encouraged to consume dietary patterns that emphasize vegetables, fruits, whole grains, legumes, and nuts; include low-and non-fat dairy products, poultry, seafood, non-tropical vegetable oils; limit sodium, saturated fat, refined grains, sugar-sweetened foods and beverages, and are lower in red and processed meats. Multiple dietary patterns can achieve these food and nutrient patterns and are beneficial for cardiovascular health, and they should be tailored to individuals' biological needs and food preferences.

Review of the Evidence

The DGAC drew evidence from SRs or MA published between January 2009 and August 2014 in English in a peer-reviewed journal, which included RCTs and/or prospective cohort studies. Participants included healthy volunteers as well as individuals at elevated chronic disease risk. The main exposure was SFA, and the main outcomes included LDL-cholesterol (LDL-C), HDL-cholesterol (HDL-C), triglycerides (TG), blood pressure (BP), and incidence of CVD and CHD, CVD- and CHD-related death, myocardial infarction, or stroke. All reviews were high-quality, with ratings ranging from 8 to 11 on AMSTAR. The Committee drew evidence on blood lipids and blood pressure outcomes from the AHA/ACC Lifestyle Guideline and the associated NHLBI Lifestyle Report, which included primarily RCTs on intermediate CVD risk factors. The Committee drew evidence on CVD endpoints and effect size estimates from seven published MA that included one or more studies not covered in these reports. Little evidence on the contribution of SFA to cardiovascular risk factors in the pediatric populations was available, and that which was published has not been systematically reviewed.

Effects of Replacing SFA on LDL-C, HDL-C, and TG

Macronutrients may affect plasma lipids and lipoproteins, which are strong predictors of CVD risk. The NHLBI Lifestyle Report summarized evidence from three feeding trials examining effects on LDL-C of dietary patterns with varying SFA levels: DASH (Dietary Approaches to Stop Hypertension), DASH-Sodium, and DELTA (Dietary Effects on Lipoproteins and Thrombogenic Activity). The results from these trials indicate that reducing total and saturated fat led to a significant reduction in LDL cholesterol in the context of the DASH dietary pattern and the National Cholesterol Education Program (NCEP) Step 1 diet. To estimate the effects of replacing SFA by specific macronutrients such as carbohydrates, MUFA, or PUFA, the NHLBI Lifestyle Report also included two MA from Mensink and Katan (n = 1,672), covering the period from 1970 to 1998 (27 controlled trials in the first MA and 60 controlled trials in the second MA) and using the same inclusion/exclusion criteria to estimate changes in plasma lipids when substituting dietary SFA with carbohydrates or other fat types and holding dietary cholesterol constant. Mensink and Katan found that replacing 1 percent of SFA with an equal amount of carbohydrates, MUFA, or PUFA led to comparable LDL-C reductions: 1.2, 1.3, and 1.8 mg/dL, respectively. Replacing 1 percent of SFA with carbohydrates, MUFA, or PUFA also lowered HDL-C by 0.4, 1.2, and 0.2 mg/dL, respectively. Replacing 1 percent of carbohydrates by an equal amount of MUFA or PUFA raised LDL-C by 0.3 and 0.7 mg/dL, raised HDL-C by 0.3 and 0.2 mg/dL, and lowered TG by 1.7 and 2.3 mg/dL, respectively. The 2003 MA by Mensink and Katan indicated that the ratio of total to HDL-C, a stronger predictor of CVD risk than total or LDL cholesterol alone, did not change when SFA was replaced by carbohydrates, but the ratio significantly decreased when SFA was replaced by unsaturated fats, especially PUFA.

In summary, strong and consistent evidence from RCTs shows that replacing SFA with unsaturated fats, especially PUFA, significantly reduces total and LDL cholesterol. Replacing SFA with carbohydrates also reduces total and LDL cholesterol, but significantly increases TG and reduces HDL cholesterol. However, the evidence of beneficial effects on one risk factor does not rule out neutral or opposite effects on unstudied risk factors. To better assess the overall effects of intervention to reduce or modify SFA intake, studies of clinical endpoints are summarized below.

The Relationship between Consumption of Total Fat and SFA and Risk of CVD

A MA by Skeaff et al. in 2009 included 28 U.S. and European cohorts (6,600 CHD deaths among 280,000 participants) and found no clear relationship between total or SFA intake and CHD events or deaths. Similarly, Siri-Tarino et al., 2010 found that SFA intake was not associated with risk of CHD, stroke or cardiovascular disease. The Siri-Tarino et al., 2010 meta-analysis included data from 347,747 participants (11,006 developed CVD) in 21 unique studies, with 16 studies providing risk estimates for CHD and 8 studies providing data for stroke as an endpoint. In the 2012 MA of trials to reduce or modify intake of SFA, Hooper et al. also found no significant associations of total fat reduction with cardiovascular events or mortality.

Consistent with these prior studies, Chowdhury et al.'s 2014 MA of total SFA also did not specify what macronutrient substituted SFA and again found no association of dietary SFA intake, nor of circulating SFA, with coronary disease. Chowdhury et al. included data from 32 observational studies (530,525 participants) of fatty acids from dietary intake, 17 observational studies (25,721 participants) of fatty acid biomarkers, and 27 RCTs (103,052 participants) of fatty acid supplementation.

The results described above do not explicitly specify the comparison or replacement nutrient, but typically it consists largely of carbohydrates (sources not defined). These results suggest that replacing SFA with carbohydrates is not associated with CVD risk. Taken together, these results suggest that simply reducing SFA or total fat in the diet by replacing it with any type of carbohydrates is not effective in reducing risk of CVD.

Effects of Replacing SFA with Polyunsaturated Fat or Carbohydrates on CVD Events

Hooper et al.'s 2012 Cochrane MA of trials of SFA reduction/modification found that reducing SFA by reducing and/or modifying dietary fat reduced the risk of cardiovascular events by 14 percent (pooled RR = 0.86; 95% CI = 0.77 to 0.96, with 24 comparisons and 65,508 participants of whom 7 percent had a cardiovascular event, I = 50%). Subgroup analyses revealed this protective effect was driven by dietary fat *modification* rather than reduction and was only apparent in longer trials (2 years or more). Despite the reduction in total cardiovascular events, there was no clear evidence of reductions in any individual outcome (total or non-fatal myocardial infarction, stroke, cancer deaths or diagnoses, diabetes diagnoses), nor was there any evidence that trials of reduced or modified SFA reduced cardiovascular mortality. These results suggest that modifying dietary fat by replacing some saturated (animal) fats with plant oils and unsaturated spreads may reduce risk of heart and vascular disease.

Emphasizing the benefits of replacement of saturated with polyunsaturated fats, Mozaffarian et al., 2010 found in a MA of 8 trials (13,614 participants with 1,042 CHD events) that modifying fat reduced the risk of myocardial infarction or coronary heart disease death (combined) by 19 percent (RR = 0.81; 95% CI = 0.70 to 0.95; p = 0.008), corresponding to 10 percent reduced CHD risk (RR = 0.90; 95% CI = 0.83 to 0.97) for each 5 percent energy of increased PUFA. This magnitude of effect is similar to that observed in the Cochrane MA. In secondary analyses restricted to CHD mortality events, the pooled RR was 0.80 (95% CI = 0.65 to 0.98). In subgroup analyses, the RR was greater in magnitude in the four trials in primary prevention populations but non-significant (24 percent reduction in CHD events) compared to a significant reduction of 16 percent in the four trials of secondary prevention populations. Mozaffarian et al. argue that the slightly greater risk reduction in studies of CHD events, compared with predicted effects based on lipid changes alone, is consistent with potential additional benefits of PUFA on other non-lipid pathways of risk, such as insulin resistance. Many of the included trials used vegetable oils containing small amounts of plant-derived n-3 PUFA in addition to omega-6 PUFA.

Consistent with the benefits of replacing SFA with PUFA for prevention of CHD shown in other studies, Farvid et al., 2014 conducted an SR and MA of prospective cohort studies of dietary linoleic acid (LA), which included 13 studies with 310,602 individuals and 12,479 total CHD events (5,882 CHD deaths). Farvid et al. found dietary LA intake is inversely associated with CHD risk in a dose-response manner: when comparing the highest to the lowest category of intake, LA was associated with a 15 percent lower risk of CHD events (pooled RR = 0.85; 95% CI = 0.78 to 0.92; I^2 = 35.5%) and a 21% lower risk of CHD deaths (pooled RR = 0.79; 95% CI = 0.71 to 0.89; I^2 = 0.0%). A 5 percent of energy increment in LA intake replacing energy from SFA intake was associated with a 9 percent lower risk of CHD events (RR = 0.91; 95% CI = 0.86 to 0.96) and a 13 percent lower risk of CHD deaths (RR = 0.87; 95% CI = 0.82 to 0.94). In the meta-analysis conducted by Chowdhury et al., there was no significant association between LA intake and CHD risk, but the analysis was based on a limited number of prospective cohort studies.

In Jakobsen et al.'s 2009 pooled analysis of 11 cohorts (344,696 persons with 5,249 coronary events and 2,155 coronary deaths), a 5 percent lower energy intake from SFAs and a concomitant higher energy intake from PUFAs reduced risk of coronary events by 13 percent (hazard ratio [HR] = 0.87; 95% CI = 0.77 to 0.97) and coronary deaths by 16 percent (hazard ratio = 0.74; 95% CI = 0.61 to 0.89).By contrast, a 5 percent lower energy intake from SFAs and a concomitant higher energy intake from carbohydrates, there was a modest significant direct association between carbohydrates and coronary events (hazard ratio = 1.07; 95% CI = 1.01 to 1.14) and no association with coronary deaths (hazard ratio = 0.96; 95% CI = 0.82 to 1.13). Notably, the estimated HRs for carbohydrate intake in this study could reflect high glycemic carbohydrate intake rather than total carbohydrate, as fiber was controlled for in the analyses. MUFA intake was not associated with CHD incidence or death.

Taken together, strong and consistent evidence from RCTs and statistical modeling in prospective cohort studies shows that replacing SFA with PUFA reduces the risk of CVD events and coronary mortality. For every 1 percent of energy intake from SFA replaced with PUFA, incidence of CHD is reduced by 2 to 3 percent. The evidence is not as clear for replacement by MUFA or replacement with carbohydrate, and likely depends on the type and source.

Methodological Issues
When individuals in natural settings reduce calories from SFA, they typically replaced them with other macronutrients, and the type and source of the macronutrients substituting SFA determine effects on CVD. For this reason, studies specifying the macronutrient type replacing SFA are more informative than those examining only total SFA intake, and the strongest and most consistent evidence for CVD reduction is with replacement of SFA with PUFA in both RCTs and observational studies.

The differing effects of the type and source of macronutrient substituted may be one reason for the limited evidence regarding whether replacing SFA with MUFA confers CVD benefits and the lack of benefit from carbohydrate substitution. The main sources of MUFA in a typical American diet are animal fats, which could confound potential benefits of SFA-replacement with plant-source MUFA, such as nuts and olive oil, which have demonstrated benefits on CVD risk. To date, evidence testing replacement of SFA by MUFA from different sources is insufficient to reach a firm conclusion. Similarly, most analyses did not distinguish between substitution of saturated fat by different types of carbohydrates (e.g., refined carbohydrate vs. whole grains).

Of the RCTs included in this evidence summary, the intervention methods used varied from long-term dietary counseling with good generalizability but variable compliance, to providing a whole diet for weeks (e.g., controlled feeding studies) with maximal compliance but limited generalizability. Though the content of the recommended or provided diet is known with greater precision in the RCTs than in observational studies, adherence to the diet is likely variable and could result in lack of compliance and high rates of dropout in long-term trials. Additionally, bias may arise from the lack of blinding in non-supplement dietary intervention trials.

In prospective observational studies, misclassification of dietary fatty acid intake could bias associations towards the null. In addition, residual confounding by other dietary and lifestyle factors cannot be ruled out through statistical adjustment. Despite these methodological issues, there is high consistency of the evidence from prospective cohort studies and RCTs in supporting the benefits of replacing saturated fat with unsaturated fats especially PUFA in reducing CVD risk.

. . .

Chapter Summary

The DGAC encourages the consumption of healthy dietary patterns that are low in saturated fat. . . . The goals for the general population are less than 10 percent of total calories from saturated fat per day. . . .

[S]aturated fat . . . is not intended to be reduced in isolation, but as a part of a healthy dietary pattern. Rather than focusing purely on reduction, emphasis should be placed on replacement and shifts in food intake and eating patterns. Sources of saturated fat should be replaced with unsaturated fat, particularly polyunsaturated fatty acids. . . .

Needs For Future Research

. . .

1. Determine the effects of replacement of saturated fat with different types of carbohydrates (e.g., refined vs. whole grains) on cardiovascular disease risk.

   Rationale: Most randomized controlled trials and prospective cohort studies compared saturated fat with total carbohydrates. It is important to distinguish different types of carbohydrates (e.g., refined vs. whole grains) in future studies.

2. Examine the effects that replacement of saturated fat with polyunsaturated fat vs. monounsaturated fat has on cardiovascular disease risk.

   Rationale: Most existing studies have examined the effects of substituting PUFA for saturated fat on cardiovascular disease risk. Future studies should also examine the potential benefits of substituting monounsaturated fat from plant sources such as olive oil and nuts/seeds for saturated fat on cardiovascular disease risk.

3. Examine lipid and metabolic effects of specific oils modified to have different fatty acid profiles (e.g., commodity soy oil [high linoleic acid] vs. high oleic soy oil).

   Rationale: As more modified vegetables oils become commercially available, it is important to assess their long-term health effects. In addition, future studies should examine lipid and metabolic effects of plant oils that contain a mix of n-9, n-6, and n-3 fatty acids, as a replacement for animal fat, on cardiovascular disease risk factors.

4. Examine the effects of saturated fat from different sources, including animal products (e.g., butter, lard), plant (e.g., palm vs. coconut oils), and production systems (e.g., refined deodorized bleached vs. virgin coconut oil) on blood lipids and cardiovascular disease risk.

   Rationale: Different sources of saturated fat contain different fatty acid profiles and thus, may result in different lipid and metabolic effects. In addition, virgin and refined coconut oils have different effects in animal models, but human data are lacking.

5. Conduct gene-nutrient interaction studies by measuring genetic variations in relevant genes that will enable evaluation of effects of specific diets for individualized nutrition recommendations.

   Rationale: Individuals with different genetic background may respond to the same dietary intervention differently in terms of blood lipids and other cardiovascular disease risk factors. Future studies should explore the potential role of genetic factors in modulating the effects of fat type modification on health outcomes.

Barbara E. Millen, founder and president of Millennium Prevention, Inc., served as chair of the 14-member 2015 Dietary Guidelines Advisory Committee.

Richard A. Passwater

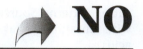 **NO**

An Interview with Professor Fred A. Kummerow, Ph.D., Cholesterol and Saturated Fats Won't Kill You, but Trans Fat May (Parts 1 and 2)

This month, I take great pride in having the legendary Professor Fred A. Kummerow, Ph.D., as our interviewee. It's not just that Dr. Kummerow was born 100 years ago on October 4, 1914 and is still hard at work, but also that he has saved many thousands of people from premature death and his research and educational efforts have paved the way to help millions more as time moves forward. It was bad enough that Dr. Kummerow nearly starved to death as a youth, but in the process of separating scientific fact from nutritional fiction, Professor Kummerow has had to endure the wrath of vested interests that gain from having you think otherwise. Readers of this column know to trust the data rather than opinions or "official procla-mations." In business, it may be "Follow the Money," but in science, it should be "Follow the Data." And, it must be the whole data—not just data hand-picked to fit a theory in spite of the fact that the total data show the theory to be wrong. Everyone can have their own opinion, but they can't have their own facts. Let's look at the facts!

Dr. Kummerow is highly regarded for his efforts to uncover the dangers of trans fats and to remove dangerous man-made fats from our food supply, but his life-saving nutritional efforts began with helping to wipe out the deadly pellagra epidemic in the United States. Today, most people have never heard of pellagra thanks to researchers including Drs. Kummerow, Joseph Goldberger and Conrad Elvehjem, but students of nutrition are familiar with the story of niacin (vitamin B3) being the anti-pellagra vita-min. What a lot of people don't know is that they had to step on quite a few toes to rid the South of pellagra.

Dr. Kummerow has published about 500 scientific articles, written two books, edited three books and contrib-uted chapters on trans fat and cholesterol in heart disease to six books. He is still publishing scientific articles to this day.

Passwater: *You were born in Berlin, Germany, on October 4, 1914. That was a very different time from what most of us know. There was no heart disease epidemic then, but there was a pellagra epidemic in the Southeast United States. Vitamins were just beginning to be discovered and World War I had just started with Austria–Hungary's war declaration on Serbia. The war lasted until November 1918. What was it like growing up poor in Germany with little food?*

Kummerow: When I was small, there was little food for my family. My mother would put my brother and me to bed during the day so we would not use up our energy and require more food. She would read to us and entertain us so that we wouldn't run around burning calories. Our food staple consisted of a slice of bread with maybe sugar on it and a little coffee for flavor.

My father's job at the railroad occasionally enabled him to bring home some extra kerosene in a flask. My mother used to exchange these small amounts of kerosene for eggs and vegetables from farmers in the area. In 1923, we were able to move to the United States.

Passwater: *I would think that almost starving gave you a special appreciation for food and nutrition.*

Kummerow: As I have written in my books, I know first-hand the impact of adding necessary ingredients to food and the difference that it makes in people's lives. I know that a vitamin lacking in the diet can kill someone, and I know this can be changed.

Passwater: *How did you become interested in chemistry?*

Kummerow: When I was 12, a relative gave me a chemistry set. I didn't learn that much from the set, but when I started high school at Boys Technical School, I took three years of chemistry. I enjoyed working in the chemistry lab and after high school I started working for a pharmaceutical company in its lab.

Passwater: *You became a biochemist at a time when there were few chemists specializing in biochemistry. How did you get started in this field?*

Kummerow: I saved enough money to start my freshman year at the University of Wisconsin in the Milwaukee Extension Division in 1936. In my sophomore year, I transferred to the University of Wisconsin in Madison. I signed up for a National Youth Administration job; money was provided by President Franklin D. Roosevelt and matched by the University. I was told to report to Dr. Steebock in Biochemistry and was assigned to work with his post-doc students for three years. I graduated with a B.S. in chemistry with honors and then in 1939 became a graduate student in biochemistry, with Dr. Steebock as my mentor. My Ph.D. research involved identifying a factor in blood that keeps blood from clotting in arteries. This factor stems from the fatty acid, linoleic acid. Today, we recognize this factor as prostacyclin. Prostacyclin is very important in heart disease to help prevent the blood clots that cause heart attacks.

I received my Ph.D. in 1943 and took a research position at Clemson University to study pellagra. In 1945, I was invited to move to Kansas State University to start a basic research program in lipid (fat) chemistry. Some of my research at Kansas State was on keeping foods from turning rancid. This was an important issue during World War II when American troops were scattered worldwide.

In 1950, I was invited to move my lipid research program to the University of Illinois in Urbana, where I have been ever since.

Passwater: *You were sought after by universities for your lipid programs. Where did you begin?*

Kummerow: My first line of research in my lipid program was the chemistry of fat and cholesterol.

Passwater: *You've seen a lot of change in the common thinking about diet and heart disease. You've seen the popular beliefs gradually change from the opposite of your research to finally come around to what you and your research had been saying all along. What were some of your early studies showing us about diet and heart disease?*

Kummerow: My early studies showed that trans fat in partially hydrogenated oils was detrimental to the health

of humans and rats. In the next phase of the study, I demonstrated that one can have a healthy heart and cardiovascular system by eating foods that contained cholesterol. Unfortunately, these foods were not recommended by physicians that served on the diet committee of the American Heart Association. Most nutritionists and biochemists did not agree with the diet these physicians recommended, however, which led to the cholesterol wars that are still going on today.

Passwater: *The popular advice was to avoid as much saturated fat and cholesterol as possible because they were thought to be the dietary culprits in heart disease. Unfortunately, in spite of overwhelming evidence to the contrary, these erroneous concepts are still being promoted today. I referenced some of your research in my paper "Dietary Cholesterol: Is It Really Related to Heart Disease?" which was published in American Laboratory in 1973. I also discussed the research by Drs. George Mann, David Kritchevsky, Edward Pinckney and many others. There was not a lack of scientific evidence showing that dietary cholesterol was not a factor.*

In 1977, I made a challenge on the back cover of my book that said, "If anyone can prove that eating cholesterol caused heart disease, I would donate all of the proceeds from my book to the American Heart Association."

That challenge earned me appearances on major television shows, but no one accepted the challenge nor did anyone even attempt to prove this belief. Instead, the experts shifted to claiming saturated fats were the dietary culprits. Is dietary cholesterol a major factor in heart disease?

Kummerow: No, it is not. You don't have to feed animals cholesterol to cause atherosclerosis.

Passwater: *Well, you certainly have presented the scientific evidence that cholesterol is not an important factor in heart disease in two of your books* Cholesterol Is Not the Culprit: A Guide to Preventing Heart Disease *and* Cholesterol Won't Kill You But Trans Fat Could.

We have covered the cholesterol myth in several interviews through the years, recently including "The Cholesterol Paradigm: The Greatest Health Scam of the Century" and "Heart Disease and the Great Cholesterol Myth."

As the renowned lipid (fat chemistry) researcher and past member of the National Academy of Sciences Food and Nutrition Board and USDA Dietary Guidelines Advisory Committees, David Kritchevsky, Ph.D., told us in 1993, "If the experts say 'A' and the data say 'B'—go with the data." The problem is that some scientists have cherry-picked the data to falsely make the scientists' incorrect theory appear to be true. We have to look at the total data and the total body of science, not just the part that seems to fit someone's pet theory.

Is high blood cholesterol the major factor in heart disease?

Kummerow: No. Michael DeBakey, M.D., who was a surgeon at Baylor University Medical School—and, by the way invented the bypass technique—stated at the 1975 Federal Trade Commission hearing on eggs that he had performed bypass surgery on patients who needed it, both with low or high cholesterol. Therefore, he didn't believe cholesterol was the problem.

Passwater: *How did this cholesterol nonsense get started?*

Kummerow: In 1913, Nikolai Anitschkov, M.D., DMedSc., performed studies on rabbits, feeding them cholesterol and eggs, and noted that it caused atherosclerosis in them. Rabbits are vegetarian animals that do not have a biochemical mechanism for handling dietary cholesterol, which comes from animal products, not vegetarian products. It is better to study the effect of cholesterol on arteries in swine, which have arteries and hearts more like humans. They are omnivores like humans.

Passwater: *People should disregard any study of dietary cholesterol or saturated fats in rabbits. Dr. Kritchevsky also told us in 1993, "In the late 1950s, two papers reported that there had been establishment of atherosclerosis in rabbits by feeding saturated fat and no cholesterol. I was one of many researchers who had fed saturated fat to rabbits for as long as a year without affecting either cholesterolemia (high blood cholesterol) or atherosclerosis. So these reports piqued my interest as to the discrepancy. I collated the available scientific literature and found that saturated fat was without effect when added to a commercial diet, but was indeed atherogenic when fed as part of a semi-purified diet. Since the fat was the same, it had to be something else, and I speculated that it was the fiber. I put this in a letter to the editors of the journal Atherosclerosis Research and it took an awfully long time to get it published. We later proved the hypothesis."*

Ancel Keys, Ph.D., published an epidemiological study that seemed to correlate fat intake with heart disease incidence. Later studies also attempted to correlate fat intake with blood cholesterol levels. He spanned a range of blood cholesterol levels (from Japan, with the lowest, to Finland, with the highest) and stated that cholesterol was responsible for heart disease.

Animal food products contain all of the eight essential amino acids, but they also contain cholesterol; vegetable food products do not contain cholesterol. Therefore, in 1961 the diet

committee of the American Heart Association stated that it was better to eat food that did not contain cholesterol. This spawned the cholesterol hypothesis. It was reinforced by the Federal Trade Commission hearing on eggs in 1975.

The epidemiological studies led by the influential Dr. Keys have been widely discounted over the years because they don't hold up to scrutiny as we will discuss shortly. Dr. Keys's series of studies evolved into additional trials called the Seven Country Studies (SCS), which were launched in 1958 and continued to be published beyond 1970. There is an official SCS Web site that explains what the studies showed and what they didn't show. The studies are basically epidemiological (population) studies and cannot show cause and effect. As the SCS Web site explains, "These graphs should not be seen as 'X causes Y' depictions, but rather as 'in groups with X, also Y is observed.'" The SCS data showed a strong cross-sectional correlation between the average saturated fat intake and average serum cholesterol level of 14 cohorts. "The following conclusion can be drawn from this graph: the cohorts with a high intake of calories from saturated fat also have a high serum cholesterol level. And cohorts with a low intake also have a low cholesterol level. This does not say that a high intake of saturated fat causes a high serum cholesterol level, but rather that there is an association at the population level which may or may not be causal."

Dr. Keys later admitted that there was "no connection whatsoever between cholesterol in food and cholesterol in the blood. None. And we've known that all along. Cholesterol in the diet doesn't matter at all unless you happen to be a chicken or a rabbit." I have read that Dr. Keys admitted to you before he died that "he was all wrong on what he was thinking."

Just about everyone has been told that the famous Framingham Study proved that cholesterol causes heart disease. The fact is that 1,000 persons in the Framingham Study were examined with a dietary review. There was no relationship between dietary habits and high blood cholesterol (cholesterolemia). Furthermore, both total mortality and cardiovascular mortality in Framingham participants increase in those with low cholesterol levels. This finding has been confirmed by multiple studies from Canada, Sweden, Russia and New Zealand. These contradictory findings have been ignored, distorted and incorrectly reported by supporters of the "Cholesterol Diet–Heart Disease" hypothesis. There have been 33 clinical trials of the Cholesterol Diet–Heart Disease hypothesis over the years and the evidence clearly shows this was not a sound hypothesis.

How did the dietary misinformation keep getting taught in spite of research showing that it was incorrect?

Kummerow: Professors, who were teaching, continued to believe it was correct because they believe in the cholesterol hypothesis. It seemed logical and it appeared that the evidence was supporting it, as meager as it was.

Passwater: *Yes, a common attitude from many scientists and politicians on the funding boards was that we need to do something now and we can't afford to wait for further studies. Everyone wanted to "do good" and they wanted to do it immediately. Heart disease had become an epidemic. A common attitude was that "we have already spent millions of dollars. Let's not get distracted by these new studies. After all, what harm can come from substituting saturated fats with partially hydrogenated oils and sugars?" They didn't see that their dietary recommendations were going to cause more harm than good. They didn't realize that they were further shifting the American diet to even more of the real culprits that cause heart disease.*

Why is cholesterol vital to our bodies?

Kummerow: Cells need cholesterol in their membranes for proper functioning and to "coat" them, which protects them from salts in the plasma.

Passwater: *How about dietary saturated fats? Last month, we discussed with Gerald P. McNeill, Ph.D., that many people have the misconception that animal fats are saturated fats and that plant fats are unsaturated fats. Natural whole foods are mixtures of both saturated and unsaturated fats. Some plant fats can be predominantly saturated fats and some animal fats can be mostly unsaturated fats. For example, beef fat is 54% unsaturated, lard is 60% unsaturated and chicken fat is about 70% unsaturated. Coconut oil, from the fruit of the coconut plant, is 85% saturated fat.*

In 1953, Dr. Keys published a paper called, "Atherosclerosis: A Problem in Newer Public Health." His paper included a graph comparing fat consumption and deaths from heart disease in men from six different countries. That paper and subsequent SCS are a massive set of inconsistencies and contradictions. First of all, we have to keep in mind that population studies contain many variables and cannot prove cause and effect. This study cannot be taken seriously by the objective and critical scientist. As one example, the mortality rate in Finland was almost seven times higher than in Mexico, although the fat consumption was identical. The so-called "French Paradox" is another example. This study intentionally left out countries where people eat a lot of fat, but have little heart disease, such as Holland and Norway. It left out countries where fat consumption is low, but the rate of heart disease is high, such as Chile. It appears that the examples selected were chosen to fit their theory, rather than looking at all the available data. Many scientists claimed that Dr. Keys did indeed cherry-pick the countries. Data were available from

22 countries at the time. If Dr. Keys had chosen Australia, Finland, Germany, Ireland, the Netherlands and Switzerland instead of Australia, Canada, England and Wales, Japan, Italy and the United States, the opposite trend would have been shown wherein a high fat intake is associated with less heart disease. These data didn't fit with Dr. Keys's theory, so maybe it was more convenient to just ignore them. Today, data are available for more countries including populations having saturated fat intake in the 60–75% range and having just about zero heart disease like the Inuit, Masai, Rendille and Todelau.

The study was widely criticized in the scientific community, but policymakers thought it was straightforward and convincing. In 1957, Drs. Jacob Yerushalmy and Herman Hilleboe scientifically rebutted the study, but they didn't have the clout to overcome the dynamic Dr. Keys. Later, as the theory still continued to gain momentum, Drs. R.L. Smith and E.R. Pinckney revealed "a massive set of inconsistencies and contradictions."

Haven't studies, including meta-studies shown that saturated fats are not associated with heart disease, but are neutral? Do they have a significant effect on cholesterol/HDL ratio or heart disease?

Kummerow: Saturated fats are heart neutral and have no effect on cholesterol/HDL ratio or heart disease. They do provide calories, though, and should not be overdone in terms of daily calories.

Passwater: *In the 1960s in the United States, fats and oils supplied around 45% of calories and only about 13% of adults were obese; less than 1% had type-2 diabetes. Now, Americans eat less fats and oils (about 33% of calories), yet 34% of adults are obese and 11% have type-2 diabetes, which seems to be becoming epidemic.*

Well, if it isn't cholesterol and saturated fats, what could it be? You have long researched dietary cholesterol. How did you come to suspect that trans fats were the heart disease culprit instead? It certainly wasn't obvious!

Dr. Kummerow replied, "In 1957, I persuaded a hospital to give me samples of arteries from patients who had died of heart attacks. When I analyzed them I found that yes, the diseased arteries were filled with fat, but it was a specific kind of fat: trans fats."

Well, he made that sound simple, but there is a whole lot more to this discovery than meets the eye. How does one recognize trans fats in arteries when so little was known about trans fats then and especially in human arteries? Let's continue the story.

Passwater: *In 1974, I attended your presentation at the annual meeting of the Federation of American Societies for*

Experimental Biology in Atlantic City. You and your colleagues presented your finding that trans fat presented a greater health risk than cholesterol-rich foods such as beef fat, butterfat and powdered eggs. In your studies, you fed the various fats to different groups of swine for eight months. Swine were used because they have aortas and hearts of similar size to humans. Your studies concluded that trans fats, which were added to margarine to make it firmer and more stable, were the most atherogenic (causing deposits in the arteries). The second worst group was the one fed an identical diet except that the calories of margarine were replaced with an equal number of calories from sugar. The animals fed the same diet except the margarine calories were replaced with butter calories had negligible changes in their arteries. The least artery disease was found in the group fed eggs. There were questions at first concerning the amount of essential fatty acids fed the swine, but your research was eventually published a few years later in the journal Artery.

This was the first time that I realized that trans fats were atherogenic. University scientists, government scientists and the food police continued to endorse trans fats as a healthier alternative to saturated fats. By 1984, food activists were pressuring fast food companies to discontinue frying food with safe, trans fats-free animal fats and tropical oils and switch to harmful trans fats-rich partially hydrogenated oils. They must be held accountable for their actions that exposed Americans to more heart disease-causing man-made trans fats. Industry groups and scientists married to the saturated fats theory continued to try to discredit your research, just as they tried to discredit the research of Mary Enig, Ph.D. But in 1990, a major study showed that trans fats increased risk factors for heart disease more than saturated fats did.

Perhaps what should have been the final nail in the coffin of the saturated fat theory came in 1993 with the Nurses' Health Study by Harvard scientists that concluded, "These findings support the hypothesis that consumption of partially hydrogenated vegetable oils may contribute to occurrence of CHD."

George Mann, M.D., called for more research on the metabolic consequences of dietary trans fatty acids. He pointed out that the epidemic of heart disease followed the introduction of partially hydrogenated fats in food and they "impair lipoprotein receptors leading to hypercholesterolemia, atherogenesis, obesity and insulin resistance."

Walter C. Willett, M.D., Dr.P.H. and Alberto Ascherio, M.D., Dr.P.H., commented in the American Journal of Public Health, "Federal regulations should require manufacturers . . . to greatly reduce or eliminate the use of partially hydrogenated vegetable fats."

What advice do you offer regarding eating eggs and butter?

Kummerow: My advice regarding eating eggs and butter is that eggs contain all of the essential amino acids and butter contains the two essential fatty acids. Both are needed for a well-balanced diet. Eggs are one of nature's most perfect foods. Besides the essential amino acids needed to build cells, whole eggs contain many vitamins and minerals.

Also, my advice is to eat less trans fat and more foods rich in magnesium, B6 and B12. Eat a balanced diet with a differing protein source every day, avoid all trans fats and don't drink sodas.

Passwater: *You mention magnesium, a much underrated nutrient. I remember your 1999 paper on magnesium reversing the artery calcification caused by trans fats.*

Kummerow: Good. In that paper, my colleagues and I showed under what conditions trans fatty acids are a risk factor to the calcification of coronary arteries, which is the beginning of atherosclerosis, and if you translate this to the human diet, it means that adequate magnesium may modify the formation of calcified streaks.

Passwater: *Getting back to eggs and butter, neither contain harmful trans fats. Please explain to our readers who may not be chemists just what is a trans fat.*

Kummerow: Trans fats are formed during the process of converting soybean oil into margarine and vegetable shortening. During this process, trans fatty acids are formed. Natural oils are extracted from natural foods and then are converted into chemicals not found in nature by a process called hydrogenation. Hydrogenation adds hydrogen atoms to partially saturate the polyunsaturated fatty acids found in the natural oils, but in doing so, hydrogenation also converts many of the natural cis fatty acids into trans fatty acids.

Unsaturated fats contain double bonds in their chemical structure whereas saturated fats do not. In chemistry, "trans" refers to identical atoms (in this case hydrogen atoms) on opposite sides of a double bond (in this case a double bond between two carbon atoms). "Cis" refers to the arrangement where the two identical atoms (hydrogen) are on the same side of the double bond.

Vegetable oils contain several fatty acids, including the recognized "dietary essential" fatty acids (EFAs) linoleic acid (omega-6) and linolenic acid (omega-3). These two EFAs have double bonds at the 9,12 or 9,12,15 positions on the carbon chain. Partial hydrogenation changes the chemical structure of these EFAs. It causes the migration of the double bonds to other positions in the chain leading to a transformation to nine different trans isomers. This is one reason why the oils can become plasticized.

The partial hydrogenation process tampered with nature by introducing 14 different fatty acids that had no business being there.

Passwater: *So, a wholesome dietary essential fat is changed by man into a different beast. The trans isomers give the fat a different molecular arrangement that converts oil into a solid, spreadable fat. The new trans configurations are more linear and not as space filling, so they have detrimental effects on membrane structure. Trans fats cause considerable harm in the body as we have discussed in previous columns with Dr. Enig dating back to 1993. Trans fats cause various alterations to cell membrane fluidity and functions. Trans fatty acids disrupt enzymes in the membranes including delta-6 desaturase.*

How do trans fats cause artery damage?

Kummerow: Trans fats become part of the endothelial cells that line the artery walls, just as they become part of all cell membranes. They cause inflammation and calcification of arterial cells—known risk factors for coronary heart disease. In the endothelial cells, trans fats interfere with the synthesis of prostacyclin, which is a compound needed in the arteries to keep the blood flowing. Trans fatty acids suppress prostacyclin production at levels found in commercial margarines, and processed foods labeled as trans-free could contribute to this effect if consumed in multiple servings or in addition to foods containing larger amounts of trans fats.

Neither cholesterol nor saturated fats are responsible for these changes. People who eat trans fats are not capable of keeping their blood flowing and can die a sudden death. They don't die immediately after eating trans fats, but they die suddenly with a heart attack years later as the trans fats build up in the arteries. In 2011, the Centers for Disease Control and Prevention reported that 275,000 Americans died of sudden death. The U.S. Food and Drug Administration (FDA) is planning to remove these trans fatty acids from the diet. According to the FDA, they are present in more than 37,000 food items in the United States.

Passwater: *Trans fats certainly are ubiquitous. What are the main dietary sources of trans fats?*

Kummerow: Margarine and vegetable shortening, which is used in the baking of cookies, cakes and bread.

Passwater: *When did trans fats begin to be significant in the American diet?*

Kummerow: About 1920. They were introduced here just before 1910.

Passwater: *The heart disease incidence grew after 1920, slowly at first, then reaching epidemic levels at a time when saturated fats and eggs were decreasing and trans fats were* increasing. *It's difficult for this generation to realize that there were few heart attacks before 1920. Coronary thrombosis was first reported in 1896 by George Doc, M.D., as a rare event. The first description of a heart attack in a medical journal may have been in 1912. When Paul Dudley White, M.D., who was one of the first cardiologists, was an intern at Massachusetts General Hospital in 1911, there was no Department of Cardiology.*

Your early research findings were not appreciated by the cholesterol gang. I believe that in the mid-70s, you testified in Federal Trade Commission (FTC) hearings that eggs don't cause heart disease, but that trans fats do. What happened to your research funding around this time?

Kummerow: I have never used university money. I lost my support from the National Institutes of Health (NIH) in 1979. I had received $200,000 a year from the NIH for my laboratory up until that point. Since I had started my research, I had received over $20 million for laboratory expenses mostly from the NIH. When I disagreed with Dr. Theodore Cooper, who was the Deputy Assistant Secretary for Health, Department of Health, Education and Welfare (HEW) and past Director of the National Heart Institute (NIH), over the cholesterol issue at the FTC Hearings in 1975, the NIH funding stopped. I was lucky to obtain other funding of $200,000 a year from the Wallace Foundation for 28 years that ended in 2008 when Mr. Wallace died. From that point, I received funding from the Weston Price Foundation. That money has now been consumed by laboratory operational expenses. It costs $25,000 a month to keep my lab operational. If you know of any funding opportunities, I would be pleased to hear of them.

Passwater: *After NIH decided to stop funding your research, millions of Americans were being exposed to harmful amounts of trans fats. Many developed heart disease. Dr. Enig, a follower of your research and an early opponent of having so much trans fatty acid in our diet spent parts of several summers in my laboratory. I witnessed some of the harassment she was subjected to by the establishment forces that tried to squelch the evidence against trans fats. You were certainly subjected to non-scientific pressures from vested interests, but you kept up your research. Eventually, you became involved with a lawsuit against the FDA to reduce the amount of trans fats in the food supply. How did this come about?*

Kummerow: Indirectly. As I mentioned, I served as an expert witness at an FTC hearing in 1975, at which I stated that eggs were a good source of protein and I didn't know, at the time, what caused heart disease. The only other witness that day, Dr. DeBakey, stated that on the basis of people he had performed bypass surgery on, he found that these patients had either high or low plasma cholesterol levels and needed the surgery.

I did not realize until years later when the entire testimony was published that Theodore Cooper, M.D., head of the NIH, testified on May 30, 1975, that eggs contained cholesterol, cholesterol caused heart disease and therefore people should not eat eggs. Reading FTC's final ruling makes it evident that only two witnesses testified that cholesterol was not the answer to heart disease. All of the other witnesses (the head of the NIH, many prominent physicians, among others) testified that cholesterol was the cause of heart disease. The final FTC ruling stated, "egg producers could not state that eggs were a good source of nutrition," without also stating that cardiologists believed eating eggs was one cause of heart disease.

In 2009, I petitioned the FDA to ban trans fats. They are supposed to act on such petitions within six months. In 2013, I received a call from a San Diego attorney named Gregory Weston asking if I had received a response from the FDA, after I had posted a docket on trans fat. Weston was concerned that after four years, I still had not received any reply from the FDA concerning this crucial matter, when the FDA was responding to other dockets concerning "white chocolate" in three months. So, Mr. Weston asked if he could represent me and we are still pushing forward to remove this deadly substance from the diet.

Passwater: *It appears that the FDA is finally taking action to reduce trans fats in foods. When do you think they will publish actual regulations?*

Kummerow: When they have answered all of the questions that were asked of them from consumers and the industry. The FDA will have to decide whether to ban trans fatty acids, or not.

Passwater: *Is the proposed regulation sufficient?*

Kummerow: It's sufficient, if the FDA will ban all trans fat. Having a little here and there in foods adds up.

Passwater: *Well, it looks as if people shouldn't wait for the FDA to act. The agency could take years to finalize its ruling and FDA can weaken it after reading the industry comments. Readers can review the comments on "Tentative Determination Regarding Partially Hydrogenated Oils; Request for Comments and for Scientific Data and Information" at* www.regulations .gov/#!documentDetail;D=FDA-2013-N-1317-0001.

What types of things can people do now to reduce their intake of trans fats?

Kummerow: Look on the label of the food products they buy, and see to it that there's no trans fat in the food product. If there is any amount of an ingredient called partially hydrogenated oil (PHO), the product contains trans fats. The largest amount of trans fats in the modern diet originates from fried and processed foods. According to the Trans Fat Task Force, up to 45% of the total fat in those foods containing artificial trans fats is formed by partially hydrogenating soybean oil. This is why we must work to remove all artificially created trans fats from the diet; consumers may be unaware of the amount of trans fat present in their food.

Passwater: *An article in the July 2013* American Journal of Cardiovascular Disease *pretty much summarizes the main aspects of your heart disease research. Please tell us a little about that paper.*

Kummerow: I discussed my findings; namely, that atherosclerosis in modern human beings is based on the biochemistry, composition and structure of three of the five phospholipids in the cell membrane of the coronary arteries. I reported my findings indicate fried foods, powdered egg yolk, excess vegetable oils, partially hydrogenated vegetable oils and cigarette smoke are the greatest culprits in heart disease. Fried foods and powdered food substitutes are dietary sources of oxysterols, which alter the phospholipid membranes of our arteries in ways that increase the deposition of calcium, a key hallmark of atherosclerosis. Consumption of excess polyunsaturated fats stimulates the formation of oxysterols within the human body. Cigarette smoke and trans fats from partially hydrogenated vegetable oils interfere with fatty acid metabolism, leading to the interruption of blood flow, a major contributor to heart attacks and sudden death. In my opinion, many of these factors have been largely ignored by the medical establishment, which has focused instead on using drugs to lower cholesterol levels.

Passwater: *This year, in* Clinical Lipidology, *you further explained that the oxysterols change the structure of the coronary arteries so that they are more susceptible to calcification and increase the synthesis of thromboxane which causes the blood to clot. The trans fatty acids inhibit prostacyclin synthesis, which prevents the blood from clotting. What about your personal diet?*

Kummerow: I eat an egg every day and drink three glasses of whole milk. I also eat meat or some kind of protein at every meal and lot of fruits and vegetables.

Passwater: *What do you eat for breakfast?*

Kummerow: I eat an egg scrambled in butter, one table-spoon of oatmeal and wheat berries (which is cooked ahead of time and kept in the refrigerator or freezer), a tablespoon of plain yogurt, a small banana, four stewed prunes and a tablespoon of chopped nuts. I also have one cup of whole milk and a glass of water.

Passwater: *Do you eat mostly natural foods?*

Kummerow: I don't eat processed or fried food. I eat fresh or frozen vegetables or fruit and meat that is baked or broiled.

Passwater: *Your new book contains lots more practical advice on reducing the risk of heart disease. It is called,* Cholesterol Won't Kill You, But Trans Fat Could.

Happy 100th birthday and thank you so much for your decades of life-saving research. Let's see now. After 70 years,

your work has saved about 250,000 people from premature death from pellagra. The number of premature deaths due to trans fats has been estimated to be between 30,000 and 325,000 and you have been warning us against this since 1957.

RICHARD A. PASSWATER has been a research biochem-ist for over 50 years and is currently research director of the Selenium Nutritional Research Center in Berlin, Maryland.

FRED KUMMEROW, emeritus professor of comparative bio-sciences, was a pioneer in establishing the connection between trans fats and heart disease, and helped discover that oxidized cholesterol, rather than cholesterol itself, is linked to heart disease. His books include *Cholesterol Won't Kill You, But Trans Fat Could* and *Cholesterol Is Not the Culprit: A Guide to Preventing Heart Disease*. Addition-ally he has published about 500 scientific articles related to lipids and health.

EXPLORING THE ISSUE

Should We Eat Less Saturated Fat?

Critical Thinking and Reflection

1. The DGAC did not include a recommendation to limit the total fat or a particular percent of calories from total fat in its technical report to HHS and USDA, nor did it mention a need for cholesterol restrictions. Describe the position that the HHS and USDA take in the actual *Dietary Guidelines for Americans (DGA) 2015* publication. Explain why you think the HHS and USDA staff chose to write the *DGA* this way.
2. In their comment letter to the secretaries of HHS and USDA, the American Society for Nutrition "encourages the government to carefully consider the recommendations within the Scientific Report to create clear, consistent messages that most effectively communicate dietary guidance to the general public and are based on the strongest evidence." As related to overall fat intake (including SFA, MUFA, and PUFA), create a two-page consumer brochure to convey this message to college students.
3. Biochemist Kummerow claims that "Consumption of excess polyunsaturated fats stimulates the formation of oxysterols within the human body." Find a peer-reviewed article that either confirms or refutes Dr. Kummerow's statement on oxysterols and summarize the article.
4. Fred Kummerow is a one of the few centenarians who continues publishing scientific papers. Write an essay explaining aspects of Kummerow's life that you think contribute to his longevity.
5. Find one research article that focuses on an area considered a "Need for Future Research" in the DGAC report. Write a two-page summation of the article including the study's purpose, methods, results, conclusions/implications, and limitations.

Is There Common Ground?

Both the DGAC and Kummerow agree that *trans* fats should be avoided in the diet to help lower cardiovascular disease risk. In their report, the DGAC simply states, "Partially hydrogenated oils containing *trans* fat should be avoided." It is very certain of its opinion about *trans* fat as does Kummerow, whose research focuses on *trans* fat; he takes great pride in being a pioneer in the area of *trans* fat research; in 2009, he even petitioned the FDA to ban *trans* fat from the U.S. food supply.

Although the DGAC did not mention dietary cholesterol, the omission of the topic may be construed as the DGAC agreeing with Kummerow, in that dietary cholesterol should not be restricted. The DGAC probably agrees strongly with the message of the title of Kummerow's book, *Cholesterol Won't Kill You, But Trans Fat Could*.

Additional Resources

Davis C, Bryan J, Hodgson J, Murphy K. Definition of the Mediterranean diet: A literature review. *Nutrients*. 2015;7(11):9139–53.

De souza RJ, Mente A, Maroleanu A, et al. Intake of saturated and *trans* unsaturated fatty acids and risk of all cause mortality, cardiovascular disease, and type 2 diabetes: Systematic review and meta-analysis of observational studies. *BMJ*. 2015;351:h3978.

Markey O, Vasilopoulou D, Givens DI, Lovegrove JA. Dairy and cardiovascular health: Friend or foe? *Nutr Bull*. 2014;39(2):161–71.

Ros E. Nuts and CVD. *Br J Nutr*. 2015;113 Suppl 2:S111–20.

Sayon-orea C, Carlos S, Martínez-gonzalez MA. Does cooking with vegetable oils increase the risk of chronic diseases?: A systematic review. *Br J Nutr*. 2015;113 Suppl 2:S36–48.

Internet References . . .

Academy of Nutrition and Dietetics (AND)

www.eatright.org

American Heart Association (AHA)

www.heart.org

Health.gov

health.gov

Whole Foods Magazine

wholefoodsmagazine.com

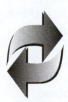

Selected, Edited, and with Issue Framing Material by:
Janet M. Colson, *Middle Tennessee State University*

ISSUE

Should We Eat Less Added Sugars?

YES: Barbara E. Millen, from "Part D. Chapter 6: Cross-Cutting Topics of Public Health Importance: Added Sugars and Low-Calorie Sweeteners," *Scientific Report of the 2015 Dietary Guidelines Advisory Committee* (2015)

NO: Andrew C. Briscoe III and P. Courtney Gaine, from "The Sugar Association's Letter Written in Response to *Scientific Report of the 2015 Dietary Guidelines Advisory Committee*," Comment ID #22978 (2015)

Learning Outcomes

After reading this issue, you will be able to:

- List the four conclusions that the Dietary Guidelines Advisory Committee (DGAC) make about the relationships between intake of added sugars and heart disease, obesity, type 2 diabetes, and dental caries.
- Outline the recommendations on added sugars or sugar-sweetened beverages from international and national organizations and how they compare to recommendations of the DGAC.
- Describe the Sugar Association's criticism of the scientific protocol followed by the DGAC and lack of objectivity used to support recommendations on limiting added sugars.

ISSUE SUMMARY

YES: The DGAC concludes that there is strong evidence that diets high in added sugars are associated with overweight, obesity, and type 2 diabetes and moderate evidence that sugars are linked to dental caries, hypertension, stroke, and cardiovascular disease. They call for an upper limit (UL) of 10 percent of energy to come from added sugars in the diet. They also recommend that additional studies need to be conducted on the roles of sugars and various health conditions.

NO: The Sugar Association, whose mission is to "monitor nutrition science . . . to provide science-based information . . . and to ensure that Federal nutrition and food policy regarding sugar is based on the preponderance of scientific evidence," asks the Secretaries of HHS and USDA to continue the same advice about added sugars that was in the *2010 DGA*. The 2010 advice is to simply reduce intake of calories from added sugars and limit refined grains that contain added sugars, without a specific upper limit recommendation based on the percent of energy.

The original *1977 Dietary Goals for the United States* set an upper limit (UL) on sugars at "about 15 percent of energy" but did not include a definition for the term "sugars." The second edition, published 11 months later in 1977, clarified the recommendation by specifying that "refined and processed sugars" be reduced to a mere 10 percent of total energy intake. Since these 1977 recommendations, none of the seven editions of the *Dietary Guidelines for Americans*

(DGA), include the "10 percent" recommendation but all have mentioned limiting added sugars to some degree. For example, the *1980 Dietary Guidelines for Americans (DGA)* simply instructed Americans to "Avoid Too Much Sugar" but did not specify an amount. The message to the public was:

> Contrary to widespread opinion, too much sugar in your diet does not seem to cause diabetes. The most common type of diabetes is seen in obese

adults and avoiding sugar, without correcting the overweight, will not solve the problem. There is also no convincing evidence that sugar causes heart attacks or blood vessel disease.

Estimates indicate that Americans use more than 130 pounds of sugars and sweeteners a year. This means the risk of tooth decay is not only increased by the sugar bowl, but also by the sugars and syrups in jam, jellies, candies, cookies, soft drinks, cakes and pies, as well as sugars found in breakfast cereals, catsup, flavored milks, and ice cream.

The *1985 DGA* continued the "Avoid Too Much Sugar" recommendation and the same messages about sugar and health. Beginning in 1990, the *DGA* instructions changed from "Avoid Too Much Sugar" to "Use Sugars Only in Moderation" and added the following message:

> Scientific evidence indicates that diets high in sugars do not cause hyperactivity or diabetes. The most common type of diabetes occurs in overweight adults. Avoiding sugars alone will not correct overweight. To lose weight, reduce the total amount of food you eat and increase your level of physical activity.

The *1995 DGA* tweaked the sugar message slightly with "Choose a diet moderate in sugars" and continued the statements about hyperactivity, diabetes, and tooth decay. The *2000 DGA* carried the message to "Choose beverages and foods to moderate your intake of sugars" and claimed that the "body cannot tell the difference between naturally occurring and added sugars because they are identical chemically." They did include the warning that "added sugars provide calories, but may have few vitamins and minerals" and included the following rather mixed message about sugar-sweetened "healthy" foods:

> Some foods with added sugars, like chocolate milk, presweetened cereals, and sweetened canned fruits, are also high in vitamins and minerals. These foods may provide extra calories along with the nutrients and are fine if you need the extra calories. Consuming excess calories from these foods may contribute to weight gain or lower consumption of more nutritious foods.

In their 2002 *Dietary Reference Intakes for Energy, Carbohydrate, Fiber, Fat, Fatty Acids, Cholesterol, Protein, and Amino Acids* report, the Institute of Medicine (IOM) suggested that the UL for added sugars be 25 percent of total calories consumed. The IOM report specifies:

> Based on the data available on dental caries, behavior, cancer, risk of obesity, and risk of hyperlipidemia, there is insufficient evidence to set a UL for total or added sugars. Although a UL is not set for sugars, a maximal intake level of 25 percent or less of energy from added sugars is suggested based on the decreased intake of some micronutrients of Americans exceeding this level.

Instead of including the IOM conclusion about sugars, the *2005 DGA* introduced the concept of "discretionary calories" (DC) which suggests the upper amount of calories from added sugars, additional fats, and alcohol. For example, a person who consumes a 2000-calorie eating plan is allowed only 267 DC per day. Therefore, if all DC come from added sugars, 14 percent of calories are the upper amount from sugar, but that leaves no calories from additional fat or alcohol—so no butter on bread and no wine or beer. A more realistic allocation of these calories is to have half of the DC from added sugar and half from fat or alcohol. This translates into a DC allowance of 7 percent (or 33 grams) of added sugars, which is less than the amount found in a typical 12-ounce sugar-sweetened soft drink.

For the *2010 DGA*, the term "discretionary calories" is replaced with the term "solid fats/added sugar" (SoFAS). (Note: SoFAS was replaced in 2011 with "empty calories" in ChooseMyPlate.) The main message on added sugars under the "Foods and Food Components to Reduce" section is simply to reduce the intake of calories from SoFAS and limit consumption of foods that contain refined grain. The *DGA* also points out that added sugars decrease the "nutrient density" of the diet and makes the following comments about sugars and solid fats:

> Although the body's response to sugars does not depend on whether they are naturally present in food or added to foods, sugars found naturally in foods are part of the food's total package of nutrients and other healthful components. In contrast, many foods that contain added sugars often supply calories, but few or no essential nutrients and no dietary fiber. Both naturally occurring sugars and added sugars increase the risk of dental caries. Added sugars contribute an average of 16 percent of the total calories in American diets. . . .
>
> As a percent of calories from total added sugars, the major sources of added sugars in the diets of Americans are soda, energy drinks, and

sports drinks (36% of added sugar intake), grain-based desserts (13%), sugar-sweetened fruit drinks (10%), dairy-based desserts (6%), and candy (6%).

Reducing the consumption of these sources of added sugars will lower the calorie content of the diet, without compromising its nutrient adequacy. . . .

For most people, no more than about 5 to 15 percent of calories from solid fats and added sugars can be reasonably accommodated in the USDA Food Patterns, which are designed to meet nutrient needs within calorie limits.

Of course, the U.S. sugar industry disagrees with the call to reduce the amount of added sugars Americans consume. The Sugar Association began efforts to convince the 2015 DGAC early during the review period. Soon after the initial DGAC meeting in June 2013, The Sugar Association sent its first letter (Comment #56) on August 30, 2013. It disagrees with the suggested sugar intake limit and points out that Americans are eating about as much added sugars as they did in 1970. Part of its letter is:

The extremely low suggested intakes of 6 to 12 teaspoons of "added sugars" in the USDA Eating Patterns have no historical basis. USDA food supply data show that Americans consumed 20.8 grams per capita of "added sugars" in 1970 and 23 grams per capita today, which is a mere 38 calories of the additional 459 calories per person per day that Americans consume today than they did in 1970.

The Sugar Association sent two more letters (Comment ID #577; July 8, 2014 and Comment ID #881; December 18, 2014) during the DGAC review period, each urging the Committee to ease the restrictions on sugar. Finally, after almost 2 years of reviewing the scientific evidence, the *2015 Scientific Report of the DGAC* was submitted to the Secretaries of USDA and HHS on January 28, 2015. The report calls for a 10 percent UL of added sugars, similar to the *1977 Dietary Goals* and they consider there is "strong evidence" to support this recommendation.

Once again, The Sugar Association sent a letter to the Secretaries of USDA and HHS expressing their disapproval of the report and to plead their case on sugar's innocence. Excerpts from their 29-page letter (Comment ID #22978; May 8, 2015) is the "NO" selection for this issue.

Other members of the sugar industry were just as displeased. One of the last letters (Comment ID #29973; May 29, 2015) about the DGAC report was from the Sugar Cane Growers Cooperative of Florida. In their letter they question if the new "sugar is evil" message will replace the "fat is evil" message in previous years and be counterproductive. Part of their letter includes:

Sugar has become the new dietary target, as was fat in the 1990s. This focus on individual components of the diet has not improved the health of the American public. As with fat guidance, dietary guidance that recommends added sugars intake of less than 10 percent of energy will be counterproductive if a reduction in total caloric intake is not achieved. There is no scientific evidence that validates the premise that by reducing sugar in a diet it will ensure energy balance to reduce obesity or chronic diseases. Further, this guidance contradicts the science-based guidance in the 2010 Dietary Guidelines that states, "Foods containing solid fats and added sugars are no more likely to contribute to weight gain than any other source of calories in an eating pattern that is within calorie limits."

Who is right about sugar and health? Is the committee of nutrition and health experts who drafted the *Scientific Report of the 2015 DGAC* right in calling for a reduction to 10 percent of energy intake or are representatives of the sugar industry, whose livelihoods are dependent on the assurance that America (and the world) will continue their dependence on and love for sugar?

YES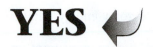

Barbara E. Millen

Part D. Chapter 6: Cross-Cutting Topics of Public Health Importance: Added Sugars and Low-Calorie Sweeteners

Added Sugars and Low-Calorie Sweeteners

Introduction

Added sugars are sugars that are either added during the processing of foods, or are packaged as such, and include sugars (free, mono- and disaccharides), syrups, naturally occurring sugars that are isolated from a whole food and concentrated so that sugar is the primary component (e.g., fruit juice concentrates), and other caloric sweeteners. Added sugars have been discussed in previous iterations of the *Dietary Guidelines*, including a key recommendation in the *2010 Dietary Guidelines* to "Reduce the intake of calories from solid fats and added sugars."

The *2010 Dietary Guidelines* also included guidance stating that, for most people, no more than about 5 to 15 percent of calories from solid fats and added sugars (combined) can be reasonably accommodated in a healthy eating pattern. However, the current intake of added sugars still remains high at 268 calories, or 13.4 percent of total calories per day among the total population ages 1 year and older.

Similar to the healthy eating patterns modeled for the 2010 DGAC, in the three healthy eating patterns modeled for the 2015 DGAC (Healthy U.S.-style Pattern, Healthy Mediterranean-style Pattern, and Healthy Vegetarian Pattern), a limited number of calories are available to be consumed as added sugars. As shown in Table D6.1, the full range of these three patterns at all calorie levels

Table D6.1.

CALORIE LEVEL	1000	1200	1400	1600	1800	2000	2200	2400	2600	2800	3000	3200
Added sugars available in the USDA Food Patterns (Healthy U.S.-style, Healthy Mediterranean-style, and Healthy Vegetarian Patterns) in calories, teaspoons, and percent of total calories per day*												
*Empty calorie limits available for **added sugars** (assuming 45% empty calories from added sugars and 55% from solid fat)*												
Healthy U.S.-style	68	50	50	54	77	122	126	158	171	180	212	275
Healthy Med-style	63	50	50	81	72	117	126	135	149	158	194	257
Healthy Vegetarian	77	77	81	81	81	131	131	158	158	158	185	234
Average	69	59	60	72	77	123	128	150	159	165	197	255
Average (tsp)	4.3	3.7	3.8	4.5	4.8	7.7	8.0	9.4	9.9	10.3	12.3	15.9
Healthy U.S.-style	7%	4%	4%	3%	4%	6%	6%	7%	7%	6%	7%	9%
Healthy Med-style	6%	4%	4%	5%	4%	6%	6%	6%	6%	6%	6%	8%
Healthy Vegetarian	8%	6%	6%	5%	5%	7%	6%	7%	6%	6%	6%	7%
Average	7%	5%	4%	5%	4%	6%	6%	6%	6%	6%	7%	8%

* See ***Part D. Chapter 1: Food and Nutrient Intakes, and Health: Current Status and Trends*** and Appendix E-3.7 for a full discussion of the food pattern modeling.

Scientific Report of the 2015 Dietary Guidelines Advisory Committee: Part D: Science Base, Chapter 6: Cross-Cutting Topics of Public Health Importance: Added Sugars and Low-Calorie Sweeteners, February 2015.

allow[s] for 3 to 9 percent of calories from added sugars, after meeting food group and nutrient recommendations. For the patterns appropriate for most people (1600 to 2400 calories), the range is 4 to 6 percent of calories from added sugars (or 4.5 to 9.4 teaspoons). The total empty calorie allowance in these patterns is 8 to 19 percent of calories, and based on current consumption patterns, 45 percent of empty calories are allocated to limits for added sugars, with the remainder (55 percent) allocated to solid fats.

Although food pattern modeling evaluates the amount of added sugars that can be consumed while meeting food group and nutrient needs, the DGAC also reviewed scientific literature examining the relationship between the intake of added sugars and health to inform recommendations. The Committee focused on the health outcomes most commonly researched related to added sugars, specifically, body weight and risk of type 2 diabetes, CVD, and dental caries.

As noted above, the Committee acknowledged that a potential unintended consequence of a recommendation on added sugars might be that consumers and manufacturers replace added sugars with low-calorie sweeteners. As a result, the Committee also examined evidence on low-calorie sweeteners to inform statements on this topic. The Committee approached this topic broadly, including sweeteners labeled as low-calorie sweeteners, non-caloric sweeteners, non-nutritive sweeteners, artificial sweeteners, and diet beverages. This work is complemented by a food safety evidence review on aspartame. As the evidence on added sugars was considered collectively, the added sugars conclusions are presented together below, and a similar approach was taken for low-calorie sweeteners.

Question: What is the relationship between the intake of added sugars and cardiovascular disease, body weight/obesity, type 2 diabetes, and dental caries?

Source of evidence: CVD: NEL systematic review; Body weight/obesity, type 2 diabetes, and dental caries: Existing reports

Conclusions

Strong and consistent evidence shows that intake of added sugars from food and/or sugar-sweetened beverages [is] associated with excess body weight in children and adults. The reduction of added sugars and sugar-sweetened beverages in the diet reduces body mass index (BMI) in both children and adults. Comparison groups with the highest versus the lowest intakes of added sugars in cohort studies were compatible with a recommendation to keep added sugars intake below 10 percent of total energy intake. **DGAC Grade: Strong**

Strong evidence shows that higher consumption of added sugars, especially sugar-sweetened beverages, increases the risk of type 2 diabetes among adults and this relationship is not fully explained by body weight. **DGAC Grade: Strong**

Moderate evidence from prospective cohort studies indicates that higher intake of added sugars, especially in the form of sugar-sweetened beverages, is consistently associated with increased risk of hypertension, stroke, and CHD in adults. Observational and intervention studies indicate a consistent relationship between higher added sugars intake and higher blood pressure and serum triglycerides. **DGAC Grade: Moderate**

The DGAC concurs with the World Health Organization's commissioned systematic review that moderate consistent evidence supports a relationship between the amount of free sugars intake and the development of dental caries among children and adults. Moderate evidence also indicates that caries are lower when free sugars intake is less than 10 percent of energy intake. **DGAC Grade: Moderate**

Review of the Evidence

Added Sugars and Body Weight/Obesity

These findings come from three recent reports, all using SRs and MA that examined the relationship between the intake of added sugars and measures of body weight. Te Morenga et al. considered "free sugars," [1] while Malik and Kaiser et al. focused on sugar-sweetened beverages. All reviews reported on body weight. The Te Morenga report also reported on body fatness. In the Te Morenga et al. study, 30 trials and 38 cohort studies were included in the analyses. In the Malik et al. study, 10 trials and 22 cohort studies were included in the analyses. Kaiser et al. provided an updated meta-analysis to a previous publication (Mattes) and included a total of 18 trials. In total, 92 articles were considered in these reviews, of which 21 were included in two or more reviews. Children and adults were included in the analyses as were females and males. Diverse demographics (race/ethnicity and geographic location) also were represented by the participants in the respective research studies. All three reviews were high-quality, with ratings of 11 out of 11 using the AMSTAR tool, and they specifically addressed the Committee's question of interest.

The reviews by Malik et al. and Te Morenga et al. were very consistent. The findings from both reports provide strong evidence that among free-living people consuming ad libitum diets, the intake of added sugars or sugar-sweetened beverages is associated with unfavorable weight status in children and adults. Increased added sugars intake is associated with weight gain; decreased added sugars intake is associated with decreased body weight. Although a dose response cannot be determined at this time, the data analyzed by Te Morenga et al. support limiting added sugars to no more than 10 percent of daily total energy intake based on lowest versus highest intakes from prospective cohort studies. Te Morenga et al. state that, "despite significant heterogeneity in one meta-analysis and potential bias in some trials, sensitivity analyses showed that the trends were consistent and associations remained after these studies were excluded." Despite these limitations the DGAC gave this evidence a grade of **Strong**, as the limitations are those inherent to the primary research on which they are based, notably inadequacy of dietary intake data and variations in the nature and quality of the dietary interventions.

The Kaiser et al. review concluded that the currently available randomized evidence for the effects of reducing sugar-sweetened beverage intake on obesity is equivocal. However, the DGAC noted methodological issues with this review, particularly the inclusion of both efficacy studies (in more controlled settings) and effectiveness studies (in real world). The outcomes from the effectiveness trials vary substantially, depending how effective the interventions are. As a result, the Committee viewed the reviews by Te Morenga et al. and Malik et al. to be stronger than the Kaiser et al. review.

Added Sugars and Type 2 Diabetes

Evidence for this question and conclusion came from five SRs and MA published between January 2010 and August 2014. Four of the reviews focused on sugar-sweetened beverages and one review examined sugar intake. Combined, a total of 17 articles were considered in these reviews, of which nine were included in two or more reviews. Increased consumption of sugar-sweetened beverages was consistently associated with increased risk of type 2 diabetes. Pooled estimated relative risks ranged from 1.20 to 1.28, and included 1.20 (95% CI = 1.12 to 1.29)/330 ml/day of sugar-sweetened soft drinks; 1.26 (95% CI = 1.12 to 1.41) for sugar-sweetened beverages, and 1.28 (95% CI = 1.04 to 1.59) for sugar-sweetened fruit juices. Comparably, a hazard ratio of 1.29 (1.02, 1.63) was identified for sugar-sweetened beverages. These consistently positive associations between sugar-sweetened beverages and type 2 diabetes were attenuated, but still existed, after adjustment for BMI, suggesting that body

weight only partly explains the deleterious effects of sugar-sweetened beverages on type 2 diabetes. Although the studies were highly heterogeneous, findings from the MA by Malik et al. tentatively showed that consumption of more than one 12-ounce serving per day of sugar-sweetened beverage increased the risk of developing type 2 diabetes by 26 percent, compared to consuming less than one serving per month. Insufficient high-quality data are available to determine a dose-response line or curve between sugar-sweetened beverage consumption and type 2 diabetes risk.

The issue of generalizability, whether the participants included in this body of evidence are representative of the general U.S. population, was not specifically addressed in the literature reviewed, but the large sample sizes of the pooled data (several hundred thousand subjects from different populations) are noteworthy.

Added Sugars and Cardiovascular Disease

This NEL systematic review included 23 articles published since 2000 that examined the relationship between added sugars and risk of CVD or CVD risk factors such as blood lipids and blood pressure. This literature included 11 intervention studies and 12 prospective cohort studies.

The majority of intervention and observational studies included in this SR provide some evidence among adults in support of an association between higher intake of added sugars, especially in the form of sugar-sweetened beverages, and higher risk of CVD or increased CVD risk factors. More consistent associations were seen between added sugars and elevated serum triglycerides, blood pressure, and increased risk of hypertension, stroke, or CHD. Evidence for associations between added sugars and dyslipidemia (i.e., low HDL, high LDL, and high total cholesterol) was not as consistent, especially among intervention studies.

The body of evidence examined in this SR had a number of limitations. For example, the intervention studies had extensive heterogeneity in terms of the types and forms of sugars used (i.e., fructose, glucose, sucrose, sugar-sweetened beverages, sweetened milk) and the type of control and/or isocaloric condition used. In addition, most intervention studies had a short duration of the intervention and a small sample size. Most of the observational studies assessed dietary intake only at baseline, and did not take assessments during follow-up. Residual confounding by other dietary and lifestyle factors in observational analyses could not be completely ruled out.

Added Sugars and Dental Caries

These findings were extracted from a World Health Organization (WHO)-commissioned SR by Moynihan et al. published in 2014 examining the association between the amount of sugars intake and dental caries. The search for SRs/MA published since completion of the WHO review did not yield any additional reviews that met the DGAC's inclusion criteria.

Moynihan et al. examined total sugars, free sugars, added sugars, sucrose, and non-milk extrinsic (NME) sugars. In the review, eligible studies reported the absolute amount of sugars. Dental caries outcomes included caries prevalence, incidence and/or severity.

Several databases were searched from 1950 through 2011. From 5,990 papers identified, 55 studies (from 65 papers) were eligible, including 3 interventions, 8 cohort studies, 20 population studies, and 24 cross-sectional studies. No RCTs were included. Data variability limited the ability to conduct meta-analysis. Of the 55 studies included in the review, the majority were in children and only four studies were conducted in adults. The terminology used for reporting sugars varied, but most were described as pertaining to free sugars or added sugars.

The findings indicated consistent evidence of moderate quality supporting a relationship between the amount of sugars consumed and dental caries development across age groups. Of the studies, 42 out of 50 studies in children and five out of five in adults reported at least one result for an association between sugars intake with increased caries. Moderate evidence also showed that caries incidence is lower when free sugars intake is less than 10 percent of energy intake. When a less than

Table D6.2.

Recommendations or statements related to added sugars or sugar-sweetened beverages from international and national organizations	
Organization	**Recommendation/Statement Related to Added Sugars and/or Sugar-Sweetened Beverages**
World Health Organization (WHO)	• WHO recommends reduced intake of free sugars throughout the life-course (*strong recommendation*). • In both adults and children, WHO recommends that intake of free sugars not to exceed 10% of total energy (*strong recommendation*). • WHO suggests further reduction to below 5% of total energy (*conditional recommendation*).
American Heart Association (AHA)	The AHA recommends reductions in added sugars with an upper limit of half of the discretionary calorie allowance that can be accommodated within the appropriate energy intake level needed for a person to achieve or maintain a healthy weight based on the USDA food intake patterns. Most American women should eat or drink no more than 100 calories per day from added sugars (about 6 teaspoons), and most American men should eat or drink no more than 150 calories per day from added sugars (about 9 teaspoons).
HealthyPeople 2020	Objective NWS-17.2: Reduce consumption of calories from added sugars (Target: 10.8%)
American Academy of Pediatrics (AAP)	Limit consumption of sugar-sweetened beverages (consistent evidence) Pediatricians should work to eliminate sweetened drinks in schools *Note: Due to limited studies in children, the American Academy of Pediatrics (AAP) has no official recommendations regarding the use of non-caloric sweeteners.*
American Diabetes Association (ADA)	Prevention Research has shown that drinking sugary drinks is linked to type 2 diabetes, and the American Diabetes Association recommends that people limit their intake of sugar-sweetened beverages to help prevent diabetes. Diabetes Management People with diabetes should limit or avoid intake of sugar-sweetened beverages (from any caloric sweetener including high fructose corn syrup and sucrose) to reduce risk for weight gain and worsening of cardiometabolic risk profile. (Evidence rating B)
NHLBI Expert Panel Guidelines for Cardiovascular Health and Risk Reduction in Childhood	Reduced intake of sugar-sweetened beverages is associated with decreased obesity measures (Grade B).

5 percent energy intake cutoff was used, a significant relationship between sugars and caries was observed, but the evidence was judged to be of very low quality. Although meta- analysis was limited, analysis of existing data indicated a large effect size (e.g., Standardized Mean Difference for Decayed/Missing/Filled Teeth [DMFT] = 0.82 [CI = 0.67-0.97]) for the relationship of sugars intake and risk of dental caries. A strength of the in-depth SR was the consistency of data, despite methodological weaknesses in many studies, which included unclear definitions of endpoints, questions about outcomes ascertainment, and lack of clarity about the generalizability of individual study results given the study populations used.

. . .

Chapter Summary

The DGAC encourages the consumption of healthy dietary patterns that are low in, added sugars, . . . The goals for the general population are: . . . a maximum of 10 percent of total calories from added sugars per day.

. . . Sources of . . . sugars should be reduced in the diet and not replaced with low-calorie sweeteners, but rather with healthy options, such as water in place of sugar-sweetened beverages. . . .

Achieving reductions in . . . added sugars, can all be accomplished and are more attainable by eating a healthy dietary pattern. [P]olicies and programs at local, state, and national levels in both the private and public sector are necessary to support reduction efforts. Similarly, the Committee supports efforts in labeling and other campaigns to increase consumer awareness and understanding of . . . added sugars in foods and beverages. The Committee encourages the food industry to continue reformulating and making changes to certain foods to improve their nutrition profile. . . . The Committee also encourages the food industry to market these improved products to consumers.

. . .

- Identify sources and names of added sugars and low-calorie sweeteners used in the food supply and quantify their consumption levels and trends in the U.S. diet.

Rationale: It is unclear whether all food and nutrient databases capture all added sugars because: 1) added sugars have varied and inconsistent nomenclature and may not be recognized as added sugars in nutrient analyses; and 2) many foods with added sugars have formulations considered proprietary by the manufacturers and for this reason actual added sugars content is difficult to obtain. Accurate assessment of added sugars in the U.S. diet is needed to quantify the population level exposure and subsequent health risks from added sugars. The lack of information on the various added sugars in the food supply hinders efforts to make policy about consumption.

- Conduct prospective research with strong experimental designs and multiple measurements of the consumption of added sugars and low-calorie sweeteners on health outcomes, such as body weight, adiposity, and clinical markers of type 2 diabetes and cardiovascular disease.

Rationale: High heterogeneity exists among published research with regard to the types and forms of added sugars and low-calorie sweeteners-containing foods/beverages used for interventions, which precludes assessing the effects of specific added sugars and low-calorie sweeteners on body weight, adiposity, and cardio-metabolic health in adults and children. Many studies use single baseline measurements of diet to reflect usual patterns and quantities of intake over time. New research should emphasize assessments within the context of usual dietary intakes and patterns of food and beverage consumption in free-living populations, along with specific added sugars and low-calorie sweeteners, especially those that are currently understudied. Large prospective studies with repeated measurements of low-calorie sweeteners are needed to monitor their long-term effects on cancer and other health outcomes.

- Design studies that emphasize assessments of relationships between the intakes of added sugars and low-calorie sweeteners and body weight, adiposity, and cardio-metabolic health in diverse subpopulations who are at high risk of obesity and related morbidities.

Rationale: Insufficient evidence exists to assess the impact of added sugars and low-calorie sweeteners contained in foods and beverages on individuals from diverse populations who have high risk for adverse health outcomes. These include (but not limited to) different race/ethnicity groups; low income groups, especially those with food insecurity; groups who live in specific geographic locations with high prevalence of obesity (e.g., inner city, rural, and Southern regions of the United States); and age and sex groups (women, children, and elderly adults).

Note

1. Free sugar is defined by WHO as "all monosaccharides and disaccharides added to foods by the manufacturer, cook, or consumer, plus sugars naturally present in honey, syrups, and fruit juices." It is used to distinguish between the sugars that are naturally present in fully unrefined carbohydrates such as brown rice, whole wheat pasta, and fruit and those sugars (or carbohydrates) that have been, to some extent, refined (normally by humans but sometimes by animals, such as the free sugars present in honey). They are referred to as "sugars" since they cover multiple chemical forms, including sucrose, glucose, fructose, dextrose, and others.

BARBARA E. MILLEN, founder and president of Millennium Prevention, Inc., served as chair of the 14-member 2015 Dietary Guidelines Advisory Committee.

Andrew C. Briscoe III and P. Courtney Gaine

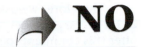 **NO**

The Sugar Association's Letter Written in Response to *Scientific Report of the 2015 Dietary Guidelines Advisory Committee*

1300 L Street NW, Suite 1001
Washington, DC 20005 (202) 785–1122
May 7, 2015

The Honorable Sylvia M. Burwell
Secretary of Health and Human Services
200 Independence Avenue, SW
Washington DC, 20201

The Honorable Thomas J. Vilsack
Secretary of Agriculture
1400 Independence Avenue, SW
Whitten Building, Room 200A
Washington DC, 20250

Dear Secretaries Burwell and Vilsack:

The Sugar Association (Association) represents United States sugar cane farmers and refiners and sugar beet farmers and processors. Association members account for over 90% of sugar/sucrose production in the United States. Founded in 1943, our mission is to monitor nutrition science, to provide science-based information on sugar to consumers and health professionals and to ensure that Federal nutrition and food policy[1][2][3][4] regarding sugar is based on the preponderance of scientific evidence. The foundation of our efforts to support and promote sugar in moderation as a safe and useful part of a balanced diet and healthful lifestyle is grounded in the totality of high-quality scientific evidence.

This comment reflects our position on sugar/sucrose. Of note, the Association has long been on the record objecting to the use of the term "added sugars" as misleading and without scientific justification.

The Association has participated in the Dietary Guidelines process since its inception and appreciates the hard work of Dietary Guidelines Advisory Committees and Federal staff to provide an advisory report to the Secretaries of Health and Human Services and the U.S. Department of Agriculture (Secretaries) every five years. We support past Dietary Guidelines' recommendations to reduce certain foods and beverages containing "added sugars" to within caloric needs. However, for the 2015 process, the Dietary Guidelines Advisory Committee (2015 DGAC) has taken "added sugars" recommendations to unchartered territory, thus raising serious concerns about the manner by which these recommendations were derived.

We emphasize that Congress in its wisdom understood that the American public is best served by dietary guidance that is based on a robust evaluation of the totality of scientific evidence. Section 301 of Public Law 101–445 (7 U.S.C. 5341, the National Nutrition Monitoring and Related Research Act of 1990, Title III) clearly mandates that the nutrition and dietary guidance in the Dietary Guidelines for Americans (DGAs) is based solely on the preponderance of science and medical knowledge current at the time of publication. The Association strongly contends that the recommendations on "added sugars" put forth in the 2015 DGAC report do not meet these important scientific standards.

The mandate of the Dietary Guidelines is to provide general dietary guidance for the American public. We contend that the 2015 DGAC has not undertaken the rigorous scientific investigation necessary to conclude links or associations between "added sugars" and serious disease outcomes. Recommendations that lead the American public to believe any dietary component is a causal factor in a serious disease outcome should only be made based on significant scientific agreement due to a robust review of the entire body of scientific literature by experts in the field of investigation. Such scientific agreement does not exist for the 2015 DGAC "added sugars" recommendations.

Therefore, we ask that the Secretaries maintain the 2010 Dietary Guidelines advice on "added sugars" and offer this comment to support this request.

We address the following issues in this comment:

- The integrity of the 2015 DGAC scientific process is in question, for the following reasons:

  - *There was a lack of fair dealing with interested parties in the 2015 DGAC process*
  - *The 2015 DGAC bypassed the established Nutrition Evidence Library (NEL) review process and, instead, subjectively selected previously published systematic reviews, raising red flags of selection bias*
  - *The 2015 DGAC conclusions contradict major, authoritative, evidence-based reviews on "added sugars" intake and health outcomes*
  - *The 2015 DGAC's reliance on pre-existing systematic reviews undermines what should be a scientifically rigorous DGA process*
  - *There was a lack of transparency in how pre-existing systematic reviews were selected*

- The 2015 DGAC used an abundance of poor-quality evidence to form conclusions, for example:

  - *A systematic review is only as strong as the studies it contains*
  - *There was a heavy reliance on observational data to inform conclusions*
  - *The use of observational data of "sugar-sweetened beverage" (SSB) consumption is an inappropriate surrogate/proxy for making conclusions about "added sugars" intake and health outcomes*
  - *The 2015 DGAC's "strong" conclusions linking "added sugars" to health outcomes is overstated, given the lack of rigorous and consistent data*

- Specific points are made below regarding the lack of objectivity by the 2015 DGAC in its overlooking of the flaws and limitations of the science used to support recommendations on "added sugars"

  - *"Added sugars" and obesity*
  - *"Added sugars" and type 2 diabetes*
  - *"Added sugars" and cardiovascular disease*
  - *"Added sugars" and dental caries*

- The 2015 DGAC provided no credible science-based evidence to support its recommendation to reduce "added sugars" intake to below 10 percent of total energy intake

  - *Calories are the real issue*
  - *Calories from "added sugars" are not a major contributing factor in increased caloric intakes or obesity*
  - *Food pattern modeling does not have the scientific underpinning to support "added sugars" intake recommendations*

- The 2015 DGAC aligning with the controversial World Health Organization's (WHO) Guideline on Sugars is a step back for U.S. standards of evidence
- The use of hypothesis-based dietary pattern studies to link or associate dietary components with serious disease outcomes or set intake recommendations is not a validated scientific methodology
- There are unintended consequences of the 2015 DGAC recommendations to reduce "added sugars" intake to historically low levels
- The 2015 DGAC "Added Sugars" policy recommendations went far beyond the Congressional mandate and DGAC Charter with no evidence-based support
- USDA has undue influence on the DGAC processes relating to its role in food patterns modeling.

The integrity of the 2015 DGAC scientific process is in question

There was a lack of fair dealing with interested parties in the 2015 DGAC process

Sugars guidance has appeared in every version of the Dietary Guidelines and the potential relationship between "added sugars" intake and health outcomes has been a source of conflicting opinions among nutrition academics for years. So, we must ask, how is it that "added sugars" were not addressed earlier in the process? Nutrition Evidence Library (NEL) questions should have been formulated early in this process with reviews conducted on the full body of scientific literature on "added sugars" to ensure recommendations on this increasingly important topic are grounded in an extensive review of the totality of high-quality scientific evidence. Instead, the DGAC waited until the very end of the process, September 2014, to announce the creation of an Added Sugars Working Group. The 2015 DGAC process ended on December 15, 2014; **this three-month timeframe was** certainly not long enough to adequately evaluate this important and large body of research, or to allow sufficient time for interested parties to respond to the Committee's conclusions.

The fact that this important topic was not given sufficient deference in this process raises serious concerns not only about fair dealing, but also the motivation of this Committee to fast-track this issue.

The 2015 DGAC bypassed the established NEL review process and, instead, subjectively selected previously published systematic reviews, raising red flags of selection bias

The 2015 Dietary Guidelines Advisory Committee Charter states:

> "The USDA Nutrition Evidence Library will assist the Committee in conducting and creating a *transparent* database of systematic reviews reflecting the *most current research* available on a wide range of food and nutrition-related topics to inform its recommendations." [Emphasis added]

Yet, for three out of four of the "added sugars" research questions, the DGAC *bypassed* the NEL process entirely.

Establishment of the NEL was a critical step in assuring that the DGAs are based *solely* on the preponderance of scientific evidence, through the process' ability to reduce bias, increase transparency and help ensure that all literature is considered. When properly employed, the NEL process yields evidence-based conclusions through a series of well-defined and pre-determined steps. The consistent use of NEL reviews across *all* research topics would have provided interested parties reasonable assurance that all subject areas were given the same consistent and unbiased consideration.

Instead, the Working Group bypassed the established NEL review process to inform its "added sugars" recommendations and almost solely used pre-existing and hand-picked systematic reviews. This raises serious concerns that *the Committee bypassed a review of the full body of science and instead* **selected science to support its predetermined conclusions.**

We question the DGAC's citing of a "short duration of time" and "limited resources" as an adequate explanation for why the Added Sugars Working Group conducted only *one* NEL review to inform its four conclusions on "added sugars," despite the known importance of the NEL process to the integrity of the DGAs.

The 2015 DGAC conclusions contradict major, authoritative, evidence-based reviews on "added sugars" intake and health outcomes

Bypassing the NEL process is of concern, particularly when doing so ultimately leads to conclusions for "added sugars" that *contradict* major evidence-based reviews by authoritative scientific bodies, including the Institute of Medicine (2002)(IOM),[5] the European Food Safety Authority (2010) (EFSA),[6] the U.K.'s Scientific Advisory Committee draft Carbohydrate and Health report (2014)(SACN)[7] and also contradict the advice in position statements of the American Diabetes Association (2014),[8] American Dental Association (2001),[9] and the American Heart Association/American Stroke Association (2014).[10]

The 2015 DGAC recommendations also differ dramatically from the conclusions of the 2010 DGAC NEL reviews[11] and contradict the advice in the 2010 Dietary Guidelines relating to "added sugars" calories not being a direct contributor to obesity, heart disease as well as its science-based advice on dental caries.

- The 2010 DGAC Carbohydrate Subcommittee identified carbohydrates as consisting of sugars, starches and fibers. The Carbohydrate Subcommittee, following the NEL review of the impact of carbohydrates on heart disease, type 2 diabetes, body weight and dental caries, stated this finding "no detrimental effects of carbohydrates as a source of calories on these or other health outcomes were reported."[12] (2010 DGAC advisory report)
- Foods containing solid fats and added sugars are no more likely to contribute to weight gain than any other source of calories in an eating pattern that is within calorie limits.[13] (2010 DGAs)

The conclusions of the 2015 DGAC contradict major evidence-based reviews on "added sugars" intake; therefore, they are already proven to *lack reproducibility.*

The fact that the conclusions from the 2015 DGAC contradict all of these other major reviews is foregone proof that external, previously published systematic reviews are too subjective to be used as the sole basis for dietary guidance and recommendations.

The 2015 DGAC's reliance on pre-existing systematic reviews undermines what should be a scientifically rigorous DGA process

There is considerable difference between the Committee subjectively selecting pre-existing systematic reviews versus relying on existing reports that are the result of a thorough evidence-based review of the full body of literature by authoritative scientific bodies, and conducted by panels that are experts in the field of investigation (i.e. the *2008 Physical Activity Guidelines for Americans*).

While systematic reviews are valuable tools in synthesizing a body of research, they are subject to multiple biases and methodological decisions of the authors; thus, systematic reviews often contradict each other even when examining the same research question.[14] So, when the NEL process is bypassed, and pre-existing reviews are selected, this means that the Committee is basing conclusions that utilize questions, search criteria, study quality, and evaluations that were determined not by the DGAC and the standardized NEL review process, but by those reports' authors. This eliminates the possibility of a review of the total body of evidence from the start, as the authors of these reviews have made study inclusion decisions for the DGAC. As it follows, this means lesser quality studies may be included and studies of high-quality containing important evidence can be left out. As such, it is widely known in the scientific community that the findings of meta-analyses differ based on the approach used by the researchers. However, when the NEL systematic review process is employed, *it is the DGAC who debates and develops the research question* and then determines these important criteria that go into the evidence-based conclusion.

Of additional concern is that in many cases the processes employed in these pre-existing reviews don't share the same rigorous scientific principles and protocols outlined in the NEL review process. As mentioned above, when using pre-existing reviews, important study inclusion determinations, such as grading of study quality and the dates of the studies to be included, are out of the DGAC's control to determine. For example, in examining the reviews used by the Added Sugars Working Group, there is significant variation with regard to study selection criteria. Using study date as an example, there are inconsistencies across the health outcomes examined with regard to the timeframe of studies included in these reviews, with studies from 1969 to present (body weight), 1950 to present (dental caries) and 1990 to present (diabetes) used to form the respective conclusions. Over time, diets change, populations change and methodologies improve; this *lack of consistency* in evidence selected by the DGAC *is* an issue.

Supporting our concerns about the 2015 DGAC's heavy reliance on prior reviews are many recently published papers that raise issues about use of systematic reviews in evidence-based dietary recommendations given the biases and errors inherent to conducting this type of analyses.[15 16 17 18]

There was a lack of transparency in how pre-existing systematic reviews were selected

We question the transparency of some of the Added Sugars Working Group's decision-making. Given that the NEL was bypassed, leaving a non-existent protocol for evidence selection, it remains unclear *how* the existing reviews were selected and how and why other studies and reviews were excluded. This is of particular concern since the Working Group identified systematic reviews that were later seemingly dismissed if their conclusions contradicted the ultimate recommendations. Throughout the process, the Working Group considered a total of four systematic reviews to address body weight, at least that the public was made aware of. The two reviews that findings differed from the Working Group's conclusion on body weight were thrown out with minimal or no explanation as to why. Below are the conclusions from the two reports that were dismissed:

> "No intervention studies were identified from which scientific conclusions could be drawn about the relationship between SSB intake and BMI or risk of obesity. The evidence for an association between SSB intake and obesity risk, when adjustment for energy and physical activity was performed, was **inconsistent** for children, adolescents, and adults."[19]
>
> "Our updated meta-analysis shows that the currently available randomized evidence for the effects of reducing SSB intake on obesity is equivocal."[20]

This is an example of the subjectivity used by the 2015 DGAC in choosing science to support its conclusions, and demonstrates the lack of transparency in evidence selection.

The 2015 DGAC used an abundance of poor-quality evidence to form conclusions

A systematic review is only as strong as the studies it contains

Not all systematic reviews, even if peer-reviewed and published, are of high quality. It is well established in the scientific literature that a high quality meta-analysis requires a homogeneous body of literature, with consistent definitions, study designs and measured outcomes.[21 22] To the contrary, the body of scientific evidence relating to "added sugars" intakes and health outcomes is known to be highly heterogeneous and often conflicting. These points are frequently cited in the literature and major factors as to why syntheses and conclusions regarding "added sugars" studies are extremely difficult.

The subjective input generally required in conducting systematic reviews was mentioned previously, but given that the studies addressing "added sugars" are so diverse, authors of these systematic reviews must make decisions on inclusion criteria that are irrefutably *subjective* in nature. For example, the Working Group ended up selecting three existing systematic reviews to form their conclusion on the relationship between "added sugars" intake and body weight. In total, there were 92 unique studies included in these three reviews. Only 21 of these studies were included in two or more of the reviews. This means that the study selection criteria defined by these authors for these three reports were so varied that 71 of the studies did not meet the criteria to be included in all three reviews *answering the same question*. This example highlights the inherent subjectivity of study selection for a systematic review, and warrants extreme caution when using these pre-existing reports as the sole basis for drawing evidence-based conclusions.

As with all studies, there are limitations that must be considered when interpreting and extrapolating findings. As such, the authors of the pre-existing reviews on "added sugars" used by the DGAC cite numerous limitations of their reviews which are found in the papers themselves. Below are some of these limitations, overlooked by the DGAC, which highlights some of the weaknesses of the science used to make the DGAC's recommendations.

- "The relatively high degree of unexplained heterogeneity observed in our analyses may limit the validity of our summary estimates."[23]
- "The studies included in our meta-analyses varied substantially with respect to study design, exposure assessment, adjustment for covariates, and specific outcomes evaluated." (Malik, 2014)
- "Assessment of dietary intake of sugars, whether by some method of recall as used in the trials, or by food frequency questionnaire as in cohort studies, was associated with a considerable degree of measurement error even when using validated methods."[24]
- "The heterogeneity of the studies, especially in terms of the consequences of altering intake of sugars in ad libitum diets, resulted in difficulties in fully explaining the effects of different dietary changes." (Te Morenga, 2013)
- "Overall, between-study heterogeneity was high. The included studies were observational, so their results should be interpreted cautiously. . . ."[25]

Not all systematic reviews are good; a systematic review is only as strong as the studies (primary research) it contains. Essentially, garbage in equates to garbage out. The Working Group did acknowledge limitations of the systematic reviews they used to support "**strong**"

recommendations for body weight (ultimately, just two); yet, they chose to ignore them, as stated in the DGAC report:

> "Despite these limitations the DGAC gave this evidence a grade of "**strong**," as the limitations are those inherent to the primary research on which they are based, notably inadequacy of dietary intake data and variations in the nature and quality of the dietary interventions."

At the bare minimum, given the weight that each of these pre-existing reviews had in the DGAC conclusions, these important limitations cited by each report's authors and acknowledged by the DGAC must be taken seriously by the Secretaries, as they are ultimately the limitations of the scientific evidence used by the 2015 DGAC to make its recommendations.

There was a heavy reliance on observational data to inform conclusions

The evidence-basis for the Added Sugars Working Group's conclusions linking "added sugars" intake with *serious* disease outcomes consists heavily of epidemiological (or observational) data and, as mentioned above, pre-selected systematic reviews. Epidemiological studies, and even meta-analyses of RCTs, are considered observational data and their findings should be interpreted as *associations* because they **do not provide proof of cause and effect.** It is widely accepted in the scientific community that caution should be applied when making and communicating recommendations that are based primarily on observational data and not confirmed through well-designed trials.[26]

One of the major issues with observational studies, such as population cohort studies, is that the dietary intake assessment tools commonly used are subject to substantial measurement error, resulting in imprecise measures of exposure, or intakes, of foods/beverages or ingredients.[27] There were numerous cohort studies used in forming the conclusions of the Added Sugars Working Group. These cohort studies predominantly examined (what are often called) sugar-sweetened beverage (SSB) intake in relation to health outcomes. The accuracy of food frequency questionnaires (FFQ) for determining SSB consumption ranges between only 30-80%, highlighting an imprecision that is well known across the nutrition field. When the intake measurement itself is this imprecise in capturing intakes, extreme caution should be employed when concluding a link between the intake of a food/beverage or ingredient with an observed health outcome.

In fact, 10 out of the 12 cohort studies used to evaluate the effects of "added sugars" on cardiovascular disease (CVD) used a FFQ tool that does not accurately capture exposure. This methodological concern was recognized and noted in the 2010 DGAC report by the Carbohydrate Working Group, stating, "Drinks can include a wide range of macronutrients and artificial sweeteners, and are difficult to assess with food frequency instruments." Adding to this established inaccurate assessment of SSB intake is the fact that in these cohort studies, dietary assessments are often performed several years (even decades) prior to the outcome measurement (i.e. blood pressure, diabetes, cholesterol, mortality), with the *assumption* that the subjects' diets did not change at all over the course of 5, 10, 20 years. This is a major assumption made worse by the fact that the initial intake assessment is only 30–80% accurate to begin with.

Given that the determination of causality between a food or nutrient and a health outcome has serious implications that are far-reaching, the Hill criteria for judging causality must be employed. These steps include an assessment of: strength and consistency of the association, evidence of dose-response, biological plausibility, and concordance with other data, particularly clinical trials.[28] This rigor was not employed by the Added Sugars Working Group in its recommendations for "added sugars."

The limitations of observational data are real and must be recognized given the magnitude of impact of the Dietary Guidelines for Americans.

The use of observational data of "sugar-sweetened beverage" (SSB) consumption is an inappropriate surrogate/proxy for making conclusions about "added sugars" intake and health outcomes

Although we contend that the science the Committee has used to support its links and association between "added sugars" and serious disease outcomes is weak, we strongly contend that without the substantial inclusion of SSB studies, there would be little or no scientific evidence to support or even imply any association between "added sugars" and disease outcomes.

"Sugar-sweetened beverages" are a class of beverages that indeed contain "added sugars," but SSBs do not represent the wide applications for sugars, reflect the intakes of "added sugars," and further, evidence exists for differential metabolic and health effects of SSBs versus "added sugars" consumed in other varieties and modes. In observational studies, SSB intake in the highest quartile or quintile can simply serve as markers of a less healthy lifestyle compared to those who never consume SSBs; these confounding factors are difficult if not impossible to tease out when analyzing data. We strongly question the scientific validity of the Added Sugars Working Group's use of SSBs as a "proxy" for all "added sugars" intake. The evidence used to evaluate health impacts from all "added sugars" intake relied heavily on studies solely assessing SSB consumption.

This reliance on SSB studies is evidenced by 10 of the 12 cohort studies and 3 of 11 trials used to evaluate CVD, 2 of the 3 systematic reviews to evaluate body weight and obesity, and 4 of 5 studies used to evaluate diabetes examining SSB intake, exclusively.

Given that SSBs are a unique source of "added sugars" intake, studies that examine potential health impacts from SSBs should not be generalized to infer similar metabolic impacts for intakes of all "added sugars." SSBs are strictly a liquid source of intake and are primarily sweetened with high fructose corn syrup (HFCS). Further, unlike the majority of foods and beverages that contain sugar (sucrose), with only a few exceptions, they do not contribute to intakes of fiber, protein and other essential micronutrients, as do cereals, other grain products and dairy products. With **less than 50% of the US population consuming SSBs on any given day,**[29] scientific conclusions based on SSBs and not "added sugars" (as consumed by the whole population) adds to the argument that relying on SSBs as a "proxy" is not valid.

The inappropriate use of SSBs as a "proxy" for "added sugars" in the DGAC's report is probably best highlighted by the findings of Sonestadt et al.,[30] one of five papers used to inform the diabetes conclusions and the only paper to measure and analyze "added sugars" and "total sugars" in addition to SSBs. The other four papers looked at SSB intake exclusively. The researchers report that none of the three studies reporting sucrose (sugar) intakes and none of the three studies reporting total sugars intake found a positive association with incident diabetes. Three of the studies even found an inverse association. These were the only data on "added sugars," and not just SSB intake, which were considered for diabetes. Yet, the DGAC report reads:

> "Strong evidence shows that higher consumption of added sugars, especially sugar-sweetened beverages, increases the risk of type 2 diabetes among adults and this relationship is not fully explained by body weight."

Quite simply, this statement is not a reflection of what the data indicate; a theme found throughout this report.

Similar to the methodology of Sonestadt et al.,[31] other attempts to answer questions around "added sugars" intake and health outcomes that the Added Sugars Working Group answered have recognized these differences and separated analyses by 'SSB' and 'added sugars' in relation to various outcomes. In fact, the 2010 DGAC performed their analyses this way, as did the recent SACN[32] review in the U.K.

The 2015 DGAC's "strong" conclusions linking "added sugars" to health outcomes is overstated, given the lack of rigorous and consistent data

The body of literature on the topic of "added sugars" is not only highly heterogeneous, as stated previously, but also lacks rigorous data, consistent definitions across studies and accurate measurement tools. These factors were concerns of the Carbohydrate Working Group of the 2010 DGAC and stated in its report[33] in the "Needs for Future Research":

"Studies of carbohydrates and health outcomes on a macronutrient level are often inconsistent or ambiguous due to inaccurate measures and varying food categorizations and definitions. The science cannot progress without further advances in both methodology and theory."

The 2010 DGAC report goes on to state that there is a need to, "Develop standardized assessment tools to determine the accurate intake of added sugars."

The methodologies for making these determinations have not changed since 2010; therefore, our ability to attribute a health effect to a type of carbohydrate remains no different or more reliable than it was in 2010. Yet, the 2015 DGAC made "**strong**" recommendations based off of these data anyway.

The lack of rigorous and consistent methodology, including poor measurement tools and inconsistencies in definitions and designs, are also critical reasons why systematic reviews for this body of literature on "added sugars" are so difficult to perform and often vary in their conclusions.

Specific points are made below regarding the lack of objectivity by the 2015 DGAC in its overlooking of the flaws and limitations of the science used to support recommendations on "added sugars"

"Added sugars" and obesity

The recommendation states that: "Strong and consistent evidence indicates that intake of added sugars from food and/or SSBs are associated with unfavorable body weight in children and adults. The reduction of added sugars and SSBs in the diet reduces BMI in both children and adults. Comparison groups with the highest versus the lowest intakes of added sugars in cohort studies were compatible with a recommendation to keep added sugars intake below 10% of total energy intake."

- These recommendations are based solely on two pre-existing systematic reviews. Four reviews were considered during the process but two, which happen to refute the ultimate conclusions, were ultimately discarded from consideration.
- It is incongruent with the evidence to conclude a relationship that is "strong and consistent" when the authors of the two reviews state such limitations as:

  - "The studies included in our meta-analyses varied substantially with respect to study design, exposure assessment, adjustment for covariates, and specific outcomes evaluated." (Malik, 2014)
  - "The data suggest that the change in body fatness that occurs with modifying intake of sugars results from an alteration in energy balance rather than a physiological or metabolic consequence of monosaccharides or disaccharides. Owing to the multifactorial causes of obesity, it is unsurprising that the effect of reducing intake is relatively small." (Te Morenga, 2013)
  - "The extent to which population based advice to reduce sugars might reduce risk of obesity cannot be extrapolated from the present findings, because few data from the studies lasted longer than ten weeks." (Te Morenga, 2013)

It has consistently been reported in the scientific literature that the observed association between "added sugars" intake, particularly SSB intake, and body weight is true only in situations of overall positive energy balance, meaning when individuals are consuming too many calories—from all sources—and *not* a unique function of sugars. This was stated by the 2010 DGAC in its report and reiterated by the author of one of the two systematic reviews used by this Committee: "We observed that isoenergetic replacement of dietary sugars with other macronutrients resulted in *no weight change*. This finding strongly suggested that energy imbalance is a major determinant of the potential for dietary sugar to influence measures of body fatness." (Te Morenga, 2013).

We contend that the 2015 DGAC recommendations oversimplify and inaccurately portray the scientific evidence that currently exists on "added sugars" and body weight.

"Added sugars" and type two diabetes (T2D):

The recommendation states that there is "**strong**" evidence for: "Higher consumption of added sugars, especially 'sugar-sweetened beverages,' increase the risk for T2D among adults and this relationship is not fully explained by body weight."

- The evidence evaluated for T2D included four systematic reviews and one cohort study. It is unclear how these five papers were selected for consideration. It is worthwhile to note that this question has not been previously evaluated by any DGAC, meaning that a formal NEL search and review of the literature on added sugars and diabetes has never occurred.
- Four of the five papers examined SSBs exclusively and the fifth was a meta-analysis that looked at both SSBs and sugars intake. *This meta-analysis concluded that "The results were limited or inconsistent on the adverse effect of intake of total sugars, glucose or fructose on the incidence of type 2 diabetes."* [Emphasis added][34] This was the only paper of the five to examine sugars other than SSBs, therefore the conclusion statement for diabetes, as written, is substantially overstating the findings.
- Two of the studies assessed the risk of T2D for *both* vartificially and "sugar sweetened beverages" and found increased risk of T2D for *both*. These findings negate the conclusion that "added sugars" intake explains the observed associations between SSBs and T2D and provide support for questioning the utility of cohort data (and FFQs to assess soda intake) and also support the case that soda drinking has collinear diet and lifestyle behaviors that can't be well controlled for, and thus impact findings.
- Importantly, this conclusion by the Added Sugars Working Group differs from those from the 2014 U.K. SACN draft report,[35] an evaluation with access to the same body of literature as the DGAC given the similar timeline of their respective evaluations. In this SACN report, no association was found between sucrose, glucose, fructose and T2D (in fact, a borderline inverse association between sucrose and T2D was found). With regard to SSBs, which were studied separately, SACN found moderate, not

"**strong**," evidence for an association with T2D. The SACN conclusion, however, was not extrapolated to include all "added sugars" as stated in the DGAC recommendation.
- By declaring "**strong**" evidence, the Working Group ignores the limitations cited in the most recent of the five papers they examined, a meta-analysis by Greenwood et al. in June 2014,[36] which states: "Overall, between-study heterogeneity was high. The included studies were observational, so their results should be interpreted cautiously. . . ."

In summary, the draft conclusion statement on "added sugars" intake and diabetes does not reflect the preponderance of science, let alone reflect the select body of science that was examined. To make such a "**strong**" recommendation linking added sugars intake to T2D based on weak scientific evidence is misleading, not evidence-based, and contradicts conclusions by other authoritative bodies and position statements of the American Diabetes Association (ADA). The ADA states that sugar is not different than starch with respect to blood glucose and lipid levels, when consumed up to 35% of calories.[37] Of note is that current intakes of "added sugars" are only ~13% of calories and the DGAC is proposing a limit of less than 10%. Again, the scientific evidence presented by the Working Group does not validate its conclusion statement and does not provide a scientific basis for any intake recommendation.

"Added sugars" and cardiovascular disease:

The recommendation states that there is "**moderate**" evidence that: "Evidence from prospective cohort studies indicates that higher intake of added sugars, especially in the form of SSBs, is consistently associated with increased risk of hypertension, stroke, and coronary heart disease in adults. Observational and intervention studies indicate a consistent relationship between higher added sugar intake and higher blood pressure and serum triglycerides."

- The majority of studies included in this evaluation examined intakes of either "added sugars" or SSB intakes that, if even reported, were at least twice as high as current mean intakes in the U.S. (~13%). Many of the studies did not even report total "added sugars" intakes, leaving actual exposure or intakes unknown.
- Over half of the studies included in this analysis were observational studies and over half of them examined SSBs exclusively, often not reporting

intakes of total "added sugars," total sugars, total carbohydrates, energy intakes, or other important dietary factors associated with CVD (i.e. fats, sodium).

- Additionally, very few of the 11 trials included employed isocaloric treatments, making evaluation of the role that sugars plays, independent of total energy or carbohydrate intake, impossible.

Ultimately, the conclusion on "added sugars" and CVD overstates what the evidence says. The study quality is generally weak, with poor control and with a heavy reliance on observational data. The CVD variables the Working Group chose to look at are numerous and a review of this nature, with studies of this quality and so few in number, is not a true evidence-based approach to making links between diet and disease. That said, even with the approach and evidence the DGAC considered, consistent associations between "added sugars" intake and any of the CVD variables studied do not exist. For example, of 11 trials, only two measured blood pressure and only one saw an effect of "added sugars" intake–at an intake of 27% energy (twice the current average in the US). As is the case with each of the DGAC recommendations, the scientific evidence does not support them.

"Added sugars" and dental caries:

The recommendation states that: "The DGAC concurs with the World Health Organization's commissioned systematic review that there is moderate consistent evidence supporting a relationship between the amount of sugars intake and the development of dental caries among children and adults. There is also evidence of moderate quality showing that caries are lower when free-sugars intake is less than 10% of energy intake."

- This conclusion was based on *one* systematic review. This review was not a meta-analysis because, according to the authors, variability in the data was too large to analyze as such.
- This one review studied only the amount of "added sugars" intake associated with dental caries and did not evaluate the role of frequency, total sugars or fermentable carbohydrates, all of which are considered to be cariogenic. This is an important point recognized in the 2010 Dietary Guidelines for Americans, where it states that, "Both naturally occurring sugars and added sugar increase the risk of dental caries." The DGAs also recognize additional factors involved in cariogenesis:

"During the time that sugars and starches are in contact with teeth, they also contribute to dental caries. A combined approach of reducing the amount of time sugars and starches are in the mouth, drinking fluoridated water, and brushing and flossing teeth, is the most effective way to reduce dental caries."

- Of note, this sole review used as the basis for this conclusion does not contain any publication more recent than 2010. This is also an important point because in 2010 EFSA concluded their review, which evaluated the role of sugars in dental caries, and made the following conclusion:

"Frequent consumption of sugar-containing foods can increase risk of dental caries, especially when oral hygiene and fluoride prophylaxis are insufficient. However, available data *does not allow setting an upper limit for intake of (added) sugars on the basis of a risk reduction for dental caries,* [Emphasis added] as caries development related to consumption of sucrose and other cariogenic carbohydrates does not depend only on the amount of sugar consumed, but is also influenced by frequency of consumption, oral hygiene, exposure to fluoride, and various other factors."[38]

In conclusion, by selecting one pre-existing review, the DGAC's shortcut to a conclusion on the role of "added sugars" and dental caries has bypassed an evidence-based approach to determine a diet and health relationship, and ignores the multifactorial nature of the role of all fermentable carbohydrates in the development of dental caries.

The 2015 DGAC provided no credible science-based evidence to support its recommendation to reduce "added sugars" intake to below 10 percent of total energy intake

The 2015 DGAC made its recommendation of "**strong**" evidence for its 10 percent of total energy from "added sugars" based on weak scientific evidence and mathematical food modeling that has not been tested for effectiveness in influencing body weight or other health outcomes. This value, 10 percent, is arbitrary and has not been scientifically tested, let alone proven.

Calories are the real issue

In fact, the body of evidence actually indicates that any observed effect of "added sugars" on body weight is a function of total calories, from all sources, and not any unique obesogenic property of "added sugars." This point is even made in the WHO-commissioned review

(Te Morenga, 2013), the nexus that has empowered the DGAC to set an "added sugars" intake level. The authors acknowledge the limitations of the evidence stating,

- "Although comparison of groups with the highest versus lowest intakes in cohort studies was compatible with a recommendation to restrict intake to below 10% total energy, *currently available data did not allow formal dose-response analysis.*" (Te Morenga, 2013) [Emphasis added]
- "The data suggest that the change in body fatness that occurs with modifying intake of sugars results from an alteration in energy balance rather than a physiological or metabolic consequence of monosaccharides or disaccharides. Owing to the multifactorial causes of obesity, it is unsurprising that the effect of reducing intake is relatively small." (Te Morenga, 2013)
- "The extent to which population based advice to reduce sugars might reduce risk of obesity cannot be extrapolated from the present findings, because few data from the studies lasted longer than ten weeks." (Te Morenga, 2013)
- "We observed that isoenergetic replacement of dietary sugars with other macronutrients resulted in **no weight change.** This finding strongly suggested that energy imbalance is a major determinant of the potential for dietary sugar to influence measures of body fatness." (Te Morenga, 2013).

The findings in the WHO commissioned review are actually consistent with the 2010 DGAs advice that clearly states, "Foods containing solid fats and added sugars are no more likely to contribute to weight gain than any other source of calories in an eating pattern that is within calorie limits."[39]

Calories from "added sugars" are not major contributing factor in increased caloric intakes or obesity

We strongly contend that the preponderance of scientific information on "added sugars" intake does not support a 10% limit or any assertion that "added sugars" intake uniquely contributes to obesity other than as a source of calories. Further, even as a source of calories, intake data do not support "added sugars" intake as a major source of increased caloric intake. In the past 40 years, U.S. per capita consumption of sugar/sucrose declined by 33% as obesity and other serious diseases increased. A recent analysis of U.S. National Health and Nutrition Examination Survey (NHANES) data found that "added sugars" consumption has declined to 14.6% percent of energy, which is a decrease of 19.3% over a period of eight years (2000 to 2008)[40] and as the 2015 DGAC noted current intake is now 13.4% of energy. More importantly, according to USDA data, Americans are consuming 425 more calories per person per day than they did in 1970 and of these 425 calories only 38 calories are attributed to "added sugars" intake (2009).[41]

The data also do not support that intakes of "added sugars" have a direct impact on body mass index (BMI). A 2010 analysis of the NHANES data verifies that intake of "added sugars" does not have a direct correlation with BMI. The authors of the study state, "The individuals with the highest mean BMI values were associated with the $\leq 0 \leq 5\%$ and $>35\%$ added sugars categories (BMI 28.9, 28.1, respectively). With each 5% increase in added sugars category above 15% of added sugars intake, we found a lower prevalence of overweight and obese individuals, with the exception of >35% added sugars for BMI ≥ 30 where the prevalence increased to 3.2%."[42]

Food pattern modeling does not have the scientific underpinning to support "added sugar" intake recommendations

The fact remains that no authoritative scientific body after a thorough review of the scientific literature has found a public health need to set an intake level or upper level for "added sugars" intake, including the IOM[43] and in 2010 the EFSA.[44] This was also the conclusion of the Food and Drug Administration (FDA) in its recent Nutrition Facts Panel (NFP) Proposed Rule stating,

". . . we have no scientifically supported quantitative intake recommendation for added sugars on which a DRV for added sugars can be derived. Therefore, we are not proposing a DRV for added sugars."

Regarding the use of USDA food modeling for setting a DRV for "added sugars" intake the FDA states,

"The solid fats and added sugars limit at each calorie level in the USDA Food Patterns is determined by calculation through food pattern modeling rather than on any biomarker of risk of disease or other public health endpoint."

Further, the 2010 DGA policy document clearly states that the USDA Eating Patterns is but one example of suggested eating patterns and that the USDA Eating Patterns *"have not been specifically tested for health benefits."*

Serious concerns must be raised regarding the scientific integrity of the 2015 DGAC's efforts to validate food pattern modeling as an evidence-based guide for food consumption or intake recommendations. At the DGAC's sixth meeting it was asserted, "The data from the intervention trials and the cohort studies provide empirical data that the USDA Food Patterns provide an evidence-based guide to food consumption." The graphs provided by the DGAC to support this assertion raise serious questions.

The table below quantifies the information provided in these graphs that depicted the correlation between intakes in *cited dietary pattern studies* and USDA Food Pattern recommendations.

Dietary Component	Studies	Within USDA Food Pattern Range	Intakes Outside USDA Food Pattern Range	Lower	Higher
Vegetables	23	9	14	6	8
Fruit	23	5	18	3	15
Dairy	19	6	13	13	
Red & Processed Meat	20	1	19	6	13
Seafood	20	5	15		15

We question how their graphical depiction can be considered evidence-based and therefore grounds for empirical support that USDA Food Patterns are an evidence-based guide for food consumption. Furthermore, this quantified table shows that in fact the majority of food group intakes from these published dietary pattern studies do not actually fall within the recommendations of the USDA Food Pattern ranges as asserted by the 2015 DGAC. Additionally, because the dietary pattern studies cited did not include "added sugars" criteria, there is no graph/empirical evidence to support the extremely low "added sugars" intake in the proposed "Healthy US-Style Patterns" or in any of the patterns in the table provided in the 2015 DGAC advisory report to support a 10 percent intake recommendation.

Until the food pattern modeling itself is tested, "empirical" evidence for its efficacy does not exist. In the interim, such creative methods of portraying the science to support "added sugars" intakes as official science-based recommendations undermines the credibility of the Dietary Guidelines process. [Emphasis added]

Therefore, we assert the use of the scientifically questionable WHO intake recommendation and hypothesis-based food modeling for recommending "added sugars" intakes undermines U.S.'s high standards in evidence-based nutrition guidance and policy.

The 2015 DGAC aligning with the controversial World Health Organization's (WHO) Guideline on Sugars is a step back for U.S. standards of evidence

The U.S. has consistently maintained a high standard of evidence-based recommendations in the development of policy. We strongly contend that the 2015 DGAC alignment with the WHO recent and controversial guideline on sugars intake[45] undermines this important standard of scientific integrity.

The WHO commissioned two systematic reviews to inform their March 2015 report, "WHO Guidelines: Sugars intake for adults and children;" one of these addressed body weight (Te Morenga, 2013) and the other dental caries.[46] Instead of conducting their own NEL reviews of these important questions, the 2015 DGAC relied heavily on the body weight review (Te Morenga, 2013) for its **"strong"** recommendation on "added sugars" and body weight and to supports its recommendation to keep "added sugars" intake below 10 percent of total energy intake. The Committee made its recommendation for dental caries solely on this WHO commissioned systematic review. It is critical to note that in the WHO report, WHO grades its own evidence for free sugars (added sugars) intake and body weight for both adults and children to be of *moderate quality, at best.* Its evidence for reducing dental caries by reducing free sugars as moderate and evidence relating to population studies as *very low quality.*[47]

The WHO has a history of controversial reports due to their recommendations being political and based on of low quality evidence. For example, regarding WHO's 2009 Report 916 free sugars recommendations in 2004, the American Dietetic Association (now the Academy of Nutrition and Dietetics) stated in its "Position of the American Dietetic Association: Use of Nutritive and Non-nutritive Sweeteners:"

"The WHO is currently in the process of designing a global strategy for making recommendations regarding diet, physical activity and health. On the basis of the opinions of a joint consultation report the WHO recommended 10% of energy from added sugars (defined as "free sugars"). The strategies used in the panel's deliberations encompass *their interpretation* of a range of epidemiologic, economic, social, and political impacts on the prevention and control of non-communicable diseases. Thus, the 10% intake recommendation may *not be based solely on scientific evidence.*"[48]

Further, highlighting a pattern of recommendations that are not grounded in strong science, a recent study published in the *Journal of Clinical Epidemiology* titled "World Health Organization recommendations are often strong based on low confidence in effect estimates" found, "Over 50% of WHO recommendations are strong and over 50% of those strong recommendations are based on low or very low confidence in effect estimates (study quality)." Regarding nutrition guidelines, this percentage jumps to 100%.[49]

In an evidence-based process, such as mandated for use in the U.S Dietary Guidelines process, the WHO report or the WHO commissioned meta-analyses (Te Morenga, 2013) does not provide the level of scientific evidence or agreement upon which the 2015 DGAC can credibly base its grade of "**strong**" evidence to associate "added sugars" intake uniquely to obesity, other than a source of calories.

Additionally, the sole use of a WHO commissioned review as evidence that "added sugars" intake is a unique contributor to dental caries is even weaker. It also undermines decades of scientific evidence and professional advice that *all* fermentable carbohydrates can cause dental caries and that dental hygiene is the most important factor in reducing tooth decay.

The use of hypothesis-based dietary patterns studies to link or associate dietary components with serious disease outcomes or set intake recommendations is not a validated scientific methodology

To further emphasize concerns that sound scientific principals were undermined in an effort to make "bold and innovative" recommendations, we strongly question the scientific validity of using hypothesis-based dietary pattern studies to link dietary components to disease outcomes. The use of hypothesis-based research to infer, or even state, cause and effect relationships between dietary components and disease outcomes that are not yet established by more traditional, experimental science is not a validated scientific process.

The "hypothesis-based" methodologies used in these dietary pattern studies do not, and cannot, accurately isolate the positive or negative effects of individual components of the dietary pattern. In this totally subjective methodology, certain components of a dietary pattern are pre-assigned negative scores based on the *presumptions* they are detrimental, resulting in outcomes that are *biased* and *predetermined*.

We contend that this methodology is not objective science and is not appropriate for use in making evidence-based recommendations. Furthermore, examination of the science cited raises concerns that the conclusions drawn by the Committee do not accurately reflect what was represented in the actual scientific studies cited (again a theme in this process). As demonstrated in the table (pg. 21) of food pattern modeling, the majority of dietary pattern studies cited by the Committee did not include a total sugars or "added sugars" criteria. Yet, the Committee implies that there is a link or association between "added sugars" and serious disease outcomes.

The DGAC "**strong**" recommendation relating to the "The Relationship Between Dietary Patterns and Risk of Cardiovascular Disease" which states that low intakes of "added sugars" reduced risks of cardiovascular disease cited 20 studies identified as having assessed the association with *individual food components* of a dietary pattern score and *CVD endpoint outcomes*. Sixteen of those studies did not even include an "added sugars," sugars-sweetened food or sweetened beverage component in their scoring methodology.

Dietary guidance that links or associates any individual component of the diet with serious disease outcomes must be supported by a thorough systematic review of the full body of science (at the highest level of evidence available) to assure recommendations are based on a preponderance of scientific evidence. In some instances, the required scientific evidence for such conclusions does not yet exist. Therefore, the science used to support these conclusions is yet another example of why serious concerns are being raised in the 2015 DGAC process that biases and not scientific evidence are influencing recommendations.

There are unintended consequences of the 2015 DGAC recommendations to reduce "added sugars" intake to historically low levels

We strongly assert that sugar is an important ingredient that contributes essential functional properties to food formulation, including safety as a natural food preservative. Additionally, historic, as well as recent analyses on "added sugars" intake confirm that sugar makes many nutrient-rich foods palatable, thus sugar is a positive factor for intake levels of many essential micronutrients.[50] [51] [52] [53] [54] [55] [56] Historic consumption data show that "added sugars" intakes have not been at these extremely low levels suggested in the USDA Food Pattern/Healthy US-Style Patterns since nutrient deficiencies were a major public health problem. The unintended consequences, including the impact on nutrient intakes, need to be strongly considered, especially for children. The American Academy of Pediatrics published a new policy statement in March 2015, which states:

"Added sugars offer no nutritional benefits. At the same time, sugars themselves are not necessarily harmful. Used along with nutrient rich foods and beverages, sugar can be a powerful tool to increase the quality of a child's diet. Used in excess, added sugars can add substantially to daily calories. Used at extreme levels (ie, more than 25% to 30% of total calories), sugars can displace other nutrients, resulting in nutrient deficiencies. Although added sugars are often presumed to be an independent cause of overweight, this claim has not been proven in studies."

"Care should be taken when prohibiting sugar-containing products to avoid compromising overall nutrition among children."

"Sugars consumed in nutrient-poor foods and beverages are the primary problem to be addressed, not simply the sugars themselves."[57]

Further, a focus on reducing "added sugars" does not necessarily translate to reduced calories. Consumers who select foods based on a reduction in grams of sugars listed in the Nutrition Facts Panel are often being misled because "added sugars" are frequently replaced by carbohydrate bulking agents, such as glycerol or maltodextrins, and/or by an increase in fat content to maintain functionality and/or taste. These sugar replacers provide no nutritional benefit or a significant caloric reduction over sugars.

Further, scientific studies have documented the inverse relationship between fat and sugars intake when expressed as percent of energy in both the United States and the European Union.[58] The current focus on reducing "added sugars" in the diet exacerbates the troubling growth in fat consumption in the United States. Despite lessening health concerns about fat, it remains a major and increasing source of calories while at the same time calories from "added sugars" consumption continuesto decline.

Reducing obesity is the number one public health objective and it is imperative that meaningfully reducing total caloric intake be the goal without compromising essential nutrient intakes. To do this effectively, all unintended consequences must be considered. Overly restrictive "added sugars" intake recommendations could have unintended negative consequences that are inconsistent with the public health goals of healthy diets and meaningfully impacting obesity.

The 2015 DGAC "Added Sugars" policy recommendations went far beyond the Congressional mandate and DGAC Charter with no evidence-based support

The 2015 DGAC went far beyond the Congressional mandate and DGAC Charter in providing specific recommendations for federal policy and regulations. Public Law 101.445 specifically states,

> "Each such report shall contain *nutritional and dietary information and guidelines for the general public*, and shall be *promoted* by each Federal agency in carrying out any Federal *food, nutrition, or health program*."

We contend that the use of dietary guidance in Federal nutrition and nutrition education programs is far different from the use of dietary guidance as a basis for establishing Federal nutrition policy, rules and regulations. We have serious concerns the interpretation of the actual language in the statute governing the DGA process has been expanded beyond its original intent. The use of dietary guidance in the Dietary Guidelines for Americans (DGA) is now being used as the sole basis to support Federal rules and regulations. However, Section 301(b)(3) of Title III of the 1990 law states,

> "LIMITATION ON DEFINITION OF GUIDANCE- For purposes of this subsection, the term `dietary guidance for the general population' does not include any rule or regulation issued by a Federal agency."

This expansion of the intent and power of the DGA has far-reaching implications for stakeholders. This is most evident by the FDA almost sole use of "selective" dietary guidance in the 2010 DGA to support is proposal to require "added sugars" labeling on the NFP, which was supported by the 2015 DGAC in its policy recommendations.

This also raises serious concern for future regulations due to the fact the Departments will have the ability to select advisory panel members that support Government initiatives and regulatory agendas. These concerns are even more relevant due to FDA's recent pronouncement that the DGA is a "consensus" document in its Proposed Rule on changes to the NFP.

Therefore, we strongly object to the use of the 2015 DGAC *"Implications"* or Federal policy recommendations in the final DGAs, especially when the 2015 DGAC provided no scientific evidence to support the efficacy of its policy recommendations.

We have strong reservations about potential implications for future changes to regulations including labeling regulation should the scientific criteria for making regulations be based solely on a single U.S. Government generated report. Our reservations are even greater in light of our concerns regarding the quality of science and biases in this 2015 DGAC process.

USDA has undue influence on the DGAC processes relating to its role in food patterns modeling

Historically, the USDA Pyramid guidance, which are now USDA Food Patterns, were developed to reflect the recommendations of the Dietary Guidelines. However, in recent Dietary Guidelines processes, the USDA Food Patterns and food modeling are being used as *the basis* for recommendations and even for setting limits and intake recommendations. Such recommendations are the purview of the IOM.

Further, the mathematical construct of USDA food modeling to develop these Food Patterns is falsely being given the weight of science, even over peer-reviewed science and reports by authoritative scientific bodies; yet, this exercise lacks such rigor. USDA, as an agency that oversees the DGAC process, and as the agency that develops the food patterns and conducts food modeling, is in a position to unduly influence the DGAC process.

We ask the Secretaries to ensure all Dietary Guidelines recommendations are based solely on a thorough review of the scientific evidence. Only then should this science-based dietary guidance be used to construct USDA Food Patterns.

In conclusion,

As participants in the Dietary Guidelines process since its inception, the Association has legitimate concerns about the scientific integrity of the 2015 DGAC process. The 2015 DGAC has taken "added sugars" recommendations to unchartered territory, contradicting decades of science on sugar and current major reviews of the scientific literature on sugar intake. This raises serious concerns about the manner by which 2015 DGAC recommendations were derived.

To this point, despite the fact there has been considerable Government investment in the establishment of the NEL systematic review process, NEL reviews were not consistently used in the 2015 process to evaluate the scientific evidence, as was done for virtually all research questions in the 2010 process. The consistent use of NEL reviews across *all* research topics would have provided interested parties reasonable assurance that all subject areas were given the same consistent and unbiased consideration.

We emphasize that the 2015 DGAC did not undertake the rigorous scientific investigation necessary to conclude links or associations between "added sugars" and serious disease outcomes. Intake recommendations that lead the American public to believe any dietary component is a causal factor in a serious disease outcome should only be made based on significant scientific agreement due to a robust review of the entire body of scientific literature by experts in the field of investigation.

Dietary Guidelines for Americans are too important not to get them right. We have seen changing scientific agreement and dietary guidance on other dietary targets over the years, i.e. dietary cholesterol (eggs) and fats. This shifting dietary guidance that targets basic staples of the American diet has an economic impact on farmers, food and beverage manufactures and ultimately causes consumer confusion and apathy. Further, it has done little to improve the health of Americans.

We respectfully ask that the Secretaries maintain the integrity of the Dietary Guidelines process and to adhere to the Congressional mandate that clearly requires changes to Dietary Guidelines for Americans to be based solely on the preponderance of scientific information, which is not the case in the 2015 DGAC advisory report for "added sugars." Therefore, we ask that the Secretaries to maintain the 2010 Dietary Guidelines advice for "added sugars" until a thorough review of the scientific literature on "added sugars" intake is conducted by an authoritative scientific body, such as the Institute of Medicine.

We thank you for your consideration of this comment.

Sincerely,

Andrew C. Briscoe III   P. Courtney Gaine, PhD, RD
President   Vice President of Scientific Affairs

Notes

1. National Nutrition Monitoring and Related Research Act of 1990, Public Law 445, 101st Congress, 2nd session (October 22, 1990). Public Law 101–445, section 301.
2. Office of Management and Budget. Guidelines for ensuring and maximizing the quality, objectivity, utility, and integrity of information disseminated by Federal agencies; republication. Federal Register 67(36): 8452–8460. Friday, February 22, 2002. Available at http://www.whitehouse.gov/omb/fedreg/reproducible2.pdf.
3. U.S. Department of Health and Human Services. HHS Guidelines for ensuring and maximizing the quality, objectivity, utility, and integrity of information disseminated by Federal agencies. Last HHS revision: Available at http://aspe.hhs.gov/infoQuality/index.shtml
4. Improving Regulation and Regulatory Review, Executive Order 13563 of January 18, 2011, Federal Register 76(14) Friday, January 21, 2011.

5. Food & Nutrition Bd., Nat'l Acad. of Sciences, Dietary Reference Intakes for Energy, Carbohydrate, Fiber, Fat, Fatty Acids, Cholesterol, Protein, and Amino Acids (2002)

6. EFSA Panel on Dietetic Products, Nutrition, and Allergies (NDA). Scientific opinion dietary reference values for carbohydrates and dietary fibre (2010). *EFSA Journal* **8**(3): 1462 [77 pp]. Available at http://www.efsa.europa.eu/en/scdocs/scdoc/1462.htm.

7. Scientific Advisory Committee on Nutrition (SACN), Draft Carbohydrates and Health Report. June 2014. (https://www.gov.uk/government/uploads/system/uploads/attachment_data/file/339771/Draft_SACN_Carbohydrates_and_Health_report_consultation.pdf)

8. Evert AB, et al. Nutrition therapy recommendations for the management of adults with diabetes. Diabetes Care. 2014 Jan;37 Suppl 1:S120–43

9. Burt BA, Pai S. Sugar consumption and caries risk: a systematic review. J Dent Edu. 2001; 65(10):1017–23

10. Meschia JF, et al. Guidelines for the primary prevention of stroke: a statement for healthcare professionals from the american heart association/american stroke association. Stroke. 2014 Dec;45(12):3754–832.

11. "The role of carbohydrates in the diet has been the source of much public and scientific interest. These include the relationship of carbohydrates with health outcomes, including coronary heart disease (CHD), type 2 diabetes (T2D), body weight, and dental caries. The 2010 DGAC conducted Nutrition Evidence Library (NEL) evidence reviews on these and other carbohydrate-related topics. The Committee also relied on evidence contained in the 2002 Dietary Reference Intakes (DRIs) report and conducted a non-NEL review of recent literature to specifically examine the relationship of carbohydrates with CHD, T2D, behavior, and cognitive performance (Colditz, 1992; Dolan, 2010; IOM, 2002; Laville, 2009; Meyer, 2000; Stanhope, 2009; Wolraich, 1995). No detrimental effects of carbohydrates as a source of calories on these or other health outcomes were reported." Dietary Guidelines Advisory Committee. 2010. Report of the Dietary Guidelines Advisory Committee on the Dietary Guidelines for Americans, 2010, to the Secretary of Agriculture and the Secretary of Health and Human Services. U.S. Department of Agriculture, Agricultural Research Service, Washington, DC.

12. *Report of the Dietary Guidelines Advisory Committee on the Dietary Guidelines for Americans, 2010 To the Secretary of Agriculture and the Secretary of Health and Human Services* May 2010 pg. 286

13. U.S Department of Agriculture and U.S. Department of Health and Human Services, Dietary Guidelines for Americans 2010, 7th Edition, Washington DC: U.S. Government Printing Office, December 2010 pg. 28

14. Berlin JS. "Meta-analysis as Evidence Building A Better Pyramid." JAMA. August 2014. Vol. 312 (6)

15. Kicinski, M. "Publication Bias in Recent Meta-Analysis." PLOS ONE. November 201: Vol. 8 (11)

16. *Op. Cit.* 14

17. Maki KC et al. "Limitations of Observational Evidence: Implications for Evidence-Based Recommendations." ASN Adv. Nutr. 5:7–15, 2014, doi:10.3945/an.113.004929

18. Rothstein HR. "Publication Bias in Meta-Analysis." *Prevention, Assessments and Adjustments.* 2005, John Wiley & Sons, Ltd.

19. Trumbo PR, Rivers CR. Systematic review of the evidence for an association between sugar-sweetened beverage consumption and risk of obesity. *Nutr Rev.* 2014.

20. Kaiser KA, Shikany JM, Keating KD, Allison DB. Will reducing sugar-sweetened beverage consumption reduce obesity? Evidence supporting conjecture is strong, but evidence when testing effect is weak. Obes Rev. 2013 Aug;14(8):620–33.

21. *Op. Cit.* 14

22. Walker E, et al. Meta-analysis: Its strength and limitations. *Clev Clin J of Med.* 2008; 75(6):431–439.

23. Malik VS, Pan A, Willett WC, Hu FB. Sugar-sweetened beverages and weight gain in children and adults: a systematic review and meta-analysis. *Am J Clin Nutr.* 2013 Oct;98(4):1084–102

24. Te Morenga L, Mallard S, Mann J. Dietary sugars and body weight: systematic review and meta-analyses of randomised controlled trials and cohort studies. Bmj. 2013;346:e7492. PMID: 23321486

25. Greenwood DC, et al. Association between sugar-sweetened and artificially sweetened soft drinks and type 2 diabetes: systematic review and dose-response meta-analysis of prospective studies. *Brit J of Nutr.* 2014, 112, 725–734.

26. *Op. Cit.* 17

27. *Ibid.*

28. Hill, Austin Bradford (1965). "The Environment and Disease: Association or Causation?". *Proceedings of the Royal Society of Medicine* **58**(5): 295–300.

29. Ogden, et al. Consumption of Sugar Drinks in the United States, 2005–2008. NCHS Data Brief. No.71, August 2011.

30. Sonestedt E, et al. Does high sugar consumption exacerbate cardiometabolic risk factors and increase the risk of type 2 diabetes and cardiovascular disease? *Food & Nut Res*. 2012. 56:19104.

31. *Ibid*.

32. *Op. Cit.* 7

33. Dietary Guidelines Advisory Committee. 2010. Report of the Dietary Guidelines Advisory Committee on the Dietary Guidelines for Americans, 2010, to the Secretary of Agriculture and the Secretary of Health and Human Services. U.S. Department of Agriculture, Agricultural Research Service, Washington, DC. Pages 311–312

34. *Op. Cit. 30*

35. *Op. Cit.* 7

36. *Op. Cit.* 25

37. *Op. Cit.* 8

38. *Op. Cit.* 6

39. U.S Department of Agriculture and U.S. Department of Health and Human Services, Dietary Guidelines for Americans 2010, 7th Edition, Washington DC: U.S. Government Printing Office, December 2010 pg. 28

40. JA Welsh, AJ Sharma, L Grellinger, MB Vos. Consumption of added sugars is decreasing in the United States. *American Journal Clinical Nutrition* (2011) **94(3)**: 726–734.

41. Available at http://www.ers.usda.gov/data/foodconsumption/FoodGuideSpreadsheets.htm; last update: February 1, 2011

42. B P Marriott et al (2010) 'Intake of Added Sugars and Selected Nutrients in the United States, National Health and Nutrition Examination Survey (NHANES) 2003–2006', Critical Reviews in Food Science and Nutrition, 50: 3, 228–258.

43. *Op. Cit.* 5

44. *Op. Cit.* 6

45. Guideline: Sugars intake for adults and children. Geneva: World Health Organization; 2015.

46. Moynihan PJ, Kelly SA. Effect on caries of restricting sugars intake: systematic review to inform WHO guidelines. *J Dent Res*. 2014 Jan; 93(1):8–18.

47. WHO evidence grading definitions, "Based on the grades of evidence set by the GRADE Working Group -moderate quality, we are moderately confident in the effect estimate: the true effect is likely to be close to the estimate of the effect, but there is a possibility that it is substantially different, low quality, our confidence in the effect estimate is limited: the true effect may be substantially different from the estimate of the effect, very low quality, we have very little confidence in the effect estimate: the true effect is likely to be substantially different from the estimate of the effect." **Citation:** Guideline: Sugars intake for adults and children. Geneva: World Health Organization; 2015.

48. American Dietetic Association, Position of the American Dietetic Association: Use of Nutritive and Nonnutritive Sweeteners, J Am Diet Assoc. Vol 4 Number 2, 255–274 Feb 2004

49. Alexander PE, et al. World Health Organization strong recommendations based on low-quality evidence (study quality) are frequent and often inconsistent with GRADE guidance. J Clin Epidemiol. 2014 Dec 19

50. Rennie KL et al "Association between added sugar intake and micronutrient intake: a systematic review" *British Journal of Nutrition* 2007; 97: 832–841

51. World Health Organization & Food and Agric. Org. of the United Nations, FAO Food and Nutrition Paper 66, Carbohydrates In Human Nutrition: Report of a Joint FAO/WHO Consultation 36(1998)

52. Frary CD et al "Children and Adolescents' Choices of Foods and Beverages High in Added Sugars Are Association with Intakes of Key Nutrients and Food Groups", *Journal of Adolescent Health* 2004; 34: 56–63

53. Murphy MM et al "Drinking flavored or plain milk is positively association with nutrient intake and is not associated with adverse effects on weight status in US children and adolescents" *J Am Diet Assoc*, 2008 Apr; 108(4):631–9

54. RA Forshee, ML Storey, Controversy and statistical issues in the use of nutrient densities in assessing diet quality. *Journal of Nutrition*, 2004 134(10): 2733–2737

55. SA Gibson, Dietary sugars intake and micronutrient adequacy: a systematic review of the evidence. *Nutrition Research Review*, 2007 20(2): 121–131

56. Johnson RK et al Dietary sugars intake and cardiovascular health: a scientific statement from the American Heart Association. Circulation. 2009;120:1011–1020

57. American Academy of Pediatrics. Policy Statement: Snacks, Sweetened Beverages, Added Sugars, and Schools. *Pediatrics*. 2015. 135;3.

58. M. Gibney et al., *Consumption of Sugars*, 62 Am. J. Clinical Nutrition 178S (Supp. 1995). This relationship was reflected in a more recent study that examined the impact of low fat interventions in school lunches—it was noted

that "[a]s percent of calories from fat or saturated fat in lunches decreased, that from sugars increased." J.T. Dwyer et al., *Fat-Sugar See-Saw in School Lunches: Impact of a Low Fat Intervention*, 32 J. Adolescent Health 428 (Supp. 6 2003) R.P. Farris, *Nutrient Intake and Food Group Consumption of 10-Year- Olds by Sugar Intake Level: The Bogalusa Heart Study*, 17 J. Am. College Nutr. 579 (1998) ;J.O. Hill and A.M. Prentice, *Sugar and Body Weight Regulation*, 62 Am. J. Clin. Nutr. 262S (Supp. 1995).

ANDREW C. BRISCOE III is current President and CEO of The Sugar Association, Briscoe served as Vice-President and past Vice-President of the Salt Institute. He also directed federal and state public affairs and public policy initiatives of Mothers Against Drunk Driving.

P. COURTNEY GAINE is Vice President of Scientific Affairs at The Sugar Association. Gaine is a registered dietitian with a PhD in nutrition, biochemistry, and exercise from the University of Connecticut.

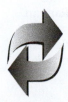

EXPLORING THE ISSUE

Should We Eat Less Added Sugars?

Critical Thinking and Reflection

1. The DGAC report concludes there is "strong evidence" that "lower intakes of *refined grains,* and *sugar-sweetened foods and beverages* . . . and moderate consumption of alcohol have beneficial outcomes on cardiovascular disease." Locate and summarize one recent peer-reviewed article that examines the relationship between alcohol and heath such as alcohol's effects on cardiovascular disease, diabetes, or gout. In your summary, include your opinion on which recommendation is better, restricting sugar-sweetened foods or consuming moderate amounts of alcohol.
2. Review and compare the recommendations or statements related to added sugars or sugar-sweetened beverages from international and national organizations found in the table of the *DGAC 2015 report.*
3. Keep a 3-day food record. Use SuperTracker.gov to determine the amount of "added sugars" in your diet. Does your intake exceed 10 percent of your energy? If so, plan a diet that will reduce your intake to 10 percent.
4. In 2015, the World Health Organization (WHO) published the new guideline, *Sugars intake for adults and children,* available on their website. The WHO strongly recommends to reduce intake of "free sugars" throughout the life-course by reducing intake to 10 percent of total energy and has a "conditional recommendation to further reduce intake to below 5 percent." Explain what WHO means by "free sugars" and describe the health benefits they believe will be achieved by a reduction to 5 percent of energy.
   The guideline is available at the WHO website at: http://www.who.int/nutrition/publications/guidelines/sugars-intake/en/
5. Describe the position that the HHS and USDA staff take in the actual *Dietary Guidelines for Americans (DGA) 2015* publication about intake of added sugars. Explain why you think they chose to write the DGA this way.

Is There Common Ground?

The DGAC conclude that there is only *moderate evidence* (instead of *strong* evidence) that added sugars are associated with increased risk of hypertension, stroke, and CHD in adults. They also acknowledge that more research is needed with "strong experimental designs and multiple measurements" to investigate the relationships between eating a diet high in added sugars and health outcomes, such as obesity, type 2 diabetes, and heart disease.

The Sugar Association agrees that more research is needed to investigate if there are relationships between added sugars and cardiovascular disease, especially hypertension. In the letter from The Sugar Association, Briscoe and Gaine point out that currently Americans average 13 percent of energy from added sugars, which is very close to the 10 percent upper limit recommendation of the DGAC. Therefore, the DGAC and The Sugar Association have areas of similarities. Obviously, this is one area where more research is needed.

Additional Resources

Dinicolantonio JJ, O'keefe JH, Lucan SC. Added fructose: A principal driver of type 2 diabetes mellitus and its consequences. *Mayo Clin Proc.* 2015;90(3):372–81.

Mazarello Paes V, Hesketh K, O'Malley C, et al. Determinants of sugar-sweetened beverage consumption in young children: A systematic review. *Obes Rev.* 2015;16(11):903–13.

Newens KJ, Walton J. A review of sugar consumption from nationally representative dietary surveys across the world. *J Hum Nutr Diet.* 2015. doi: 10.1111/jhn.12338.

Wittekind A, Walton J. Worldwide trends in dietary sugars intake. *Nutr Res Rev.* 2014;27(2):330–45.

Zheng M, Allman-Farinelli M, Heitmann BL, Rangan A. Substitution of sugar-sweetened beverages with other beverage alternatives: A review of long-term health outcomes. *J Acad Nutr Diet.* 2015;115(5):767–79.

Internet References . . .

Academy of Nutrition and Dietetics (AND)

www.eatright.org

American Diabetes Association (ADA)

www.diabetes.org

Health.gov

health.gov

The Sugar Association

www.Sugar.org

World Health Organization

www.who.int

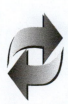

Unit 2

UNIT

Nutrition and Health

*E*veryone agrees that what we eat has an important effect on health, but arguments begin when the discussion focuses on the exact affect of specific foods or nutrients. The issues in this unit focus on the relationship that diet and supplements have on health, and how dietary intake is assessed. For many years, debates have persisted about fat and sugar and the recognition that intakes of the two parallel increases in obesity, type 2 diabetes, cardiovascular disease, and certain cancers. Fat and sugar have both been a part of the American diet for years; however, the forms of sugars and fats are different than in the past. More recently, new products have hit the market with many health claims, such as soy and heart health or extra virgin coconut oil reducing incidence of seizures and Alzheimer's disease. Over the last 50 years, we have been bombarded with advice warning us that eating certain foods may have a catastrophic impact on health. As a result, some people have developed diet-related psychological disorders.

The opinions expressed in the selections are from a variety of perspectives. Some are based on opinions of health and nutrition professionals and others are from representatives from the food industry, advocacy groups or individuals, governmental entities, and journalists. As you read the selections, keep in mind the possible motives of the authors and their stakes in the claims. Consider, "what's in it for them" as you compare their opinions. Also, keep in mind that only two positions are presented in each issue—other professionals and advocacy groups might have totally different stances on the topic.

Selected, Edited, and with Issue Framing Materials by:
Janet M. Colson, *Middle Tennessee State University*

ISSUE

Can an Overemphasis on Eating Healthy Become Unhealthy?

YES: Lindsey Getz, from "Orthorexia: When Eating Healthy Becomes an Unhealthy Obsession," *Today's Dietitian* (2009)

NO: Chris Woolston, from "What's Wrong with the American Diet?" *Consumer Health Interactive* (2009)

Learning Outcomes

After reading this issue, you will be able to:

- Identify the messages that professional health and nutrition associations, government agencies, and registered dietitians promote about healthy eating.
- Explain what orthorexia is and what causes the condition.
- Discuss how "healthy eating" messages may lead to orthorexia.
- Differentiate between orthorexia nervosa and anorexia nervosa.
- Outline how to recognize a person with symptoms of orthorexia and the recommended treatment for the condition.

ISSUE SUMMARY

YES: Writer Lindsey Getz describes "orthorexia" as the condition that makes a person strive for a perfect diet. People with orthorexia avoid sugar, *trans* fat, cholesterol, sodium, and anything they believe is "unhealthy" and take pride in being in total control of the foods they eat.

NO: Health and medical writer Chris Woolston believes the typical American diet is excessive in calories, fat, and sugar. He says we would be much healthier if we ate more "fish, poultry, cruciferous vegetables (i.e., cabbage and broccoli), greens, tomatoes, legumes, fresh fruits, and whole grains." He also believes we should "skimp on fatty or calorie-rich foods such as red meats, eggs, high-fat dairy products, French fries, pizza, mayonnaise, candy, and desserts."

The 1960s was the birth of the "negative nutrition" era when people were told certain foods are bad and to avoid eating them. During this time, reports hit the news telling people that foods high in saturated fat and cholesterol cause heart disease; sugary foods increase chances of getting diabetes and cause cavities; salt increases blood pressure; and artificial flavors and coloring increase the risk of cancer.

Perhaps the negative nutrition craze also has roots to the "prudent diet," developed in 1956 by Dr. Norman

Jolliffe, former Director of the New York City Health Department. The diet was originally developed for cardiac health, and stressed the importance of avoiding fat and cholesterol. Jean Nidetch, founder of Weight Watchers, was one of the early followers of the prudent diet, and used it as the basis for Weight Watchers' original food plan.

Adding to the negativism, the *U.S. Dietary Goals for Americans* were developed in 1977 and 3 years later, the first *Dietary Guidelines for Americans* were published. Both convey messages telling us not to eat certain foods. At the same time, organizations like the American Heart Association and American Cancer Society published dietary recommendations with similar messages.

The organic food movement began in the late 1970s and has increased dramatically since then, especially after the passage of the Organic Food Production Act of 1990. Proponents of organic foods say that organics are better than conventionally grown foods because the pesticides in conventionally grown products cause health problems or the chemicals used in conventional fertilizers are harmful.

Today, we are bombarded with messages that tell us to eat better. Websites, newsletters, and newspaper columns are dedicated to the "right" way to eat. Magazine covers stress healthy eating, and there is even one called *Eating Well*. The web address for the Academy of Nutrition and Dietetics says it all, *"www.eatright.org."*

In 1997, after years of working with patients who were obsessed with healthy diets, physician Steven Bratman wrote the article "The Health Food Eating Disorder" (October, *Yoga Journal*.) In the article, he describes a new condition where people are obsessed with healthy foods. In the following paragraphs, he outlines his definition and description of the disorder:

> Many of the most unbalanced people I have ever met are those who have devoted themselves to healthy eating. In fact, I believe some of them have actually contracted a novel eating disorder for which I have coined the name "orthorexia nervosa." The term uses "ortho," meaning straight, correct, and true, to modify "anorexia nervosa." Orthorexia nervosa refers to a pathological fixation on eating proper food.
>
> Orthorexia begins, innocently enough, as a desire to overcome chronic illness or to improve general health. But, because it requires considerable willpower to adopt a diet that differs radically from the food habits of childhood and the surrounding culture, few accomplish the change gracefully. Most must resort to an iron self-discipline bolstered by a hefty dose of superiority over those who eat junk food. Over time, what to eat, how much, and the consequences of dietary indiscretion come to occupy a greater and greater proportion of the orthorexic's day."

Orthorexia is not considered a medically defined eating disorder by the American Psychiatric Association (APA). Tim Walsh, who led the group of psychiatrists that worked on the 2013 edition of APA'S *DSM-5 (Diagnostic and Statistical Manual of Mental Disorders)* manual told *Time* magazine (Feb 12, 2010) that the condition will not be included in the manual. "We're not in a position to say it doesn't exist or it's not important," Walsh told *Time* magazine. "The real issue is significant data. Getting listed as a separate entry in the DSM requires extensive scientific knowledge of a syndrome and broad clinical acceptance, neither of which orthorexia has."

More research has been conducted in Europe than the United States about orthorexia. Donini and colleagues published a report in *Eating and Weight Disorders* (June, 2004) where they found that 6.9 percent of the 400 Italians he observed have the condition. So, based on his report, the condition is relatively common.

The National Eating Disorders Association (NEDA) developed a list of questions to help a person self-diagnose his- or herself. The more questions a person responds to as "yes," the more likely he or she is dealing with orthorexia. The NEDA questions are:

1. Do you wish that occasionally you could just eat and not worry about food quality?
2. Do you ever wish you could spend less time on food and more time living and loving?
3. Does it seem beyond your ability to eat a meal prepared with love by someone else—one single meal—and not try to control what is served?
4. Are you constantly looking for ways foods are unhealthy for you?
5. Do love, joy, play, and creativity take a back seat to following the perfect diet?
6. Do you feel guilt or self-loathing when you stray from your diet?
7. Do you feel in control when you stick to the "correct" diet?
8. Have you put yourself on a nutritional pedestal and wonder how others can possibly eat the foods they eat?

Many nutritionists and other health professionals believe that it is a true disorder. So what has caused the condition? Have the messages to improve our eating caused some people to eat too healthfully? Lindsey Getz describes orthorexia as a real condition that dietitians should be concerned about. Chris Woolston promotes healthy eating focusing on the importance of a prudent diet in which "people eat relatively large amounts of fish, poultry, cruciferous vegetables (i.e., cabbage and broccoli), greens, tomatoes, legumes, fresh fruits, and whole grains." Woolston even considers this type of diet as "a nutritionist's dream." So, has America's obsession with healthy eating caused orthorexia? After reading the two articles, decide for yourself.

TIMELINE

1956 Dr. Norman Jolliffe, Director of the New York City Health Department, develops the "prudent diet" that begins negativism against fat and cholesterol.

1961 Weight Watchers is launched using the prudent diet as its model.

1977 *U.S. Dietary Goals* are published that recommend for all Americans to limit fat to 30 percent of total caloric intake.

1979 The first *Healthy People: The Surgeon General's Report on Health Promotion and Disease Prevention* is published that tells people to eat less fat, sugar, and salt.

1980 First *Dietary Guidelines for Americans* is published that recommends limiting fat, sugar, and sodium—as do the 1985, 1990, 1995, 2000, 2005, 2010, and 2015 editions of the *Dietary Guidelines*.

1990 The Organic Food Production Act is passed.

1997 "Orthorexia" is first defined by Steven Bratman.

DEFINITIONS

Diagnostic and Statistical Manual of Mental Disorders (DSM) Manual published by the American Psychiatric Association that defines various mental disorders.

"Negative nutrition" Harmful foods and practices.

Obsessive-compulsive disorder (OCD) Anxiety disorder characterized by recurrent unwanted thoughts (obsessions) and/or repetitive behaviors (compulsions).

Orthos Greek word meaning "correct or right."

Orexis Greek word meaning "appetite."

Orthorexia A fixation of eating only pure, healthy, and natural foods.

YES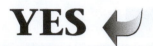

Lindsey Getz

Orthorexia: When Eating Healthy Becomes an Unhealthy Obsession

There's a fine line between including foods deemed healthy in your diet and eating nothing but! Teaching your clients the value of all foods can help them forge a healthy relationship with eating and may prevent them from taking their diet to a potentially dangerous extreme.

What could be wrong with a desire to eat healthy? After all, promoting healthy eating is part of a dietitian's job description. But when the urge to eat healthy foods becomes more of an obsession, there may be an eating disorder in the works—and the consequences can be dangerous.

Although it is not yet a clinically recognized term or disorder, orthorexia is gaining wider recognition as cases continue to emerge and capture media attention. Steven Bratman, MD, author of *Health Food Junkies—Orthorexia Nervosa: Overcoming the Obsession with Healthful Eating,* coined the term to denote an eating disorder characterized by an obsession with eating foods deemed healthy.

Bratman began studying the condition after personally becoming obsessed with health foods. "I suffered from a psychological obsession with food," he said in a *20/20* interview last year. "When I was involved with this, it took up way too much of my life experiences when there were other things I could have been doing."

Like other eating disorders, orthorexia starts to negatively impact many areas of an individual's life and, in some cases, can even lead to severe malnutrition or death, as the person increasingly eliminates food types from his or her diet.

"It's not an official diagnostic term, but I think it's something that's important for dietitians to know about," says Evelyn Tribole, MS, RD, owner of a California-based nutrition counseling practice and author of seven books, including *Healthy Homestyle Cooking* and *Intuitive Eating.* "If a client likes to always eat healthy, the question is whether it's helping or hurting them. Is it something that affects their social life? For instance, are they no longer seeing their friends because they can't go out to dinner?

This is the type of indication that eating healthy is becoming an unhealthy obsession."

Orthorexia could easily begin as simple healthy habits but then spiral out of control, adds Sondra Kronberg, MS, RD, CDN, a national liaison for the National Eating Disorders Association and the cofounder and nutritional director of the Eating Disorder Associates Treatment & Referral Centers and Eating Wellness Programs of New York. "The person takes something that's normally considered healthy and good for their body and takes it to the extreme," she says. "They wind up with disordered thinking and psychological torment. The behavior becomes restrictive to the degree that it begins to interfere with the person's quality of life. And what starts out as something they are controlling becomes something that controls them."

Unlike anorexia or bulimia, orthorexia is not about the desire to become thin. "The driving force seems to be a desire to eat a perfectly healthy or even 'pure' diet," says Deborah Kauffmann, RD, LDN, owner of Mindfulness Based Nutrition Counseling in Baltimore. "For instance, organically grown vegetables and fruits may be thought of as 'safe foods' [for both those with anorexia and orthorexia] because they are seen as healthy and low in calories. But artificial sweeteners and diet frozen meals, which usually seem acceptable to someone with anorexia, would not be seen as acceptable to someone with orthorexic tendencies. Conversely, expeller-pressed canola oil may be acceptable to someone with orthorexia but not someone with anorexia because of the fear of weight gain due to eating fat."

Impressionable Minds

Perhaps one of the most alarming trends associated with orthorexia is that children are picking up some of these tendencies. Kids who watch their parents obsess over certain foods may mimic that behavior. And well-intentioned parents who strictly limit their children's sugar intake or try to feed them only organic foods may instill a sense of fear in their children that other foods are "bad" or that scary things could happen if they eat them.

"A few years ago, I had a 10 year old who was terrified of trans fats," says Tribole. "Part of her treatment was me sitting down and eating a Ding Dong with her. Can you imagine a dietitian eating a Ding Dong with her client? But she needed a healthier relationship with food. She had to realize that you don't eat one Ding Dong and end up with a clogged artery."

"I believe many well-meaning parents, teachers, pediatricians, and even dietitians are passing on their beliefs about unhealthy foods to children," says Kauffmann. "This can create not only orthorexia but eating disorders like anorexia, bulimia, and compulsive eating. Recently, I have seen children in my practice afraid to eat all kinds of foods because of things they have learned at home or in school regarding foods being unhealthy or fattening. In my practice, I often use the program in the book *Preventing Childhood Eating Problems* [*A Practical, Positive Approach to Raising Children Free of Food & Weight Conflicts*] by Jane Hirschmann and Lela Zaphiropoulos to teach parents how to help their children become healthy, intuitive eaters. Parents also need to understand that healthy bodies come in all shapes and sizes. Ellyn Satter's book *Your Child's Weight: Helping Without Harming* includes a wonderful appendix which reviews the literature regarding the actual relationship between weight and health in children."

Parents must be especially careful with the behavior they exhibit around their kids and also keep an eye on whether they are too involved with their children's diet, says D. Milton Stokes, MPH, RD, CDN, owner of One Source Nutrition, LLC in Connecticut. Parents can easily make the transition from being helpful and healthy to giving their children a complex about what they're eating. "Kids have a natural appetite regulation," says Stokes. "They eat when they're hungry and stop when they're full. That gets interrupted when mom starts pushing more or less food. Everyone should rely more on that physiological hunger rather than turning eating into something emotional."

Developing a healthy relationship with food certainly seems to be a key to preventing these tendencies, and that means not tying words with heavy meaning to food. "In our society, food is constantly painted as this moral dilemma," says Tribole. "A low-fat food may be termed 'guilt free,' for instance. But eating shouldn't make you feel guilty. And we are constantly calling foods 'good' or 'bad.' Putting all of this weight onto what we eat, as though it actually affects who you are as a person, is where the problem is stemming from. And kids pick up on that."

Instead, parents should teach their children about moderation. Frequently eating trans fatty foods such as French fries or processed snacks is not healthy behavior, but neither is becoming obsessive about avoiding them or being scared to be around such foods.

Warning Signs

Because orthorexia is not an officially recognized disorder and is somewhat controversial, many dietitians may be unfamiliar with it. Some physicians and other health professionals say orthorexia does not require its own classification because they believe it is a form of anorexia or obsessive-compulsive disorder.

Still, regardless of what orthorexia is called or how it is classified, dietitians should be aware of potential warning signs that could indicate something is wrong with the way a client views and eats food. The "worry factor" is one of the biggest indicators, suggests Tribole. "If a client has too much anxiety over what they eat, then that stress may be worse for their health than what they're actually eating and can lead to these orthorexic tendencies," she says.

If you have a client who follows a particularly restrictive diet, try to gain a sense of their feelings about food and whether they're behaving obsessively. "In other words, if they go to a party and they're only serving fried foods, are they going to be devastated? Are they not going to eat all night? These are signs that their behavior is extreme," warns Tribole.

"Also look for any patterns that your client has become overly ritualistic when it comes to their diet," adds Stokes. "If you find out it takes them an extraordinary amount of time to shop for food, that could be another indicator."

Like other eating disorders, orthorexia may also have a lot to do with control. Those with orthorexia often want to be able to heavily regulate the health food they consume. Kronberg says this may be particularly true of clients who have an unmanageable illness and have become desperate to take control of their situation.

"If they have some illness or disease that medicine could not cure, they may become obsessed with their diet, something they feel they can control even when they can't control the disease," she explains. "Maybe they have cancer and they follow a macrobiotic diet extremely rigidly. Or maybe they have multiple sclerosis and they read a book that said to eliminate animal protein. These behaviors can start with good intentions but can lead to a restrictive diet, which isn't healthy for the client."

But a person's desire to gain control doesn't have to be the result of an illness. Orthorexia may stem from someone hearing about a negative effect of a food type or group and ultimately eliminating it from his or her diet. Fat is a good example, says Stokes.

"Some people may have this intense fear that fat is bad and will kill them, so they avoid it at all costs," he says. "But in fact, fat can be healthy, particularly unsaturated fats, [which] may actually be able to protect our heart and lower our cholesterol. We don't need much fat, but we do need some. It's important for the health of our skin and our hair. And we also have fat deposits throughout sensitive places in the body, such as on the temples to protect the skull from impact or around the kidneys to provide some cushioning" should someone fall.

Some with orthorexia are focused more on what they do eat than on what they don't. This could mean, for instance, eating only organic foods. But in many cases, orthorexic tendencies may drive a person to eliminate those foods that he or she believes to be bad—commonly carbohydrates, trans fats, animal products, dyes, and sugars. Doing so can ultimately lead to malnutrition.

A recent article on orthorexia that appeared in *The New York Times* reported on an 18-year-old girl who began her struggle with food when she started eliminating all carbohydrates, meats, refined sugars, and processed foods from her diet. By the time she had gotten rid of all of the foods that she thought were not "pure," she had brought her daily calorie intake down to only 500. Her weight fell to 68 lbs, and she was repeatedly hospitalized until she finally received help and restored her weight. Which food(s) your client may obsess over depends largely on his or her own experiences. "It's all based on information," says Kronberg. "People may have become carb restrictive because of the Atkins diet or fat phobic because of some various theories they've heard. It's all about what they read or what they hear, and the obsession differs from person to person."

How to Help

Dietitians who specialize in eating disorders are most likely the best match for someone dealing with orthorexia. However, all dietitians can learn to recognize early signs and perhaps even prevent orthorexic tendencies from developing. "In general, dietitians need to take the leading role in helping patients to 'legalize' all foods by educating about the nutritional value of all foods, as well as teaching mindful eating techniques and empowering individuals to use primarily internal cues when making eating decisions," says Kauffmann.

Tribole adds that it's important for dietitians to be careful that they do not generate or enable a client's fear of certain foods or food types. While the average person may take advice about avoiding trans fats and apply it meaningfully to the diet, an individual who is bordering on developing an eating disorder may distort that information. "You may be giving out very ordinary nutritional advice, but if they have an eating disorder brewing and you don't know it, then it could be taken the wrong way," says Tribole. "It's just important to pay attention to the way we give out orders to our clients."

"Dietitians can end up being an ally to the disorder without even recognizing it," agrees Kronberg. "Clients could come to you seeking assistance for their disorder, ways that they can be more obsessively healthy. It's our job to recognize when it's become a problem and balance things back out."

Orthorexia may be an emerging condition, but dietitians should realize that they have the power to prevent it from becoming a more widespread issue. Kronberg notes, "We're on the front line, so it's crucial that we're able to recognize early on when there's a problem."

Lindsey Getz is a full-time, freelance writer who has written for dozens of magazines, both local and national, as well as many trade publications for a variety of industries. She is a graduate of Muhlenburg College.

Chris Woolston   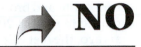 **NO**

What's Wrong with the American Diet?

What's wrong with the typical American diet? This is what the experts have to say:

"Too many calories," says Marion Nestle, PhD, MPH, Professor of Nutrition and Food Studies at New York University.

"Too many calories," asserts Melanie Polk, registered dietitian and former director of nutrition education for the American Institute of Cancer Research.

Barbara Gollman, a registered dietitian who used to be the spokesperson for the American Dietetic Association, weighs in with her own theory: "Too many calories."

Perhaps it's time to stop talking about fatty foods and admit that we simply eat too many calories. Twenty-five years ago, the average American consumed about 1,850 calories each day. Since then, our daily diet has grown by 304 calories (roughly the equivalent of two cans of soda). That's theoretically enough to add an extra 31 pounds to each person every year. Judging from the ongoing obesity epidemic, many Americans are gaining those pounds—and then some.

Take the latest national surveys on weight. More than sixty-six percent of all Americans are considered overweight, according to the Centers for Disease Control and Prevention. (This means they have a Body Mass Index greater than 25.)

But calories don't tell the whole story. To truly understand what's wrong with the American diet, you have to know how we manage to consume all those calories. There are two possible ways to go overboard: You can eat too many calorie-dense foods, or you can eat too much food or beverages in general. Many people choose to do both.

Our fondness for fast food is taking a particularly heavy toll. Although the federal government recommends that we have at least two to five cups of fruits and vegetables a day, for example, surveys show that the average American eats only three servings a day, and 42 percent eat fewer than two servings a day.

Here's a closer look at our love affair with calories—and the health crisis it has created.

The Carnival Mirror

Of course, there is no single American diet. We all have our individual tastes, quirks, and habits. Still, experts see clear patterns in our food choices. In fact, most American diets fall into one of two broad categories: "Western" or "prudent."

The prudent diet is a nutritionist's dream. People in this category tend to eat relatively large amounts of fish, poultry, cruciferous vegetables (i.e., cabbage and broccoli), greens, tomatoes, legumes, fresh fruits, and whole grains. They also skimp on fatty or calorie-rich foods such as red meats, eggs, high-fat dairy products, french fries, pizza, mayonnaise, candy, and desserts.

The Western diet is the prudent diet reflected in a carnival mirror. Everything is backwards: Red meat and other fatty foods take the forefront, while fruits, vegetables, and whole grains are pushed aside. In addition to fat and calories, the Western diet is loaded with cholesterol, salt, and sugar. If that weren't bad enough, it's critically short on dietary fiber and many nutrients—as well as plant-based substances (phytochemicals) that help protect the heart and ward off cancer.

Put it all together and you have a recipe for disaster. In a 12-year study of more than 69,000 women, published in the *Archives of Internal Medicine,* a Western diet was found to significantly raise the risk of coronary heart disease. Other studies have shown that a high-fat, low-nutrient diet increases the likelihood of colon cancer, diabetes, and a host of other ailments.

Portion Distortion

The Western diet is nothing new. The typical American family in the 1950s was more likely than we are to sit down to a meal of pork chops and mashed potatoes than stir-fried tofu and broccoli. So why has the obesity epidemic exploded in the last 20 years? It's a matter of size. "Twenty years ago, the diet wasn't as varied as it is today, and people didn't eat nearly enough fruits and vegetables," Gollman says. "But the portions were more in line with what people really need."

From bagel shops to family restaurants to vending machines to movie theater concession stands to the dining room table, our meals and snacks are taking on gargantuan proportions. "Everyone in the food industry decided they had to make portions larger to stay competitive, and people got used to large sizes very quickly," Nestle says. "Today, normal sizes seem skimpy."

The hyperinflation of our diet is especially obvious away from home. "Look through the window of any of the big chain restaurants, and you'll see huge platters of food coming out of the kitchen," Polk says. One of those platters could easily pack 2,000 calories, enough to last most people all day.

Convenience Culture

Despite our national obsession with weight loss, the obesity epidemic continues to be a national health concern. The human craving for fats and sweets will never go away, and it's getting easier than ever to satisfy those cravings. With 170,000 fast-food restaurants and 3 million soft-drink vending machines spread across the country, huge doses of calories are never far away—especially when those soda machines are sitting right in the middle of public schools.

In 1978, for example, the typical teenage boy in the United States drank about seven ounces of soda a day, according to *Fast Food Nation* author Eric Schlosser. Today, he drinks nearly three times that much, getting a whopping 9 percent of his daily calories from soda. Teenage girls are close behind.

Perhaps not surprisingly, studies show that childhood obesity has hit epidemic proportions over the last decade. One study, published in the *Journal of the American Medical Association*, notes that from 1986 to 1998 the number of overweight white children doubled. Among Latino and African American kids, there's a 120 percent increase. More recent data shows no significant changes in the past few years, though the number of overweight kids remains high. The main culprits, according to experts: high-fat foods, sodas, and too little exercise.

However, the obesity epidemic has moved some to take action. In 2006, the Alliance for a Healthier Generation

struck a deal with the American Beverage Association to eliminate high-calorie soft drinks from public schools by the 2009–2010 academic year. While government agencies and private industry grapple with implementing new policies, ultimately it will be up to us individually to improve the way we eat and increase the amount of exercise we get.

Taking Control

Fatty, unbalanced, and oversized: That, in a nutshell, is the American diet. But it doesn't have to be your diet. "People think eating healthy is a difficult task, but small things make a big difference," Polk says. "You just have to employ some important strategies. It's called taking charge."

If you eat more than four meals away from home each week, you can start by making healthy choices as you dine. "As we eat at restaurants more and more, we have to take control of these outlandish meals," Polk says. Order foods that have been baked, steamed, or grilled instead of deep-fried. Have your salad dressing or other fatty toppings served on the side, and if mayonnaise isn't low-fat, skip it entirely. Consider ordering a salad and an appetizer instead of an entree. If you do order an entree, plan to take at least half of it home with you. For more information on portion control, see Downsize This!. ["Downsize This: The Fun of Smaller Portions" by Chris Woolston (updated on Sept. 18, 2009) is available at: http://www.cvshealthresources .com/topic/portions]

No matter where you eat, try to stick to a few basic guidelines. The amount you should eat depends on your age and activity level—teenage boys and men need to eat more than young children, for example. Aim for three to eight ounces of bread, cereal, rice, or pasta each day, the more whole grains the better. This isn't quite as daunting as it sounds—one cup of rice counts as two ounces, and a single slice of bread counts as one ounce. Two to five cups of fruits and vegetables each day will give you fiber and vital nutrients. (One serving is a medium piece of fruit, a half cup of chopped fruit, a half cup of chopped vegetables, or a cup of fresh greens.) Taken together, fruits, vegetables, and grains can satisfy your hunger and fuel your body without blowing your calorie budget.

Meat isn't forbidden, but try to think of it as a complement to your meals, not the main attraction. According to the U.S. Department of Agriculture (USDA) food pyramid, you only need two servings (up to six and a half ounces) from the "meat group" each day. The group includes meat, poultry, fish, dry beans, eggs, and nuts. It goes without saying that six ounces of salmon, pinto beans, or chicken breast is preferable to six ounces of marbled steak (a serving of meat, by the way, should be about the size of a deck of cards).

Much of the advice can be boiled down to one word: moderation. By eating different foods from every part of the pyramid and watching your portion size, you can make your own personal American diet healthy and nutritious. We have more choices and more temptations than ever before, but ultimately, we also have the final say over what we eat. Take control, and enjoy.

CHRIS WOOLSTON is a freelance health, science, and travel writer from Billings, Montana. He writes "The Healthy Skeptic" column in the *Los Angeles Times* and has articles in *Prevention, Health,* and *Reader's Digest.* He received a degree in biology and completed the science writing program at UC Santa Cruz.

EXPLORING THE ISSUE

Can an Overemphasis on Eating Healthy Become Unhealthy?

Critical Thinking and Reflection

1. List the typical eating habits of a person who has orthorexia.
2. Outline the nutrition messages from USDA, professional health associations such as AMA and ADA, and registered dietitians related to healthy eating.
3. Compare characteristics of a person with orthorexia nervosa to one with anorexia nervosa.
4. Do you think the dietary messages and advice to "eat right" that many nutrition experts and government agencies encourage may cause orthorexia? Explain your answer.
5. Currently, the APA does not include orthorexia nervosa as a clinical mental disorder in their *DSM-5*. Why do you think it is not currently in their manual? Do you think it should be considered a clinical mental disorder? Explain your answer.

Is There Common Ground?

Writer Lindsey Getz describes how people with orthorexia avoid sugar, *trans* fat, cholesterol, sodium, and anything they believe is "unhealthy" and take pride in being in total control of foods they eat. Health and medical writer Chris Woolston believes the typical American diet is excessive in calories, fat, and sugar. He says we would be much healthier if we ate more "fish, poultry, cruciferous vegetables (i.e., cabbage and broccoli), greens, tomatoes, legumes, fresh fruits, and whole grains." He also believes we should "skimp on fatty or calorie-rich foods such as red meats, eggs, high-fat dairy products, french fries, pizza, mayonnaise, candy, and desserts."

The issue centers on society's overemphasis on healthy eating and questions if it has caused people to develop orthorexia. Over the last 40 years, we have been bombarded with "don't eat this" and "that food is not good for you." Even the new *Dietary Guidelines* focus on controlling, reducing, limiting—they basically tell us not to eat certain foods, eat other "healthy" foods, and take control of what we eat. And this is what a person with orthorexia does. Getz defines the condition as "an eating disorder characterized by an obsession with eating foods deemed healthy."

The term "orthorexia" was coined by Dr. Steven Bratman, who admits that he suffered from the condition. Currently, the American Psychiatric Association does not include orthorexia nervosa as a clinical mental disorder in their DSM-5. Getz writes that children and adolescents

have "impressionable minds" and the role that parents have on what kids eat and their attitudes about food.

Woolston describes "what's wrong with the American diet" and recommends that we all need to "take control" of what we eat. He points out the many problems of the typical American diet and stresses that we need to eat more prudently. By "prudent" he means to cut back on red meats, cheese and ice cream, fried potatoes, pizza, candy, and sugary desserts. In other words, his recommendations could lead some susceptible people, especially youth, to go to the extreme about eating—and develop orthorexia.

Additional Resources

Brytek-Matera A, Rogoza R, Gramaglia C, Zeppegno P. Predictors of orthorexic behaviours in patients with eating disorders: A preliminary study. *BMC Psychiatry*. 2015;15(1):252.

Håman L, Barker-ruchti N, Patriksson G, Lindgren EC. Orthorexia nervosa: An integrative literature review of a lifestyle syndrome. *Int J Qual Stud Health Well-being*. 2015;10:26799.

Koven NS, Abry AW. The clinical basis of orthorexia nervosa: Emerging perspectives. *Neuropsychiatr Dis Treat*. 2015;11:385–94.

Moroze RM, Dunn TM, Craig Holland J, Yager J, Weintraub P. Microthinking about micronutrients: A case of transition from obsessions about healthy eating to near-fatal "orthorexia nervosa" and proposed diagnostic criteria. *Psychosomatics*. 2015;56(4):397–403.

Musolino C, Warin M, Wade T, Gilchrist P. "Healthy anorexia": The complexity of care in disordered eating. *Soc Sci Med*. 2015;139:18–25.

Segura-Garcia C, Ramacciotti C, Rania M, et al. The prevalence of orthorexia nervosa among eating disorder patients after treatment. *Eat Weight Disord*. 2015;20(2):161–6.

Internet References . . .

Academy of Nutrition and Dietetics

www.eatright.org

American Psychiatric Association

www.psychiatry.org/

The National Eating Disorder Association (NEDA)

www.nationaleatingdisorders.org

Selected, Edited, and with Issue Framing Materials by:
Janet M. Colson, *Middle Tennessee State University*

ISSUE

Does a Diet High in Fructose Increase Body Fat?

YES: Joseph Mercola, from "This Harmful Food Product Is Changing Its Name—Don't Get Swindled," *Mercola.com* (2010)

NO: Corn Refiners Association, from "Questions & Answers About High Fructose Corn Syrup," *SweetSurprise .com* (2008)

Learning Outcomes

After reading this issue, you will be able to:

- Differentiate between high fructose corn syrup (HFCS) and sucrose (table sugar).
- Compare the trends in consumption of HFCS to regular sugar.
- Describe how fructose metabolism differs from glucose metabolism and why fructose is considered "lipogenic."
- Compare the health effects of a diet high in HFCS to a diet high in regular sugar.

ISSUE SUMMARY

YES: Osteopathic physician Joseph Mercola considers that HFCS is more deadly than sugar and explains how the body converts fructose to fat. He accuses the Corn Refiners Association of trying to convince us that their product is equal to table sugar.

NO: The Corn Refiners Association claims that HFCS has no adverse health effect and is the same as sucrose and honey. They also include the many benefits that HFCS provides to food.

Corn syrup has been on the market for about 100 years. It is made from breaking down corn starch to free glucose. In the late 1950s, the enzyme glucose isomerase was developed. The enzyme rearranges (isomerizes) the carbons that make up glucose so it becomes fructose, changing plain corn syrup into high fructose corn syrup (HFCS). The name "high fructose" leads many to believe it is mainly fructose, but in reality, most HFSC is either 42 percent or 55 percent fructose with the other part glucose. In the mid-1970s, when the cost of sugar cane and sugar beet imports became very high, the food industry began looking for alternative sweeteners and realized that HFCS, made from American-grown corn, was the solution. Soft drink manufacturers quickly began to replace expensive sugar with cheap HFCS; by 1985 virtually all non-diet soft drinks were sweetened with it.

With the help of U.S. government subsidies, corn farmers have managed to keep the price of corn (and HFCS) about 25 to 30 percent below production costs. This translates into a win-win situation for farmers and the food industry. Because the price of HFCS is low, beverage manufacturers have been able to make large 20- and 32-ounce bottles of pop while charging the consumer just a little more than for the typical price of the 12-ounce can. And with the cheap cost, many people drink more and more of it. HFCS is hidden in many other foods; even canned and frozen vegetables, cereals, and breads contain it. An important question to ask is, what is this doing to our health?

The average American consumes 52 grams of HFCS per day, which translates into about 200 kcalories. And most of it is from HFCS-sweetened beverages. The increase in HFCS consumption has not only paralleled increases in diabetes, but also obesity, high blood lipids, and other metabolic problems common today. Should we blame these health problems on HFCS? In a 2010 *Am J Clin Nut* article, "Are Refined Carbohydrates Worse than Saturated Fat?," Frank Hu predicts that "refined carbohydrates are likely to cause even greater metabolic damage than saturated fat."

Most experts consider that HFCS is definitely a "refined" carbohydrate; whereas, the Corn Refiners Association (CRA) considers HFCS to be a "natural" ingredient. They point out that "under FDA rules, 'natural' means that nothing artificial or synthetic has been included." The Association had their hands slapped by the FDA because HFCS has several chemicals added during processing. Additionally, the CRA petitioned the FDA to allow use of the term "corn sugar" instead of HFCS on labels, but the FDA denied the request.

In 2011, a battle between the regular sugar industry and the CRA began. Representatives of the sugar industry sued the CRA, claiming that the public education campaign that HFCS is natural is false and misleading. This was the beginning of a multiyear battle after the CRA countersued claiming infringement of their first amendment rights to promote HFCS.

From a chemical standpoint, because the fructose and glucose in HFCS are "unbound," many scientists report they form chemicals (called reactive carbonyls) that cause tissue damage which could lead to diabetes, especially in children. These damaging chemicals are not found in beverages made with sucrose, because its glucose and fructose are "bound."

Numerous other studies have been published on the health effects of HFCS, and on regular sugar. In the following selections, Joseph Mercola claims that HFCS is more deadly than regular sugar (sucrose). The CRA counters that HFCS has no adverse health effect and is the same as sucrose or honey, because all three have about the same one-to-one ratio of fructose to glucose.

TIMELINE

1921   Corn syrup (made of glucose) developed in the United States.

1950s   The enzyme glucose isomerase developed that converts glucose to fructose.

1970s   High fructose corn syrup (HFCS) use in the United States began.

1980s   HFCS used in all soft drinks in the United States.

2011   The sugar industry sues the Corn Refiners Association (CRA) for false and misleading claims about HFCS.

2012   The CRA countersues the sugar industry claiming they are deceiving consumers into believing that processed sugar is safer and more healthful than HFCS.

DEFINITIONS

Glucose isomerase   Enzyme that changes the structure of glucose to fructose.

Government subsidies   Money given by the government to an individual or business to support an enterprise regarded as being needed by the general public.

Reactive carbonyls   An unstable carbonyl, which is a carbon double bonded to an oxygen; high levels are associated with diabetes.

YES ↩

Joseph Mercola

This Harmful Food Product Is Changing Its Name—Don't Get Swindled

The Corn Refiners Association (CRA) has petitioned the U.S. FDA to allow manufacturers the option of using the term "corn sugar" instead of "high fructose corn syrup."

In their press release on the subject, they claim that "independent research demonstrates that the current labeling is confusing to American consumers."

They blame "inexact scientific reports and inaccurate media accounts" for the current stigma associated with high fructose corn syrup.

In reality, as opposed to the CRA's dream world, if you need to lose weight, or if you want to avoid diabetes and heart disease, high-fructose corn syrup is one type of sugar you'll want to avoid.

Part of what makes HFCS such an unhealthy product is that it is metabolized to fat in your body far more rapidly than any other sugar.

Source: PR Newswire September 14, 2010

Dr. Mercola's Comments

As I've stated on many occasions, the number one source of calories in the United States is high-fructose corn syrup (HFCS), mainly in the form of soda.

This dangerous sweetener is also in many processed foods and fruit juices.

Even seemingly "health-conscious" beverages like Vitamin Water, Jamba Juice and Odwalla SuperFood contain far more added sugar and/or fructose than many desserts!

The corn industry persistently claims that it is not much different than sugar and is perfectly safe, but we know otherwise.

The primary reason it's so dangerous is that it is quite cheap to produce, so it has been added to nearly all processed foods. The excessive consumption of fructose, such as HFCS, is a primary driving factor behind a number of health epidemics, including obesity, diabetes and heart disease.

Don't Get Confused By the Latest Smoke and Mirror Tactics

Americans' consumption of corn syrup has fallen to a 20-year low, probably due to consumer concerns that it is more harmful or more likely to cause obesity than ordinary sugar.

This is why the corn industry wants to sugar coat the fact that their product may be prematurely killing hundreds of thousands of Americans each year, and rename it to confuse people to keep using it—all in the name of trying to "clear up" confusion!

You have probably seen their new marketing campaign on television. Two new commercials try to alleviate shopper confusion, showing people who say they now understand that "whether it's corn sugar or cane sugar, your body can't tell the difference."

This is an absolutely brilliant marketing strategy and will work as the average consumer will not be smart enough to realize the difference.

However with your help, spreading the message through your Facebook accounts, your blogs and websites, and sharing it with your friends and family, we can sabotage their plans to manipulate and deceive you and the rest of the public.

Their latest strategy is aimed at seeking to defend their market and their profits, and your health depends on whether or not you buy into their smoke and mirrors routine.

The corn industry is still holding fast to the claim that all sugars are metabolized by your body in the same way, even though this outdated belief has been entirely SHATTERED in more recent years by a number of scientific studies.

This research has devastated the image of high fructose corn syrup which is why they are doing this massive makeover, to do an end-run around the science.

The CRA claims that "a continuing series of inexact scientific reports and inaccurate media accounts about high fructose corn syrup and matters of health and nutrition have . . . increased consumer uncertainty."

Folks, there's nothing inexact about the evidence against fructose. It's very clear. If you want to improve your health, you need to avoid fructose in all its forms, especially HFCS, which is a highly processed, unnatural form of fructose.

Why the ADA's Support of Fructose as 'Safe and Equivalent to Other Sugar' Means NOTHING . . .

The industry has one ace up their sleeve that they pull out again and again—the 2008 report by the American Dietetic Association (ADA), which concluded that HFCS is "nutritionally equivalent to sucrose (table sugar)."

But, could that report possibly have had anything at all to do with the fact that the ADA partnered with Coca-Cola Company earlier that same year?

The press release declaring this unholy union states:

> "The Coca-Cola Company's Beverage Institute for Health & Wellness team of physicians, PhD-level nutrition scientists and registered dietitians serve as a resource for health professionals and others interested in the science of beverages and their role in health and living well.
>
> The Coca-Cola Company will share research findings with ADA members in forums such as professional meetings and scientific publications, to augment the body of knowledge around consumer motivation and health behaviors. To improve understanding of consumer behavior and motivation around healthy living, The Coca-Cola Company will also share its consumer research and expertise with ADA members."

How nice. I'm sure we can all sleep better knowing that one of the authorities for dietary recommendations in the US is getting their scientific information from such a health-minded group of corporate scientists.

And while we're at it, who are some of the *other* ADA sponsors?

Let's see . . . there's PepsiCo . . . and sugary-snack giants Hershey and MARS Inc . . . oh, and SoyJoy, along with a couple of sugary-cereal giants.

All in all, I'm not impressed. In fact, it's downright frightening to see how many corn syrup-reliant companies support the ADA.

Financial alliances such as these are a major part of why it is virtually impossible to get honest, impartial, factual information about health from conventional media, medicine, and government health agencies.

The Truth about High Fructose Corn Syrup

The truth is, scientists HAVE linked the rising HFCS consumption to the epidemics of obesity, diabetes and metabolic syndrome in the U.S., and medical researchers HAVE pinpointed various health dangers associated with the consumption of HFCS specifically, compared to regular sugar.

This is why the corn industry is now scrambling to save face and profits—NOT because it's *really okay* to consume an average of 59 pounds of HFCS a year.

If you haven't yet read the impressive scientific analysis on fructose in one of my favorite nutritional journals, I would strongly encourage you to do so as it will open your eyes to some of the major problems with this sweetener. [Sharon S. Elliott and colleagues, from "Fructose, Weight Gain, and the Insulin Resistance Syndrome," *The New England Journal of Medicine* (November 2002)]

And for an in-depth review of just how different fructose and HFCS really is from regular sugar, please read through this article [Joseph Mercola, from "This Common Food Ingredient Can Really Mess Up Your Metabolism," *Mercola.com* (January 26, 2010)] and watch the lecture given by Dr. Robert Lustig. ["Sugar: The Bitter Truth" is available on the UCTV site at http://www.uctv.tv/search-details.aspx?showID=16717]

If you have not yet taken the time to see it, you owe it to yourself to do so. It's a real eye-opener!

Another expert on fructose is Dr. Richard Johnson, who has also written the best book on the market on the dangers of fructose, called *The Sugar Fix*.

The information presented by Drs. Lustig and Johnson is exactly why I am so passionate about educating you about the dangers of fructose!

I am thoroughly convinced it's one of the leading causes of a great deal of needless suffering from poor health and premature death.

If you received your fructose only from vegetables and fruits (where it originates) as most people did a century ago, you'd consume about 15 grams per day—a far cry from the 73 grams per day the typical adolescent gets from sweetened drinks today. And, in vegetables and fruits, the fructose is mixed in with fiber, vitamins, minerals, enzymes, and beneficial phytonutrients, all which moderate its negative metabolic effects.

The main factor that makes fructose so dangerous is the fact that people are consuming it in absolutely

MASSIVE DOSES. This is largely related to technology advances in the mid 70s that made it so cheap to produce. The vast majority of processed and restaurant foods are now loaded with it, so it is very difficult to avoid.

How Fructose Wrecks Your Health

Contrary to industry claims, your body does NOT recognize and treat all sugars the same.

HFCS is a *highly processed* product that contains similar amounts of unbound fructose and glucose.

Fructose and glucose are metabolized in very different ways in your body.

Glucose is metabolized in every cell of your body and is converted to blood glucose, while all fructose is metabolized in your liver, where it's quickly converted to fat and cholesterol. (When a diet includes a large amount of fructose, it can therefore create fatty liver, and even cirrhosis.)

Sucrose, on the other hand, is a larger sugar molecule that is metabolized into glucose and fructose in your intestine.

Fructose is metabolized to fat in your body far more rapidly than any other sugar, and, because most fructose is consumed in liquid form (soda), its negative metabolic effects are further magnified.

Why does it turn to fat more readily than other sugar?

Most fats are formed in your liver, and when sugar enters your liver, it decides whether to store it, burn it or turn it into fat. However, researchers have discovered that fructose *bypasses this process* and turns directly into fat.

According to Dr. Elizabeth Parks, associate professor of clinical nutrition at UT Southwestern Medical Center, and lead author of a recent study on fructose in the *Journal of Nutrition*:

> "Our study shows for the first time the surprising speed with which humans make body fat from fructose. Once you start the process of fat synthesis from fructose, it's hard to slow it down. The bottom line of this study is that fructose very quickly gets made into fat in the body."

It is also this uncontrolled movement of fructose through these metabolic pathways that causes it to contribute to greater triglyceride [i.e. fat] synthesis. There are over 35 years of hard empirical evidence that refined man-made fructose like HFCS metabolizes to triglycerides and adipose tissue, not blood glucose.

The metabolic pathways used by fructose also generate uric acid. In fact, fructose typically generates uric acid within minutes of ingestion. When your uric acid level exceeds about 5.5 mg per dl, you have an increased risk for a host of diseases, including:

- Hypertension
- Kidney disease
- Insulin resistance, obesity, and diabetes
- Fatty liver
- Elevated triglycerides, elevated LDL, and cardiovascular disease
- For pregnant women, even preeclampsia

Other specific health problems associated with excessive fructose consumption include:

- Metabolic syndrome
- Diabetes
- High blood pressure
- Obesity
- An increase in triglycerides and LDL (bad) cholesterol levels
- Liver disease

Name virtually any disease, and you will find elevated insulin levels is a primary risk factor. This is why, if you want to be healthy, let alone optimally healthy, you simply MUST restrict your fructose consumption.

And if you're currently eating a diet full of processed foods, sodas and sweetened drinks, that restriction will need to be quite severe, because you're ingesting *massive amounts* of fructose in the form of HFCS and other forms of corn syrup, such as crystalline fructose.

Please understand that if you eat processed foods, there's fructose in practically every single bite of food you put in your mouth.

Ironically, diet foods are clear culprits here as well.

Yes, the very products that most people rely on to lose weight—low-fat diet foods—are often those that contain the most fructose!

The downside of this is that fructose does not stimulate your insulin secretion, nor enhance leptin production. (Leptin is a hormone thought to be involved in appetite regulation.) Because insulin and leptin act as key signals in regulating how much food you eat, as well as your body weight, this suggests that dietary fructose may contribute to increased food intake and weight gain.

So, any "diet" food containing fructose will not help you lose any weight. And neither will diet foods containing artificial sweeteners for that matter. . . .

Another significant health concern of HFCS is that the majority of it is made from genetically modified corn, which is fraught with its own well documented side effects. And, adding insult to injury, last year nearly 50 percent of tested HFCS-containing foods and beverages were found to be contaminated with mercury.

What about Fructose from Fruit?

Fresh fruits also contain fructose, although an ameliorating factor is that whole fruits also contain fiber, vitamins, and antioxidants that reduce the hazardous effects of the fructose.

Nearly every canned or bottled commercial juice, on the other hand, are actually worse than soda, because a glass of juice is loaded with fructose, and a lot of the antioxidants are lost. Additionally the processed juice has methanol which has its own toxicities.

It is important to remember that fructose in and of itself isn't evil as fruits are certainly beneficial. (HFCS, however, is far from natural. It's a highly processed product that does not exist anywhere in nature. Changing the name to 'corn sugar' will not change this fact.)

But when you consume high amounts of fructose—regardless of its source—it will absolutely devastate your biochemistry and physiology.

Remember the AVERAGE fructose dose is 70 grams per day which exceeds the recommended limit by 300 percent.

So, I urge you to be careful with your fruit consumption as well—especially if you eat processed foods of any kind.

I recommend limiting your total fructose consumption to 25 grams per day, and your fructose from fruit to below 15 grams, since you are virtually guaranteed to consume plenty of "hidden" fructose in other foods.

Keep in mind, 15 grams of fructose is not much—it represents two bananas, one-third cup of raisins, or just two Medjool dates! (For comparison, however, the average 12-ounce can of soda contains 40 grams.)

If you're a raw food advocate, have a pristine diet, and exercise very well, then perhaps you could be the exception that could exceed this limit and stay healthy. Dr. Johnson has a handy chart, included below, which you can use to estimate how much fructose you're getting in your diet.

In his book, *The Sugar Fix,* Dr. Johnson includes detailed tables showing the content of fructose in different foods—an information base that isn't readily available when you're trying to find out exactly how much fructose is in various foods. I encourage you to pick up a copy of this excellent resource. It is important to note however, that Dr. Johnson does promote the use of artificial sweeteners in this book—which I do not recommend, under any circumstances.

Fruit	Serving Size	Grams of Fructose
Limes	1 medium	0
Lemons	1 medium	0.6
Cranberries	1 cup	0.7
Passion fruit	1 medium	0.9
Prune	1 medium	1.2
Apricot	1 medium	1.3
Guava	2 medium	2.2
Date (Deglet Noor style)	1 medium	2.6
Cantaloupe	1/8 of med. melon	2.8
Raspberries	1 cup	3.0
Clementine	1 medium	3.4
Kiwifruit	1 medium	3.4
Blackberries	1 cup	3.5
Star fruit	1 medium	3.6
Cherries, sweet	10	3.8
Strawberries	1 cup	3.8
Cherries, sour	1 cup	4.0
Pineapple	1 slice (3.5" × .75")	4.0
Grapefruit, pink or red	1/2 medium	4.3
Boysenberries	1 cup	4.6
Tangerine/mandarin orange	1 medium	4.8
Nectarine	1 medium	5.4
Peach	1 medium	5.9
Orange (navel)	1 medium	6.1
Papaya	1/2 medium	6.3
Honeydew	1/8 of med. melon	6.7
Banana	1 medium	7.1
Blueberries	1 cup	7.4
Date (Medjool)	1 medium	7.7
Apple (composite)	1 medium	9.5
Persimmon	1 medium	10.6
Watermelon	1/16 med. melon	11.3
Pear	1 medium	11.8
Raisins	1/4 cup	12.3
Grapes, seedless (green or red)	1 cup	12.4
Mango	1/2 medium	16.2
Apricots, dried	1 cup	16.4
Figs, dried	1 cup	23.0

One of the Simplest Ways to Improve Your Health NOW!

I recommend that you avoid sugar as much as possible, particularly fructose in all its forms.

This is especially important if you are overweight or have diabetes, high cholesterol, or high blood pressure as fructose will clearly worsen all of these conditions.

However, I also realize we don't live in a perfect world, and following rigid dietary guidelines is not always practical or even possible.

If you want to use a sweetener occasionally, this is what I recommend:

1. Use the herb stevia. My favorites are the flavored liquid bottles.
2. Use organic cane sugar in moderation.
3. Use organic raw honey in moderation, but remember, honey is also very high in fructose so it is not an ideal replacement.
4. Avoid ALL artificial sweeteners, which can damage your health even more quickly than fructose.
5. Avoid agave syrup since it is a highly processed sap that is *almost all fructose*. Your blood sugar will spike just as it would if you were consuming regular sugar or HFCS. Agave's meteoric rise in popularity is due to another great marketing campaign, but any health benefits present in the original agave plant are eliminated during processing.
6. Avoid so-called energy drinks, sports drinks, and vitamin-enriched waters because they are loaded with sugar, sodium and chemical additives. Rehydrating with pure, fresh water is your best choice.

   If you or your child is involved in athletics, I recommend you read my article "Energy Rules" for some great tips on how to optimize your child's energy levels and physical performance through optimal nutrition.

As a last precaution, if you have high fasting insulin levels (anything above 3), high blood pressure, high cholesterol, diabetes, or if you're overweight, I strongly recommend avoiding ALL sweeteners, including stevia, until you've normalized your condition.

This is because any sweetener can decrease your insulin sensitivity, which as I've mentioned before, drives up your risk of nearly every disease there is, from diabetes to cancer.

Joseph Mercola is an osteopathic physician, health activist, and author practicing in Hoffman Estates, Illinois. He advocates dietary and lifestyle approaches to health and says that his passion is "to transform the traditional medical paradigm in the United States." Dr. Mercola received his medical degree from Chicago College of Osteopathic Medicine.

Corn Refiners Association   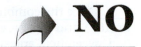 **NO**

Questions & Answers About High Fructose Corn Syrup

Since its introduction in the 1970s, high fructose corn syrup has become a widely accepted American sweetener made from corn. This brochure offers answers to some frequently asked questions about this highly versatile sweetener.

What Is High Fructose Corn Syrup?

High fructose corn syrup (HFCS) is a sweetener made from corn and can be found in numerous foods and beverages on grocery store shelves in the United States. HFCS is composed of either 42 percent or 55 percent fructose, with the remaining sugars being primarily glucose and higher sugars. In terms of composition, HFCS is nearly identical to table sugar (sucrose), which is composed of 50 percent fructose and 50 percent glucose. Glucose is one of the simplest forms of sugar that serves as a building block for most carbohydrates. Fructose is a simple sugar commonly found in fruits and honey.

HFCS is used in foods and beverages because of the many benefits it offers. In addition to providing sweetness at a level equivalent to sugar, HFCS enhances fruit and spice flavors in foods such as yogurt and spaghetti sauces, gives chewy breakfast bars their soft texture and also protects freshness. HFCS keeps products fresh by maintaining consistent moisture.

What Is the Difference Between HFCS and Sugar?

Sugar and HFCS have the same number of calories as most carbohydrates; both contribute 4 calories per gram. They are also equal in sweetness.

Sugar and HFCS contain nearly the same one-to-one ratio of two sugars—fructose and glucose:

- *Sugar is 50 percent fructose and 50 percent glucose.*

- *HFCS is sold principally in two formulations—42 percent and 55 percent fructose—with the balance made up of primarily glucose and higher sugars.*

HIGH FRUCTOSE CORN SYRUP QUICK FACTS

- Research confirms that high fructose corn syrup is safe and no different from other common sweeteners like table sugar and honey. All three sweeteners contain nearly the same one-to-one ratio of two sugars—fructose and glucose.
- High fructose corn syrup has the same number of calories as table sugar and is equal in sweetness. It contains no artificial or synthetic ingredients.
- The U.S. Food and Drug Administration granted high fructose corn syrup "Generally Recognized as Safe" status for use in food, and reaffirmed that ruling in 1996 after thorough review.
- High fructose corn syrup offers numerous benefits. It keeps food fresh, enhances fruit and spice flavors, retains moisture in bran cereals, helps keep breakfast and energy bars moist, maintains consistent flavors in beverages and keeps ingredients evenly dispersed in condiments.

Comparison of Caloric Sweetener Compositions

Component Percentage	HFCS-42	HFCS-55	Table Sugar	Invert Sugar*	Honey**
Fructose	42	55	50	45	49
Glucose	53	42	50	45	43
Other Sugars	5	3	0	10	5

* Hydrolyzed sugar comprised equally of free fructose and glucose.
** Does not sum to 100 because honey also contains some proteins, amino acids, vitamins and minerals.
For more information on different types of sweeteners, see www.SweetSurprise.com.

Once the combination of glucose and fructose found in HFCS and sugar are absorbed into the blood stream, the two sweeteners appear to be metabolized similarly in the body.

In terms of chemical structure, table sugar and HFCS differ by the bonding of their sugars. Table sugar is a disaccharide, in which fructose and glucose are linked by a chemical bond. Fructose and glucose are not bonded in HFCS, and so are sometimes referred to as "free" sugars.

Is HFCS a "Natural" Sweetener?

HFCS is made from corn, a natural grain product. HFCS contains no artificial or synthetic ingredients or color additives and meets the U.S. Food and Drug Administration's (FDA) requirements for use of the term "natural."

Is HFCS Sweeter Than Sugar?

No. When HFCS was developed, it was specifically formulated to provide sweetness equivalent to sugar. In order for food and beverage makers to use HFCS in place of sugar, it was important that it provide the same level of sweetness as sugar so that consumers would not perceive a difference in product sweetness and taste.

HFCS-55 has sweetness equivalent to sugar and is used in many carbonated soft drinks in the United States. HFCS-42 is somewhat less sweet and is used in many fruit-flavored noncarbonated beverages, baked goods and other products in which its special characteristics such as fermentability, lower freezing point, surface browning and flavor enhancement add value to the product.

Is there a Correlation Between the Introduction of HFCS and the Rise of Obesity in the Past 30 Years?

Many factors contribute to the development of obesity, yet nutritionists, health experts and researchers generally agree that the chief cause is an imbalance between calories consumed and calories burned. Excessive calories can be consumed as fats, proteins, alcohol or carbohydrates. The American Dietetic Association notes, "Excess body fat [obesity] arises from the energy imbalance caused by taking in too much energy and expending too little energy. . . . Obesity is a complex problem and its cause cannot be simply attributed to any one component of the food supply such as sweeteners."

Further, the prevalence of obesity is increasing around the world, according to the International Obesity Task Force—even though use of HFCS outside of the United States is limited or nonexistent. In fact, sugar accounts for about 92 percent of caloric sweeteners consumed worldwide.

Scientific studies continue to find that HFCS does not contribute to obesity any differently than sugar.

An expert panel, led by Richard Forshee, Ph.D. of the University of Maryland Center for Food, Nutrition and Agriculture Policy, concluded that "the currently available evidence is insufficient to implicate HFCS per se as a causal factor in the overweight and obesity problem in the United States." The panel's report was published in the August 2007 issue of *Critical Reviews in Food Science and Nutrition.*

The report found that there are many other "plausible explanations for rising overweight and obesity rates" in the United States, listing such factors as "a decrease in smoking; an increase in sedentary occupations; an increase in two-income households and single-parent households; transportation and infrastructure changes that discourage physical activity; a decrease in PE classes and extracurricular sports programs in schools; an increase in sedentary forms of entertainment (i.e. TV/movie viewing, video games, etc.); demographic changes (i.e. aging population, immigration, etc.); a decrease in food costs with increase in food availability; and changes in food consumption patterns."

Another peer-reviewed study summized that those who frequently consume sweetened soft drinks do not have a higher obesity rate than those who rarely drink them. The study found higher obesity rates correlated with several other factors, such as the amount of time in front of the computer or TV, or the consumption of high amounts of dietary fat.

Further, the November/December 2005 issue of *Nutrition Today* includes a report from the Center for Food, Nutrition and Agriculture Policy and its Ceres Workshop, which was compiled by scientists who reviewed a number of critical commentaries about HFCS. Their analysis found that HFCS is not a unique contributor to obesity, concluding "there is currently no convincing evidence to support a link between HFCS consumption and overweight/obesity."

Is HFCS Known to Cause Diabetes?

No. Many parts of the world, including Australia, Mexico and Europe, have rising rates of obesity and diabetes despite having little or no HFCS in their foods and beverages, which supports findings by the U.S. Centers for Disease Control and the American Diabetes Association that the primary causes of diabetes are obesity, advancing age and heredity.

U.S. Department of Agriculture (USDA) data show that per capita consumption of HFCS has been declining in recent years, yet the incidence of obesity and diabetes in the United States remains on the rise.

Has the Use of HFCS in the Food Supply Increased the Amount of Fructose in the Diet?

No. Many press reports note the dramatic increase of HFCS in the food supply since its introduction in the 1970s. However, it is important to note that as HFCS consumption increased, sugar consumption decreased. USDA data show that the per capita use of HFCS in the U.S. food supply was matched with an almost equal decline, on a one-to-one basis, in the per capita use of sugar. In fact, consumption of HFCS has declined since its peak in 1999. The USDA estimates per capita sugar consumption in 2007 was 44.2 lbs per year and 40.1 lbs per year for HFCS.

As HFCS use increased in the United States, it replaced sugar in various foods and beverages on a nearly one-for-one basis. Yet because sugar and HFCS share a common composition, the ratio of fructose-to-glucose in the diet has remained relatively unchanged over time. This confirms that the approximate overall sugars mixture in the foods and beverages we consume—principally glucose and fructose—is nearly the same today as it was 30 years ago, before HFCS was introduced.

Is HFCS Considered a Safe Food Ingredient?

Yes. In 1983, the FDA listed HFCS as "Generally Recognized as Safe" (known as GRAS status) for use in food and reaffirmed that ruling in 1996. In its 1996 GRAS ruling, the FDA noted that "the saccharide composition (glucose to fructose ratio) of HFCS is approximately the same as that of honey, invert sugar and the disaccharide sucrose [table sugar]." GRAS recognition by FDA is important because it is only assigned to food ingredients that are recognized by experts as having a long history of safe use

or as having their safety shown through adequate scientific studies.

According to the American Dietetic Association, "Consumers can safely enjoy a range of nutritive and nonnutritive sweeteners when consumed in a diet that is guided by current federal nutrition recommendations . . . as well as individual health goals."

Does Consumption of HFCS, as Compared to Sugar, Reduce the Ability of the Body to Produce Insulin?

No. Both have largely the same effect on insulin production. Insulin is essentially responsible for the uptake of glucose into cells and the lowering of blood sugar. All caloric sweeteners trigger an insulin response to a greater or lesser extent. Among common sweeteners, pure glucose triggers the greatest insulin release, while pure fructose triggers the least. Both table sugar and HFCS trigger about the same intermediate insulin release because they contain nearly equal amounts of glucose and fructose.

It is extremely rare for pure fructose to be consumed alone in the diet. Fructose is usually consumed together with glucose, as it is in HFCS, table sugar and honey. It is important to remember that no matter the source of the ingredients—whether from sugar or HFCS—the human body produces insulin in response to the whole meal consumed.

Kathleen J. Melanson, *et al.*, at the University of Rhode Island reviewed the effects of HFCS and sugar on circulating levels of glucose, leptin, insulin and ghrelin in a study group of lean women. All four tested substances have been hypothesized to play a role in metabolism and obesity. The study found "no differences in the metabolic effects" of HFCS and sugar in this short-term study, and called for additional studies of obese individuals and males.

Does the Body Process HFCS Differently Than Other Sugars?

No. HFCS contains approximately equal ratios of fructose and glucose, as does table sugar, honey and many fruits.

Once the combination of glucose and fructose found in HFCS and sugar are absorbed into the blood stream, the two sweeteners appear to be metabolized similarly in the body.

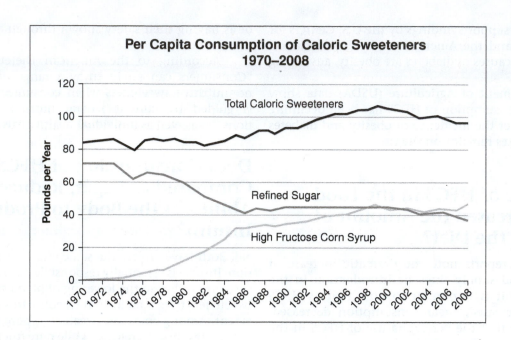

Leptin and Ghrelin

Kathleen J. Melanson, *et al.*, at the University of Rhode Island reviewed the effects of HFCS and sugar on circulating levels of glucose, leptin, insulin and ghrelin in a study group of lean women. The study found "no differences in the metabolic effects" of HFCS and sugar.

Triglycerides

A study by Linda M. Zukley, *et al.*, at the Rippe Lifestyle Institute reviewed the effects of HFCS and sugar on triglycerides in a study group of lean women. This short-term study found "no differences in the metabolic effects in lean women [of HFCS] compared to sucrose," and called for additional studies of obese individuals or individuals at risk for the metabolic syndrome.

The metabolic syndrome is a collection of metabolic risk factors including abdominal obesity, atherogenic dyslipidemia, raised blood pressure, insulin resistance, prothrombotic state and proinflammatory state, which increase the chance of developing vascular disease.

Uric Acid

Joshua Lowndes, *et al.*, at the Rippe Lifestyle Institute reviewed the effects of HFCS and sugar on circulating levels of uric acid in a study group of lean women. Uric acid is believed to play a role in the development of the metabolic syndrome.

This short-term study found "no differences in the metabolic effects in lean women [of HFCS] compared to sucrose," and called for additional studies of obese individuals and males.

Does HFCS Affect Feelings of Fullness?

No credible research has demonstrated that HFCS affects calorie control differently than sugar. A study by Pablo Monsivais, *et al.*, at the University of Washington found that beverages sweetened with sugar and HFCS, as well as 1% milk, all have similar effects on feelings of fullness.

Stijn Soenen and Margriet S. Westerterp-Plantenga, researchers at the Department of Human Biology at Maastricht University in The Netherlands, studied the effects of milk and beverages sweetened with sugar and HFCS on feelings of fullness. The researchers found "no differences in satiety, compensation or overconsumption" between the three beverages.

Tina Akhavan and G. Harvey Anderson at the Department of Nutritional Sciences, Faculty of Medicine, University of Toronto studied the effect of solutions containing sugar, HFCS and various ratios of glucose to fructose on food intake, average appetite, blood glucose, plasma insulin, ghrelin and uric acid in men. The researchers found that sugar, HFCS, and 1:1 glucose/fructose solutions do not differ significantly in their short-term effects on subjective and physiologic measures of satiety, uric acid and food intake at a subsequent meal.

Further, research by Almiron-Roig and co-workers in 2003 showed that a regular soft drink, orange juice and low-fat milk were not significantly different in their effects on hunger or satiety ratings, or in calories consumed at a subsequent meal.

Does HFCS Have a High Glycemic Index?

The Glycemic Index (GI) is a ranking of foods, beverages and ingredients based on their immediate effect on blood glucose levels. The GI measures how much blood sugar increases over a period of two or three hours after a meal. Some scientists believe that selecting foods with a low GI helps in diabetes management.

Carbohydrate foods that break down quickly during digestion have the highest GI. The benchmark in many indexes is glucose, with a GI of 100. Compared with glucose, the GI of fructose is very low with a value of 20. Sugar and honey, both with similar compositions to HFCS, have moderate GI values that range from 55 to 60. Although it has not yet been specifically measured, HFCS would be expected to have a moderate GI because of its similarity in composition to honey and sugar.

It must be kept in mind that the body does not respond to the GI of individual ingredients, but rather to the GI of the entire meal. Since *added sugars* (principally sugar and HFCS) typically contribute less than 20 percent of calories, it is clear that HFCS is a minor contributor to the overall GI in a normal diet.

Is HFCS Allergemic?

A number of cereal grains are known to cause allergic reactions (e.g., wheat, rye, barley), but corn is not among them. In fact, the prevalence of corn allergy in the U.S. is extremely low—estimated to affect no more than 0.016 percent of the general population. Food allergies are caused by certain proteins in foods. Nearly all of the corn protein is removed during the production of HFCS. Moreover, the trace protein remaining in HFCS likely bears little immunological resemblance to allergens in the original kernel.

Facts About Caloric Sweeteners

Sweeteners that contribute calories to the diet are called caloric or nutritive sweeteners. All common caloric sweeteners have the same composition: they contain fructose and glucose in essentially equal proportions. All caloric sweeteners require processing to produce a food-grade product.

Fructose	a simple sugar commonly found in fruits and honey
Glucose	a simple sugar that serves as a building block for most carbohydrates
High fructose corn syrup (HFCS)	free (unbonded) fructose and glucose in liquid (syrup) form; produced from corn
Sucrose	crystalline white table sugar; produced from sugar cane or sugar beets; fructose and glucose bonded together
Invert sugar	free fructose and glucose in liquid (syrup) form; produced from the breakdown of sugar
Hydrolyzed cane juice	free fructose and glucose in liquid (syrup) form; produced from the breakdown of cane juice
Honey	liquid (syrup) product; principally free fructose and glucose with minor levels of other sugars and some trace minerals
Fruit juice concentrate	concentrated, filtered, clarified fruit juice; fructose-to-glucose ratio varies by fruit source, but generally equivalent to other nutritive sweeteners (orange juice and grape juice have a fructose to glucose ratio of 1 to 1, while apple juice has a ratio of 2 to 1)

For more information on different types of sweeteners, see www.SweetSurprise.com.

Nutritional Characteristics

Common caloric sweeteners share the same general nutritional characteristics:

- each has roughly the same composition—equal proportions of the simple sugars fructose and glucose;
- each offers approximately the same sweetness on a per-gram basis;
- one gram (dry basis) of each adds 4 calories to foods and beverages;
- each is absorbed from the gut at about the same rate;
- similar ratios of fructose and glucose arrive in the bloodstream after a meal, which are indistinguishable in the body.

Since caloric sweeteners are nutritionally equivalent, they are interchangeable in foods and beverages with no measurable change in metabolism.

What if caloric sweeteners are removed from foods?

To replace one caloric sweetener with another provides no change in nutritional value. To remove sweeteners entirely from their commonly used applications and replace them with high intensity sweeteners would drastically alter product flavor and sweetness, require the use of chemical preservatives to ensure product quality and freshness, result in a reduction in perceived food quality (bran cereal with the caloric sweeteners removed would have the consistency of sawdust), and would likely require the addition of bulking agents to provide the expected texture, mouth feel or volume for most baked goods.

Why is HFCS used in specific applications?

If consumers are sometimes surprised to find HFCS in particular foods or beverages, it may be because they do not have a full appreciation of its versatility and value. HFCS often plays a key role in the integrity of food and beverage products that has little to do with sweetening. Here are some examples in popular products:

Baked goods	HFCS gives a pleasing brown crust to breads and cakes; contributes fermentable sugars to yeast-raised products; reduces sugar crystallization during baking for soft-moist textures; enhances flavors of fruit fillings
Yogurt	HFCS provides fermentable sugars; enhances fruit and spice flavors; controls moisture to prevent separation; regulates tartness
Spaghetti sauces, ketchup and condiments	HFCS enhances flavor and balance – replaces the "pinch of table sugar grandma added" to enhance spice flavors; balances the variable tartness of tomatoes
Beverages	HFCS provides greater stability in acidic carbonated sodas than sucrose; flavors remain consistent and stable over the entire shelf-life of the product
Granola, breakfast and energy bars	HFCS enhances moisture control, retards spoilage and extends product freshness; provides soft texture; enhances spice and fruit flavors

WWW.HFCSfacts.com

Corn Refiners Association, 1701 Pennsylvania Ave, NW, Suite 950, Washington, DC 20006-5806, phone: (202) 331-1634 fax: (202) 331-2054

How Is HFCS Made?

The corn wet milling industry makes HFCS from corn starch using a series of unit processes that include steeping corn to soften the hard kernel; physical separation of the kernel into its separate components—starch, corn hull, protein and oil; breakdown of the starch to glucose; use of enzymes to invert glucose to fructose; removal of impurities; and blending of glucose and fructose to make HFCS-42 and HFCS-55. . . .

Corn Refiners Association is the national trade association representing the corn refining industry of the United States since 1913.

EXPLORING THE ISSUE

Does a Diet High in Fructose Increase Body Fat?

Critical Thinking and Reflection

1. List foods that contain high fructose corn syrup (HFCS) and the type HFCS (42 percent or 55 percent) they contain.
2. Based on the Mercola article, explain how fructose increases lipid levels in the body.
3. Compare the health effects of HFCS outlined by Mercola to the claims made by the Corn Refiners Association.
4. The rates of obesity, type II diabetes, and metabolic syndrome have increased since HFCS was introduced 30 years ago. Do you feel that HFCS has caused these problems? Justify your answer.
5. Select 10 processed foods in your kitchen cabinets. Determine which foods contain HFCS. Go to the grocery store and identify HFCS-free foods you could use in place of the items that contain HFCS and compare the prices of the two.

Is There Common Ground?

It might be hard to find the common ground between the two selections. Numerous studies have been published on HFCS and health. These two selections include claims by the Corn Refiners Association (CRA), who justify that HFCS is just as safe and healthful to consume as regular table sugar. The CRA also claims that HFCS has no adverse health effects and is the same as sucrose and honey, as all three have about the same one-to-one ratio of fructose to glucose. Their selection begins by explaining what HFCS is and how it is used in the food industry. They then explain why it is no different than sucrose, including claims that the body does not process it any differently than regular table sugar. They point out that it does not raise blood triglyceride levels, uric acid, hunger, or blood glucose levels like many critics of the product claim.

Joseph Mercola claims that HFCS is much worse than sugar and that the CRA are "swindling" the nation and even petitioned the FDA to "allow manufacturers the option of using the term 'corn sugar' instead of 'high fructose corn syrup'." He contends that the rise in obesity, diabetes, and metabolic syndrome in the United States parallels HFCS consumption. Mercola briefly outlines how fructose is metabolized and lists various conditions that are aggravated by fructose. He ends by recommending that people should limit fructose to 25 grams per day and provides a list of the fructose content of various fruits. Perhaps the main common ground is that both selections emphasize the relationship between fructose (or HFCS) and health—but they do not agree on the effect that fructose has on health.

Additional Resources

Hu FB. Are refined carbohydrates worse than saturated fat? *Am J Clin Nutr.* 2010;91(6):1541–2.

Kolderup A, Svihus B. Fructose metabolism and relation to atherosclerosis, type 2 diabetes, and obesity. *J Nutr Metab.* 2015;2015:823081.

Lowette K, Roosen L, Tack J, Vanden Berghe P. Effects of high-fructose diets on central appetite signaling and cognitive function. *Front Nutr.* 2015;2:5.

Malik VS, Hu FB. Fructose and cardiometabolic health: What the evidence from sugar-sweetened beverages tells us. *J Am Coll Cardiol.* 2015;66(14):1615–24.

White JS, Hobbs LJ, Fernandez S. Fructose content and composition of commercial HFCS-sweetened carbonated beverages. *Int J Obes.* 2015;39(1):176–82.

Internet References . . .

Corn Refiners Association

www.corn.org

The Sugar Association, Inc

www.sugar.org

Sweet Surprise

sweetsurprise.com

Selected, Edited, and with Issue Framing Material by:
Janet M. Colson, *Middle Tennessee State University*

ISSUE

Do Americans Need Vitamin D Supplements?

YES: Jane Brody, from "What Do You Lack? Probably Vitamin D," *The New York Times* (2010)

NO: Institute of Medicine, from "Dietary Reference Intakes for Calcium and Vitamin D," *The National Academies Press* (2010)

Learning Outcomes

After reading this issue, you will be able to:

- Identify the possible health problems associated with vitamin D deficiency.
- Differentiate between the blood levels of vitamin D considered to be deficient by the nutrition experts mentioned by Brody and the level proposed by the Institute of Medicine (IOM).
- Compare the amount of vitamin D recommended in the Brody selection compared to the EAR and RDA established by the IOM.
- Describe possible problems associated with excessive vitamin D intake.

ISSUE SUMMARY

YES: Best-selling author Jane Brody says that a huge part of the population is deficient in vitamin D and studies indicate that deficiency increases risk of cancer, heart disease, arthritis, and a host of other conditions. She also reports that the "experts" recommend a supplement of 1000 to 2000 IU each day.

NO: The 14-member committee appointed by the Institute of Medicine (IOM) of the National Academy of Sciences to establish the Recommended Dietary Allowance (RDA) disagrees. After reviewing over 1000 studies and listening to testimonies from scientists and other stakeholders, the committee set the RDA for people up to age 70 years at 600 IU and at 800 IU for those over age 70. They conclude that few people are deficient in vitamin D and the only health benefit is the vitamin's role in bone health.

Jane Brody is on target when she writes that vitamin D is "the most talked-about and written-about supplement of the decade." From the 1930s until the late 1990s, it was generally agreed that most healthy people had ample vitamin D. We synthesize the vitamin when our skin is exposed to sun, hence, the vitamin is commonly known as "the sunshine vitamin." During warm months, if our arms and legs are exposed to sun, we make plenty. According to the Vitamin D Council, "Caucasian skin produces approximately 10,000 IU vitamin D in response to 20 to 30 minutes summer sun exposure." However, during colder months, when our skin is covered in warm clothing, additional vitamin D may be needed. People with dark skin and those who just don't go outside may also need additional D.

In the early 1920s, scientists found that rickets could be corrected by giving a fat soluble substance that was found in cod liver oil. It was originally called the "antirachitic factor" and later named vitamin D. In those days, a daily dose of cod liver oil was given to ward off rickets. The first recommendation about the amount of vitamin D needed was published with the initial edition of the RDA in 1941. It was set at 400 IU since that is approximately the amount found in one teaspoon of cod liver oil. The RDA remained at this level until 1997, when the IOM expanded the RDA to the

Dietary Reference Intakes (DRI). The DRI are composed of four different nutrient recommendation levels:

- **Estimated Average Requirements (EAR):** The amount expected to satisfy the needs of 50 percent of people.
- **Recommended Dietary Allowances (RDA):** The daily intake level of a nutrient considered sufficient to meet the requirements of nearly all (97–98 percent) healthy individuals.
- **Adequate Intake (AI):** Used when no RDA has been established; the amount believed to be adequate for all healthy people.
- **Tolerable Upper Intake Levels (UL):** The highest amount that should be consumed; higher intakes may be harmful.

The 1997 IOM committee that developed the new guidelines did not find adequate scientific studies to base an actual RDA on so they established an AI. The AI for people up to age 50 years was 200 IU, from ages 51 to 70 the AI was 400 IU, and for those over age 70 it increased to 600 IU.

For most of the 20th century, vitamin D was thought to only be involved in bone formation. In the 1980s, a few researchers began looking at other functions of the vitamin and the fact that many cells contain vitamin D receptors. Since that time, reports of new research have exploded. In fact, the IOM reviewed over 1000 studies to base their 2010 recommendations. Even though many of the studies conclude that we need 1000 to 2000 IU each day and supplements are the only way to achieve the level needed for optimal health, the IOM report disagrees. They report that the majority of Americans and Canadians are receiving adequate vitamin D. While the IOM did increase the RDA to 600 IU for people up to age 70 years and to 800 IU for those over 70, the amount is lower than what most scientists recommend.

You may be wondering what food provides vitamin D. Actually, hardly any food contains it naturally. A few oily fishes are the main sources. Recently, the mushroom industry has developed a portabella mushroom that contains about 400 IU of the vitamin. They found that exposing the mushrooms to UV light stimulates vitamin D synthesis, similar

Vitamin D Content of Selected Foods		
Food	Serving	IU Vit. D
Salmon, sockeye canned with bones	3 oz	667
Salmon, pink canned with bones	3 oz	466
Cod liver oil	1 tsp	450
Mushroom, portabella exposed to UV light	1 cup	384
Tuna, light canned in oil	3 oz	229
Sardines, canned in oil	3 oz	164
Tuna, canned in water	3 oz	154
Orange juice, fortified with vitamin D	8 oz	137
Milk, low fat	8 oz	120
Flounder	3 oz	103
Total Raisin Bran Cereal	1 cup	100
Froot Loops Cereal	1 cup	41
Mushrooms, shitake	1 cup	41
Cod, Atlantic	3 oz	40
Egg, medium	1	36
Mushrooms, canned	1 cup	12
Mushrooms, portabella not exposed to UV light	1 cup	9
Butter	1 tbsp	9
Cheddar cheese	1 oz	7
Mushrooms, white button	1 cup	7
Ice cream, vanilla	½ cup	5

Source: USDA Nutrient Database (Retrieved January 8, 2011)

to the way our bodies produce it. Studies are still being conducted to see the bioavailability of the UV-produced vitamin D in mushrooms to humans. Most milk processors fortify fluid milk with 100 IU per 8 ounces. This, combined with the small amount of natural vitamin D in milk, translates into about 120 IU per 8 ounces. Notice in the table below that fluid milk is the only significant dairy source of the vitamin. Also, look at the amount found in various types of mushrooms—only those exposed to UV light are significant sources. With recent interest on the vitamin, more cereal and juice manufacturers fortify their products.

The debate of this issue focuses on how much vitamin D is needed and if supplements are required to get this amount. The new RDA is higher than it was in previous years, but it is still much lower than the amount many researchers recommend. Even Harvard's nutrition faculty recommends a supplement of vitamin D for most people in their Healthy Eating Pyramid. A criticism of the new IOM RDA was posted on Harvard's *The Nutrition Source*. They consider that the new guidelines are:

. . . overly conservative about the recommended intake, and they do not give enough weight to some of the latest science on vitamin D and health. For bone health and chronic disease prevention, many people are likely to need more vitamin D than even these new government guidelines recommend.

The Vitamin D Council, which is sponsored by four companies that market vitamin D supplements or sell tanning beds, considers that adults may need 5000 IU per day and that blood levels should be between 50 and 80 ng/ml. Both of these levels are much higher than the IOM recommendations. (The IOM considers blood levels of 20 ng/ml to be adequate.) The Council also recommends 20 to 30 minutes of midday sun exposure from spring to fall and to use a tanning bed during the winter months.

What do you think? Do you agree with the IOM that few people are deficient in vitamin D and intakes of 600 IU are adequate? Or do you think we need to take supplements of vitamin D for optimal health?

YES ←

Jane Brody

What Do You Lack? Probably Vitamin D

Vitamin D promises to be the most talked-about and written-about supplement of the decade. While studies continue to refine optimal blood levels and recommended dietary amounts, the fact remains that a huge part of the population—from robust newborns to the frail elderly, and many others in between—are deficient in this essential nutrient.

If the findings of existing clinical trials hold up in future research, the potential consequences of this deficiency are likely to go far beyond inadequate bone development and excessive bone loss that can result in falls and fractures. Every tissue in the body, including the brain, heart, muscles and immune system, has receptors for vitamin D, meaning that this nutrient is needed at proper levels for these tissues to function well.

Studies indicate that the effects of a vitamin D deficiency include an elevated risk of developing (and dying from) cancers of the colon, breast and prostate; high blood pressure and cardiovascular disease; osteoarthritis; and immune-system abnormalities that can result in infections and autoimmune disorders like multiple sclerosis, Type 1 diabetes and rheumatoid arthritis.

Most people in the modern world have lifestyles that prevent them from acquiring the levels of vitamin D that evolution intended us to have. The sun's ultraviolet-B rays absorbed through the skin are the body's main source of this nutrient. Early humans evolved near the equator, where sun exposure is intense year round, and minimally clothed people spent most of the day outdoors.

"As a species, we do not get as much sun exposure as we used to, and dietary sources of vitamin D are minimal," Dr. Edward Giovannucci, nutrition researcher at the Harvard School of Public Health, wrote in *The Archives of Internal Medicine*. Previtamin D forms in sun-exposed skin, and 10 to 15 percent of the previtamin is immediately converted to vitamin D, the form found in supplements. Vitamin D, in turn, is changed in the liver to 25-hydroxyvitamin D, the main circulating form. Finally, the kidneys convert 25-hydroxyvitamin D into the nutrient's biologically active form, 1,25-dihydroxyvitamin D, also known as vitamin D hormone.

A person's vitamin D level is measured in the blood as 25-hydroxyvitamin D, considered the best indicator of sufficiency. A recent study showed that maximum bone density is achieved when the blood serum level of 25-hydroxyvitamin D reaches 40 nanograms per milliliter or more.

"Throughout most of human evolution," Dr. Giovannucci wrote, "when the vitamin D system was developing, the 'natural' level of 25-hydroxyvitamin D was probably around 50 nanograms per milliliter or higher. In modern societies, few people attain such high levels."

A Common Deficiency

Although more foods today are supplemented with vitamin D, experts say it is rarely possible to consume adequate amounts through foods. The main dietary sources are wild-caught oily fish (salmon, mackerel, bluefish, and canned tuna) and fortified milk and baby formula, cereal and orange juice.

People in colder regions form their year's supply of natural vitamin D in summer, when ultraviolet-B rays are most direct. But the less sun exposure, the darker a person's skin and the more sunscreen used, the less previtamin D is formed and the lower the serum levels of the vitamin. People who are sun-phobic, babies who are exclusively breast-fed, the elderly and those living in nursing homes are particularly at risk of a serious vitamin D deficiency.

Dr. Michael Holick of Boston University, a leading expert on vitamin D and author of *The Vitamin D Solution* (Hudson Street Press, 2010), said in an interview, "We want everyone to be above 30 nanograms per milliliter, but currently in the United States, Caucasians average 18 to 22 nanograms and African-Americans average 13 to 15 nanograms." African-American women are 10 times as likely to have levels at or below 15 nanograms as white women, the third National Health and Nutrition Examination Survey [NHANES III] found.

Such low levels could account for the high incidence of several chronic diseases in this country, Dr. Holick maintains. For example, he said, in the Northeast, where sun exposure is reduced and vitamin D levels consequently are lower, cancer rates are higher than in the South. Likewise, rates of high blood pressure, heart disease, and prostate cancer are higher among dark-skinned Americans than among whites.

The rising incidence of Type 1 diabetes may be due, in part, to the current practice of protecting the young from sun exposure. When newborn infants in Finland were given 2,000 international units a day, Type 1 diabetes fell by 88 percent, Dr. Holick said.

The current recommended intake of vitamin D, established by the Institute of Medicine, is 200 I.U. a day from birth to age 50 (including pregnant women); 400 for adults aged 50 to 70; and 600 for those older than 70. While a revision upward of these amounts is in the works, most experts expect it will err on the low side. Dr. Holick, among others, recommends a daily supplement of 1,000 to 2,000 units for all sun-deprived individuals, pregnant and lactating women, and adults older than 50. The American Academy of Pediatrics recommends that breast-fed infants receive a daily supplement of 400 units until they are weaned and consuming a quart or more each day of fortified milk or formula.

Given appropriate sun exposure in summer, it is possible to meet the body's yearlong need for vitamin D. But so many factors influence the rate of vitamin D formation in skin that it is difficult to establish a universal public health recommendation. Asked for a general recommendation, Dr. Holick suggests going outside in summer unprotected by sunscreen (except for the face, which should always be protected) wearing minimal clothing from 10 a.m. to 3 p.m. two or three times a week for 5 to 10 minutes.

Slathering skin with sunscreen with an SPF of 30 will reduce exposure to ultraviolet-B rays by 95 to 98 percent. But if you make enough vitamin D in your skin in summer, it can meet the body's needs for the rest of the year, Dr. Holick said.

Can You Get Too Much?

If acquired naturally through skin, the body's supply of vitamin D has a built-in cutoff. When enough is made, further exposure to sunlight will destroy any excess. Not so when the source is an ingested supplement, which goes directly to the liver.

Symptoms of vitamin D toxicity include nausea, vomiting, poor appetite, constipation, weakness and weight loss, as well as dangerous amounts of calcium that can result in kidney stones, confusion and abnormal heart rhythms.

But both Dr. Giovannucci and Dr. Holick say it is very hard to reach such toxic levels. Healthy adults have taken 10,000 I.U. a day for six months or longer with no adverse effects. People with a serious vitamin D deficiency are often prescribed weekly doses of 50,000 units until the problem is corrected. To minimize the risk of any long-term toxicity, these experts recommend that adults take a daily supplement of 1,000 to 2,000 units.

JANE BRODY, award-winning author and health columnist for *The New York Times*, graduated from Cornell with a degree in biochemistry and a degree in science writing from the University of Wisconsin. Brody has authored over a dozen books including two best-sellers, *Jane Brody's Nutrition Book* and *Jane Brody's Good Food Book*.

Institute of Medicine

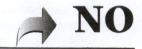

Dietary Reference Intakes for Calcium and Vitamin D

Calcium and vitamin D are two essential nutrients long known for their role in bone health. Over the last ten years, the public has heard conflicting messages about other benefits of these nutrients—especially vitamin D—and also about how much calcium and vitamin D they need to be healthy.

To help clarify this issue, the U.S. and Canadian governments asked the Institute of Medicine (IOM) to assess the current data on health outcomes associated with calcium and vitamin D. The IOM tasked a committee of experts with reviewing the evidence, as well as updating the nutrient reference values, known as Dietary Reference Intakes (DRIs). These values are used widely by government agencies, for example, in setting standards for school meals or specifying the nutrition label on foods. Over time, they have come to be used by health professionals to counsel individuals about dietary intake.

The committee provided an exhaustive review of studies on potential health outcomes and found that the evidence supported a role for these nutrients in bone health but not in other health conditions. Overall, the committee concludes that the majority of Americans and Canadians are receiving adequate amounts of both calcium and vitamin D. Further, there is emerging evidence that too much of these nutrients may be harmful.

Health Effects of Vitamin D and Calcium Intake

The new reference values are based on much more information and higher-quality studies than were available when the values for these nutrients were first set in 1997. The committee assessed more than one thousand studies and reports and listened to testimony from scientists and stakeholders before making its conclusions. It reviewed a range of health outcomes, including but not limited to cancer, cardiovascular disease and hypertension, diabetes and metabolic syndrome, falls, immune response, neuropsychological functioning, physical performance, preeclampsia, and reproductive outcomes. This thorough review found that information about the health benefits beyond bone health—benefits often reported in the media—were from studies that provided often mixed and inconclusive results and could not be considered reliable. However, a strong body of evidence from rigorous testing substantiates the importance of vitamin D and calcium in promoting bone growth and maintenance.

Dietary Reference Intakes

The DRIs are intended to serve as a guide for good nutrition and provide the basis for the development of nutrient guidelines in both the United States and Canada. The science indicates that on average 500 milligrams of calcium per day meets the requirements of children ages 1 through 3, and on average 800 milligrams daily is appropriate for those ages 4 through 8 (see table for the Recommended Dietary Allowance—a value that meets the needs of most people). Adolescents need higher levels to support bone growth: 1,300 milligrams per day meets the needs of practically all adolescents. Women ages 19 through 50 and men up to 71 require on average 800 milligrams daily. Women over 50 and both men and women 71 and older should take in 1,000 milligrams per day on average to ensure they are meeting their daily needs for strong, healthy bones.

Determining intake levels for vitamin D is somewhat more complicated. Vitamin D levels in the body may come from not only vitamin D in the diet but also from synthesis in the skin through sunlight exposure. The amount of sun exposure one receives varies greatly from person to person, and people are advised against sun exposure to reduce the risk of skin cancer. Therefore, the committee assumed minimal sun exposure when establishing the DRIs for

Dietary Reference Intakes for Vitamin D

Life Stage Group	Vitamin D		
	Estimated Average Requirement (IU/day)	Recommended Dietary Allowance (IU/day)	Upper Level Intake (IU/day)
Infants 0 to 6 months	*	*	1,000
Infants 6 to 12 months	*	*	1,500
1–3 years old	400	600	2,500
4–8 years old	400	600	3,000
9–13 years old	400	600	4,000
14–18 years old	400	600	4,000
19–30 years old	400	600	4,000
31–50 years old	400	600	4,000
51–70 years old males	400	600	4,000
51–70 years old females	400	600	4,000
>70 years old	400	800	4,000
14–18 years old, pregnant/lactating	400	600	4,000
19–50 years old, pregnant/lactating	400	600	4,000

*For infants, adequate intake is 400 IU/day for 0 to 6 months of age and 400 IU/day for 6 to 12 months of age.

vitamin D, and it determined that North Americans need on average 400 International Units (IUs) of vitamin D per day (see table for the Recommended Dietary Allowances—values sufficient to meet the needs of virtually all persons). People age 71 and older may require as much as 800 IUs per day because of potential changes in people's bodies as they age.

Questions About Current Intake

National surveys in both the United States and Canada indicate that most people receive enough calcium, with the exception of girls ages 9–18, who often do not take in enough calcium. In contrast, postmenopausal women taking supplements may be getting too much calcium, thereby increasing their risk for kidney stones.

Information from national surveys shows vitamin D presents a complicated picture. While the average total intake of vitamin D is below the median requirement, national surveys show that average blood levels of vitamin D are above the 20 nanograms per milliliter that the IOM committee found to be the level that is needed for good bone health for practically all individuals. These seemingly inconsistent data suggest that sun exposure currently contributes meaningful amounts of vitamin D to North Americans and indicates that a majority of the population is meeting its needs for vitamin D. Nonetheless, some subgroups—particularly those who are older and living in institutions or who have dark skin pigmentation—may be at increased risk for getting too little vitamin D.

Before a few years ago, tests for vitamin D were conducted infrequently. In recent years, these tests have become more widely used, and confusion has grown among the public about how much vitamin D is necessary. Further, the measurements, or cut-points, of sufficiency and deficiency used by laboratories to report results have not been set based on rigorous scientific studies, and no central authority has determined which cut-points to use. A single individual might be deemed deficient or sufficient, depending on the laboratory where the blood is tested. The number of people with vitamin D deficiency in North America may be overestimated because many laboratories appear to be using cut-points that are much higher than the committee suggests is appropriate.

Tolerable Upper Levels of Intake

The upper level intakes set by the committee for both calcium and vitamin D represent the safe boundary at the high end of the scale and should not be misunderstood as amounts people need or should strive to consume. While these values vary somewhat by age, as shown in the table, the committee concludes that once intakes of vitamin D surpass 4,000 IUs per day, the risk for harm begins to increase. Once intakes surpass 2,000 milligrams per day for calcium, the risk for harm also increases.

As North Americans take more supplements and eat more of foods that have been fortified with vitamin D and calcium, it becomes more likely that people consume high amounts of these nutrients. Kidney stones have been associated with taking too much calcium from dietary supplements. Very high levels of vitamin D (above 10,000 IUs per day) are known to cause kidney and tissue damage. Strong evidence about possible risks for daily vitamin D at lower levels of intake is limited, but some preliminary studies offer tentative signals about adverse health effects.

Conclusion

Scientific evidence indicates that calcium and vitamin D play key roles in bone health. The current evidence, however, does not support other benefits for vitamin D or calcium intake. More targeted research should continue. However, the committee emphasizes that, with a few exceptions, all North Americans are receiving enough calcium and vitamin D. Higher levels have not been shown to confer greater benefits, and in fact, they have been linked to other health problems, challenging the concept that "more is better."

Institute of Medicine (IOM) is an independent, nonprofit organization that works outside of government to provide unbiased and authoritative advice to decision makers and the public. It is the health arm of the National Academy of Sciences.

EXPLORING THE ISSUE

Do Americans Need Vitamin D Supplements?

Critical Thinking and Reflection

1. List the health problems associated with low levels of vitamin D.
2. State the blood levels of vitamin D that Brody considers are desirable compared to the levels considered adequate by the Institute of Medicine (IOM).
3. Explain the controversies related to blood levels of vitamin D used to determine vitamin D status.
4. Plan a one-day menu that provides the RDA for vitamin D for an 80-year-old female. Use either MyPyramid (http://www.mypyramid.gov) or the USDA Nutrient Data Base (http://www.nal.usda.gov/fnic/foodcomp/search/) to determine the vitamin D content of the foods.
5. Select 20 types of fish or other seafood. Using the USDA Nutrient Data Base, compile a table with the amount of vitamin D in a 3-ounce serving of each.

Is There Common Ground?

Best-selling nutrition author Jane Brody believes that a huge part of the population is deficient in vitamin D. She even cites studies that indicate vitamin D deficiency increases risk of cancer, heart disease, arthritis, and a host of other conditions. In her article, she points out that many "experts" recommend a supplement of 1000 to 2000 IU each day. The IOM committee disagrees; after reviewing over 1000 studies and listening to testimonies from scientists and other stakeholders, the committee set the Recommended Dietary Allowance (RDA) for people up to age 70 years at 600 IU and at 800 IU for those over age 70. They conclude that few people are deficient in vitamin D and the only health benefit is the vitamin's role in bone health.

It is interesting to note that Brody wrote the *New York Times* article 4 months before the IOM report was published in November 2010. Brody mentions that the IOM was (in July 2010) working on a revision for the recommended intake for the vitamin, and she forecasted that it "will err on the low side." And Brody was correct in her prediction. The IOM did increase the RDA, in fact they tripled the RDA for young and middle-age adults (up to age 50 years) from 200 IU to 600 IU. They stress that there was not enough scientific evidence to "support other benefits for vitamin D" and that "research should continue" on the benefits of the vitamin related to the variety of health claims that have surfaced over the last few years. They continue that "with a few exceptions, all North Americans are receiving enough vitamin D." They challenge the concept that "more is better" and consider that consuming excessive amounts have been linked to other health problems.

Not only does Brody have a graduate degree in science writing, she also has a degree in biochemistry, therefore she understands the science around vitamin D and interviewed some of the leading vitamin D researchers in the United States. The IOM report was developed by 14 of the leading experts on vitamin D in America including some of the top medical and nutrition researchers. In the process, they reviewed virtually all studies conducted on the vitamin over the lasts 10 years and comments from leading scientists involved in vitamin D research. So a common ground is that all 15 authors are very knowledgeable about vitamin D; they agree that the RDA of 200 to 600 IU is too low, but they disagree on what the RDA should be. The IOM considers 600 to 800 IU to be an adequate intake, which can be consumed from foods. In contrast, Jane Brody thinks we need a vitamin D supplement of 1000 to 2000 IU each day.

Additional Resources

Balvers MG, Brouwer-Brolsma EM, Endenburg S, DeGroot LC, Kok FJ, Gunnewiek JK. Recommended intakes of vitamin D to optimise health, associated circulating 25- hydroxyvitamin D concentrations, and dosing regimens to treat deficiency: Workshop report and overview of current literature. *J Nutr Sci.* 2015;4:e23.

Cashman KD. Vitamin D: Dietary requirements and food fortification as a means of helping achieve adequate vitamin D status. *J Steroid Biochem Mol Biol*. 2015;148:19–26.

Saraff V, Shaw N. Sunshine and vitamin D. *Arch Dis Child*. 2015. doi:+10.1136/archdischild-2014-307214.

Taylor CL, Thomas PR, Aloia JF, Millard PS, Rosen CJ. Questions about Vitamin D for primary care practice: Input from an NIH conference. *Am J Med*. 2015;128(11):1167–70.

Internet References . . .

The Institute of Medicine (IOM)

iom.nationalacademies.org

**The Office of Dietary Supplements
of the National Institutes of Health**

https://ods.od.nih.gov/factsheets/list-all/VitaminD

The Vitamin D Council

vitamindcouncil.org

The Vitamin D Society

vitamindsociety.org

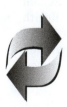

Selected, Edited, and with Issue Framing Material by:
Janet M. Colson, *Middle Tennessee State University*

ISSUE

Does Coconut Oil Provide Health Benefits?

YES: The Coconut Research Center, from "The Coconut Oil Miracle: Where Is the Evidence?" Coconutresearchcenter.org (2015)

NO: William A. Correll, from "FDA Warning Letter to Carrington Farms," Office of Compliance, Center for Food Safety and Applied Nutrition, Food and Drug Administration (2015)

Learning Outcomes

After reading this issue, you will be able to:

- Describe the fatty acid profile of coconut oil.
- Outline the studies conducted on coconut oil since the 1930s.
- Identify the specific violations in FDA's warning letter to Carrington Farms and the instructions FDA provided to Carrington Farms.

ISSUE SUMMARY

YES: Authors of the Coconut Research Center website boast of the various health benefits of coconut oil related to seizures, dementia, ALS, and cardiovascular disease. They describe the number of studies available through a PubMed search that support the health benefits of coconut oil and the medium-chain fatty acids found in the oil.

NO: After reviewing claims that Carrington Farms includes on the labels of coconut oil, William Correll, FDA Director Office of Compliance, Center for Food Safety and Applied Nutrition, issues a warning letter to the company pointing out the therapeutic claims on their website about coconut oil classify it as a drug, not a food, and points out other violations on the labels.

The scientific name for coconut trees is *Cocos nucifera*. According to the University of Queensland's Coconut Project, the word *"cocos"* is Macau Portuguese for monkey, "because the 3 germination pores (the 'eyes') look like a monkey's face." The term *"nucifera"* means "bearing coconuts."

Based on Index Mundi's 2015 data, most of the world's coconuts are grown in the Philippines, Indonesia, and India. The Philippine's Department of Agriculture describes coconuts as "The Tree of Life" because of the "endless list of products and by-products derived from its various parts." Coconuts are important to the Philippine economy because about one-third of the Philippine's population is dependent on the coconut industry for its livelihood. However, in November 2013, Typhoon Haiyan struck the Philippines destroying many of the islands' coconut trees resulting in a significant reduction in the islanders' income. To produce coconuts, trees must be about 10 years old; therefore, the world's supply of coconuts might be low for the next few years.

In the United States, coconut oil got a bad reputation during the 1970s and 1980s when the nation was told to avoid all tropical oils because of their high saturated fat content and the cholesterol-raising, artery-clogging problems that result. At that time, all saturated fats were lumped into one category and the concept of medium-chain versus long-chain fats had not been introduced to the general public. *New York Times* journalist Melissa Clark describes her bafflement about coconut oil's new reputation in her 2011 article "Once a Villain, Coconut Oil Charms the Health Food World."

> So given all this greasy baggage, what was coconut oil doing in a health food store? In fact, it has recently become the darling of the natural-foods world. Annual sales growth at Whole Foods "has been in the high double digits for the last five years," said Errol Schweizer, the chain's global senior grocery coordinator.
>
> Two groups have helped give coconut oil its sparkly new makeover. One is made up of scientists, many of whom are backtracking on the worst accusations against coconut oil. And the other is the growing number of vegans, who rely on it as a sweet vegetable fat that is solid at room temperature and can create flaky pie crusts, crumbly scones and fluffy cupcake icings, all without butter.

The food industry is taking advantage of coconut oil's new popularity and promoting it as a healthy option. Promoters claim that our bodies use the medium-chain fats in coconut oil differently than the longer chain fats found in other oils. Also, many promote the benefits of the natural phytochemicals in "virgin" coconut oil as being heart healthy and providing a host of other benefits. This leaves many consumers feeling like Melissa Clark when she first found the oil in a health food store.

The public's opinions about the healthiness of foods can be easily swayed by the savvy and misleading marketing schemes of some companies. And that is what the U.S. Food and Drug Administration (FDA) thinks is true about one company that sells coconut oil.

The FDA, currently housed under the U.S. Department of Health and Human Services, is the oldest federal consumer protection agency. Although it was not known as "FDA" until 1930, most historians trace FDA's beginning to the Patent Office in the mid-1800s, whose main function was to chemically analyze agricultural products. In 1906, the Pure Food and Drugs Act was passed; the law prohibits interstate commerce in misbranded and adulterated foods, drinks, and drugs. FDA's current mission is to "protect consumers and enhance public health by maximizing compliance of FDA regulated products and minimizing risk associated with those products."

Today, in addition to regulating foods and drugs, the FDA is also responsible for medical devices; biologics such as vaccines; electronics that give off radiation; cosmetics; and tobacco products. Foods are regulated under the direction of the Center for Food Safety and Applied Nutrition. If the FDA finds that a manufacturer has significantly violated FDA regulations, a representative from the FDA notifies the manufacturer, often in the form of a "warning letter." The focus of this issue is an FDA warning letter to Carrington Farms about claims in their coconut oil labels paired with a web article by the Coconut Research Center.org website boasting about the health benefits of coconut oil.

YES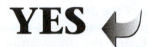

Coconut Research Center

The Coconut Oil Miracle: Where Is the Evidence?

Christine Tomlinson, MD, director of the National Candida Society, in the UK believes in the antibacterial properties of coconut oil, and advises candida sufferers (those with a yeast overgrowth) to include it in their diet. Mary Newport, MD, director of the neonatology unit at Spring Hill Regional Hospital in Florida, is a firm believer in the power of coconut for the treatment of neurological disorders, such as Alzheimer's and Parkinson's. She should, her husband suffered with Alzheimer's for five years before she discovered coconut oil. With the aid of coconut oil he's making a remarkable comeback. Others claim that it can help with diabetes, cancer, kidney and liver function, vitamin and mineral absorption, digestive problems, immune function, and weight loss. From all the glowing reports coconut oil appears to be a super food with a multitude of nutritional and medicinal uses.

In recent years coconut oil has shot to superstardom in the world of health foods. Celebrities are using it, nutritionists are recommending it, and patients are extolling its many virtues.

Yet, despite the growing popularity, some people are skeptical. How could one thing have so many health benefits? It sounds too good to be true. In addition, many doctors, dieticians, and other health care professionals have been reluctant to accept coconut oil as a health food. Coconut oil contains a high percentage of saturated fat. Saturated fats have been condemned for so many years, that they find it hard to change their opinions even when faced with evidence to the contrary.

The objection they state is always the same: there is not enough evidence to prove that coconut oil is harmless or that it has any health benefits. "If it has any health benefits," they bellow, "show me the evidence!" They demand peer-reviewed studies published in respected medical journals. By crying "show me the evidence" they are implying that there is little evidence and that there are no such studies available.

In recent years doctors and editors of health journals are frequently being asked about coconut oil. Most don't know anything about it and consider it just another passing fad. Their answers reflect this view.

A letter sent to the editors of the *Journal of the American Dietetic Association* asks: "Is there science to support claims for coconut oil?" The editor's reply begins by inferring that all the so-called health claims come from websites selling coconut oil and then states, "According to these sources, the health benefits of coconut oil help to prevent or mitigate a wide range of medical conditions. However . . . there is insufficient evidence to support the claims."[1]

A similar question was posed to bestselling author Andrew Weil, MD. "We don't have any evidence suggesting that coconut oil is better for you than other saturated fats," he states on his website. "The benefits of coconut oil in the diet, if any, are likely to be minimal, and until we have *more and better evidence* about coconut oil's effect . . . I do not recommend using it.[2]

Readers of Dr. John McDougall's newsletter asked him the same question. "Coconut oil is the newest miracle food promoted on the Internet and at health food stores for rejuvenation and cure of 'whatever ails you,'" responds Dr. McDougall. "Advocates of coconut oil claim this sensational food has anti-microbial, anti-heart disease, anti-cancer, and anti-obesity benefits. Furthermore, this fat is sold as a cure for low thyroid function (hypothyroidism). This is a huge turnaround for a substance that has traditionally been thought of as an artery-clogging saturated fat. *Testimonials provide most of the evidence* for the miraculous effects these oils have on people, rather than *well thought out and carefully designed experiments* [italics mine]. Thus, most of these claims are based on a little truth overblown into a sales pitch for sellers of coconut oil."[3]

The answers are all the same; the health claims are attributed to people selling coconut oil and that there is little or no evidence to back up their claims. Obviously, these doctors did not bother to take the time to research the question but simply gave their uneducated, biased opinions. That's the problem with those who refuse to acknowledge new advances in science and medicine. They don't take the time to find out and belittle those who have.

Celebrity doctor Mehmet Oz, MD, wrote an article a couple of years ago lambasting coconut oil in the same vein as those above. However, recently Dr. Oz reversed his stance and acknowledged that coconut oil is a healthy food and admitted that he himself now takes it every day. He even included several segments of his TV show to the benefits of coconut oil. (You can view them at http://www.doctoroz.com/videos/coconut-oil-super-powers-pt-1) If these other doctors were open minded enough and had taken the time to do just a little investigation, like Dr. Oz, they would have seen the overwhelming evidence and become believers too.

"Show me the evidence." That's the universal battle cry of the critics. Is there sufficient evidence to justify the safety and value of coconut oil? There is actually plenty of evidence, if you know where to look. On the Internet there is a website sponsored by U.S. National Institutes of Health called PubMed (www.pubmed.gov). This is a research tool that indexes nearly 6,000 medical and biological journals published around the word.

If you key in the word "coconut oil" you get a listing of all the studies in the database that involve coconut oil. Currently there are 1,315 studies listed. Over thirteen hundred studies, that's a lot of evidence! New studies are continually being added. We can say to the critics are these enough studies? They would probably say "no, we want more studies." OK, well you can find additional studies by looking up similar search terms like "virgin coconut oil," "medium chain fatty acids," "medium chain triglycerides," "lauric acid," "capric acid," "caprylic acid," and so forth. When you have done that, you will get a listing of over 17,000 studies! How's that for evidence! This would blow their minds. Some of these studies, however, will be listed twice. So if we take into account some duplication, that still leaves about 10,000 studies on coconut oil.

Ten thousand studies should be enough to convince any skeptic, especially when you consider that the FDA grants approval to new drugs if only *two* positive studies are published. The arthritis drug Vioxx, had only four published studies before it was approved. When new drugs are approved for distribution to the public, why don't doctors stand up and scream for more evidence? When Vioxx, Baycol, and Darvon were approved why didn't the medical community rise up in protest asking for more evidence for their efficiency and safety? They should have, since each of these drugs were later taken off the market because they were crippling and killing people

When the Alzheimer's drug, Apricept, was approved by the FDA in 1996 there were less than 10 studies available, not all of them positive. The effects of the drug have been less than impressive. A few of the studies suggested that some patients may benefit from taking the drug, while others failed to show any benefit. In general, less than half of those taking the drug demonstrate any benefit. When improvement does occur, it lasts only a few months and is not great enough to have any worthwhile effect on the patient's symptoms or day-to-day functioning. The results have been generally disappointing, nevertheless, the drug was approved and is currently the most wildly used treatment for Alzheimer's.

What price does the patient pay for the possibility of a few months of minor improvement? The price can be measured in terms of the adverse reactions from taking the drug, which may include any number of the following: diarrhea, dizziness, muscle cramps, nausea, fatigue, insomnia, vomiting, weight loss, seizures, and death. Is it worth it? While the benefits are only expected to last a few months, patients often continue the drug for years. Where are the voices calling for more studies on Apricept? Where are the voices challenging its safety? Is it because it is a chemical created in a laboratory that gives it acceptance among the medical community, while coconut oil being a product of nature is looked upon with suspicion?

Coconut oil has caused no deaths or harm of any type. It's been used safely for thousands of years. There is no risk in using it. Thousands of studies have proven its therapeutic worth and tens of thousands satisfied users can attest to its health promoting properties. Coconut oil has proven to be far more effective at treating Alzheimer's than Apricept.[4] Yet, critics still call for more studies on coconut oil.

Admittedly, not all of the 10,000 studies involving coconut oil are of equal value, some provide little or no useful information. However, the same is true for drug studies as well, not all of them are useful either. Nevertheless, there are ample studies on coconut oil to clearly demonstrate its many nutritional and medicinal properties. Let's take a brief look at the evidence behind the modern medical uses for coconut oil.

The basic chemistry of coconut oil was figured out back in the 1920s and 1930s. Back then it was discovered that coconut oil was distinctly different from other fats and oils. Coconut oil was found to be composed predominately of a unique family of fats called medium chain fatty acids. In coconut oil these fatty acids are in the form of medium chain triglycerides (MCTs).

In the 1930s and 1940s. It was discovered that when coconut oil was added into the diet it improved the absorption of various nutrients. For example, W.D. Salmon and J.G. Goodman at the Alabama Polytechnic Institute (now

Auburn University) studied the effects of vitamin B-1 deficiency in animals given different types of fats. Vitamin B-1 deficiency leads to a fatal disease called beriberi. The fats and oils evaluated included olive oil, butter, beef fat, linseed oil (flaxseed), cottonseed oil, and other oils. When rats were given a vitamin B deficient diet, coconut oil was by far the most efficient in preventing the disease and extending lifespan. In fact, those receiving coconut oil actually gained weight, indicating continued growth even though the diet was nutritionally poor.[5] None of the tested oils, including coconut oil, contains vitamin B-1. However, coconut oil makes what little of the vitamin that is in the diet more biologically available, thus preventing the deficiency disease.

A number of studies over the years have found similar effects. Coconut oil improves the absorption of not only the B vitamins but also vitamins A, D, E, K, beta-carotene, CoQ10, and other fat soluble nutrients, minerals such as calcium, magnesium, and some amino acids—the building block for protein.[6] (Please note that for readability only a very few references will be included in this article. If all available references were listed, this article would swell to well over 30 pages in length.)

The fact that coconut oil improved absorption of a wide variety of nutrients led researchers to investigate its use in treating malnutrition and malabsorption syndrome in children and infants. Eventually it was included in hospital feeding formulas for the sick and in infant formulas, especially for premature and low birth weight babies. When compared to other dietary fats, coconut oil produced faster growth, weight gain, and improved nutritional status.[7] Coconut oil became a standard ingredient in all commercial infant formulas and still is today. Coconut oil or MCTs are also still used in hospital IV and feeding formulas to treat sick patients of all ages. Adding the oil reduces the patients' recovery time and improves nutritional status.[8]

In the 1950s researchers began investigating the nutritional and medicinal uses for MCTs. Harvard researcher Vigen K. Babayan, PhD is credited with developing the process of distilling coconut oil down into pure MCT oil. He called the purified oil *fractionated coconut oil* or *MCT oil*.[9] A great deal of research followed and it was soon evident that MCTs possessed unique biological properties with a number of important nutritional and medical applications.

It was soon discovered that MCTs digest differently than other fats. When swallowed, most fats travel down the esophagus (throat), through the stomach, and into the small intestine where they are broken down by digestive enzymes and bile into individual fatty acids (long chain fatty acids). These fatty acids are then absorbed into the intestinal wall where they are repackaged into bundles of fat, cholesterol, and protein called lipoproteins. These lipoproteins pass into the bloodstream. As they circulate in the bloodstream they release little particles of fat and cholesterol that are utilized by the cells or stored as body fat.

The process is completely different with MCTs. When MCTs are consumed, they digest very rapidly and begin breaking down immediately. When they pass from the stomach into the small intestine, they are already completely separated into individual fatty acids (medium chain fatty acids) and, therefore, do not need pancreatic digestive enzymes or bile for digestion, thus relieving stress on the digestive system. Since they are already in the form of fatty acids when they enter the small intestine they are immediately absorbed into the portal vein and sent directly to the liver. In the liver they are metabolized into energy.[10]

The difference in the way MCTs are digested is very important because it provides a means to treat a number of medical conditions. Extensive research and clinical work in the 1960s and 1970s led to the use of MCTs for the treatment of a variety of malabsorption syndromes including obstructive jaundice,[11] cystic fibrosis,[12] tropical sprue,[13] a-beta-lipoprotenaemia,[14] intestinal lymphangiectasia,[15] pancreatic insufficiency,[16] and to speed recovery after intestinal surgery.[17]

Because of the unique way in which MCTs are digested and metabolized they produce an increase in energy and boost metabolism. For this reason, MCTs are used by athletes to improve performance. MCTs or coconut oil are commonly found in commercially produced energy bars and sports drinks marketed to people with active lifestyles.

This metabolic boosting effect diminishes fat deposition. This led researchers in the 1980s to begin investigating the use of MCTs as a means for weight management.[18] Researchers from McGill University in Quebec, Canada and elsewhere are now recommending the use of MCTs as a means to treat obesity.[19]

In the 1960s Jon J. Kabara, PhD, a professor of pharmacology at Michigan State University, discovered that MCTs possess potent antimicrobial properties. In his search for a safe means to protect foods from fungal and bacterial contamination he found that MCTs fit the bill. Over the years he and other researchers found that MCTs can kill a wide variety of disease-causing bacteria, fungi, viruses, and parasites.[20] MCTs were not only useful in preserving foods, but could be used topically and internally as antimicrobial agents to prevent and fight off infectious disease. Many common disease-causing microbes as well as potentially deadly ones like HIV and drug-resistant bacteria are vulnerable to MCTs.[21-22] This aspect of MCTs is extensively researched. There are literally hundreds of studies on this topic and even entire books describing the antimicrobial effects of MCTs.

Because coconut oil is composed predominately of MCTs, it possesses the same antimicrobial power, as evidenced in many clinical and laboratory studies.[23]

In the 1970s it was discovered that while the liver burns some MCTs immediately to produce energy, others are converted into ketones. Ketones are a super potent form of energy that are used specifically by the brain, but can be used by all the tissues in the body except the liver.

Ketones not only provide a high quality source of energy for the brain but trigger the activation of special proteins that function in brain cell maintenance, repair, and growth, thus providing a therapeutic effect on the brain. Since the 1970s MCTs have been used in ketogenic diets to treat epilepsy. Today modified ketogenic diets, using MCTs, are the standard dietary treatment for drug-resistant epilepsy.[24]

Besides epilepsy, ketones have been successfully used to treat a number of other neurological disorders such as Alzheimer's disease, Parkinson's disease, Huntington's disease, ALS, stroke, narcolepsy, brain trauma, and brain cancer. The consumption of coconut oil can increase blood ketone levels to therapeutic levels that can successfully treat all of these conditions. Many patients with Alzheimer's and other forms of dementia are currently being treated with coconut oil and are achieving far better results than the medications currently approved for these conditions. Studies show that MCTs can effectively mitigate the effects of Alzheimer's and a dietary supplement designed for this purpose was approved by the Food and Drug Administration (FDA) in 2009 for the treatment of Alzheimer's.

Coconut oil is known to aid those with diabetes by balancing blood sugar levels. MCTs improve insulin secretion and insulin sensitivity, thus reversing the underlying cause of diabetes.[25]

Coconut oil has very potent anti-cancer properties. When cancer is chemically induced in lab animals the addition of coconut oil into their diets can completely negate the carcinogenic effects of the chemicals.[26]

Coconut oil can prevent and even reverse liver disease caused by a variety of toxic agents such as alcohol, bacteria, drugs, and chemicals.[27] It does the same for other organs in the body such as the intestines, colon, kidneys, and pancreas.[28-30]

Even heart health is improved with the use of coconut oil. While much criticism has been cast on coconut oil because of its saturated fat content, the evidence supports its heart friendly nature. MCTs are readily used by the heart as fuel. In fact, it uses MCTs in preference to glucose or polyunsaturated fatty acids as a source of energy. Ketones, as well, which are produced from MCTs act as a superfuel for the heart, increasing oxygen delivery by 39 percent and heart function by 28 percent. In fact, researchers at University François Rabelais in France are now recommending the use of MCTs for the treatment of heart diseases.

They have shown that the diseased heart is energy deficient and by improving oxygen and fuel delivery, heart function and survival is dramatically improved.[31] The fact that coconut oil is not harmful to the heart and may even be therapeutic is substantiated by numerous studies on coconut eating populations where heart disease rates are among the lowest in the world.[32] Many other degenerative diseases are also much lower in these populations such as cancer, diabetes, colitis, liver disease, gallbladder disease, and dementia. Could it be due to the coconut in their diets?

Coconut oil has the potential to aid in the protection and treatment of a number of health problems due to its documented antimicrobial, antioxidant, anti-inflammatory, antiulcerogenic, antimutagenic, analgesic, and antipyretic activities.[33-34] Scientists and pharmaceutical companies have recognized the importance of MCTs and have filed numerous patents for their therapeutic use in the treatment of Alzheimer's disease, cancer, dental caries, periodontal disease, skin diseases, and various bacterial, viral, and fungal infections. Apparently the researchers at these companies feel there is ample scientific evidence to invest their time and money in procuring the legal rights to use them therapeutically.

The health benefits of MCTs are so well documented that the critics cannot argue against their nutritional and medicinal value or safety. However, some will argue that many of the studies were done using fractionated coconut oil or MCT oil, not coconut oil, and therefore, are not representative of the effects of coconut oil. This argument is just a smokescreen to justify the demand for "more evidence."

Since coconut oil is predominately a medium chain triglyceride oil (63%), "the biological effects of coconut oil are a consequence of the presence of these acids," says Hans Kaunitz, MD, professor of pathology at Columbia University Medical School and long time MCT researcher.[35] Because coconut oil is composed predominately of MCTs, it influence on the body is characterized by these fatty acids.

While critics may question if coconut oil has the same therapeutic effects as MCT oil, they will acknowledge that soybean oil is characterized by linoleic acid because it contains 51 percent of this polyunsaturated fatty acid, or that olive oil is a monounsaturated oil because it is 77 percent oleic acid (a monounsaturated fatty acid), or that fish oil (salmon oil in this case) is characterized by omega-3s because it contains 38 percent omega-3 fatty acids, yet it also contains saturated fat (22 percent) and cholesterol (485 mg/100 g).

Likewise, soybean oil and olive oil also contain saturated fats, so they are not pure either, but their character is defined by their predominate fatty acids and their saturated fat content is ignored as inconsequential. Conclusion: coconut oil is an MCT oil and its effects on the body are characterized by these fatty acids. This has been observed time and time again in studies and in clinical settings.

Some of the nutritional and therapeutic benefits of coconut oil come from the saturated fats in the oil, such as its resistance to oxidation, long shelf life, and superior cooking properties. Some come from MCTs such as the antimicrobial effects and its unique mode of digestion and nutrient delivery. However, most of its medicinal benefits undoubtedly come from the ketones produced from the MCTs. The protective effects on the heart, brain, kidneys, colon, pancreas, and other organs, its metabolic boosting and energizing effects, and its anti-cancer, anti-diabetes, anti-Alzheimer's and other effects come principally from ketones.

If you do a search on PubMed for ketones, as they relate to MCTs and diet, you will find about 25,000 studies. Combining these studies with the 10,000 on coconut oil and MCTs, we have a total of over 35,000 studies describing the effects of coconut oil on health. Is that enough evidence? There is far more evidence demonstrating the safety and efficiency of coconut oil than there are for most FDA approved drugs.

Of course, additional studies are welcomed and encouraged, but to state that there is little or no evidence demonstrating the safety and value of coconut oil is simply not true. Coconut oil has been used successfully in traditional medicine for thousands of years, and in western medicine for at least 60 years with no adverse effects. It's been granted GRAS (i.e., generally recognized as safe) status by the FDA.

Regardless of the number of studies available, the real test for the value of coconut oil is how it affects people's lives. Coconut oil is helping thousands of people with various health problems. Here is a typical example. "I was once diagnosed with lupus, lichen planus (lost all 20 nails), ADD, depression, COPD, allergies, atherosclerosis with chest pain, metabolic syndrome, rapidly progressing to full blown diabetes, high CRP, high cholesterol, high triglycerides, chronic fatigue, and fibromyalgia," says Peggy M. "I was living on inhalers, antibiotics, prednisone, antidepressants, sleeping pills, allergy meds and more . . . I began to try

alternative things. I am sooooo thankful to say, I have been using organic coconut oil for several years . . . My thyroid meds continue to be decreased, and I no longer have to take any allergy meds besides shots. I'm afraid to quit them. My breathing problems are totally gone. I have healthy nails, no fibromyalgia, metabolic syndrome, or diabetes."

While testimonies like this may not provide "scientific" proof, tens of thousands of people can attest that coconut oil has changed their lives for the better. Medications may give good results in laboratory settings, yet in real life prove disastrous (i.e., Vioxx). Coconut oil has proven its worth in real life.

Whenever someone says, "Show me the evidence," give him a copy of this article and say "here is the evidence check it out if you want to learn the truth." If they demand more evidence, refer them to books such as *Coconut Cures* or *Stop Alzheimer's Now*. Every health claim made in regard to coconut is backed up by published research and historical facts. Each book includes hundreds of references to medical studies.

You can also send them to www.coconutresearchcenter .org and have them look under the heading "Medical Studies" to access a 25 page listing of some of the 10,000 studies on coconut oil.

References

1. Cunningham, E. Is there science to support claims for coconut oil? *J Am Diet Assoc* 2001;111:786.
2. http://www.drweil.com/drw/u/id/QAA316479
3. McDougall, J. The newest food-cure: Coconut oil for health and vitality. *The McDougall Newsletter* 2006;5:5.
4. Newport, M. Case study: Dietary intervention using coconut oil to produce mild ketosis in a 58 year old APOE4+ male with early onset Alzheimer's disease. 25th International Conference of Alzheimer's Disease International (ADI), March 10–13, 2010, Greece.
5. Salmon, W.D. and Goodman, J.G. Alleviation of vitamin B deficiency in the rat by certain natural fats and synthetic esters. *Journal of Nutrition* 1936;13:477–500.
6. Tantibhedhyangkul, P. and Hashim, S.A. Medium-chain triglyceride feeding in premature infants: Effects on calcium and magnesium absorption. *Pediatrics* 1987;61:537–545.
7. Vaidya, U.V., et al. Vegetable oils fortified feeds in the nutrition of very low birthweight babies. *Indian Pediatr* 1992;29:1519–1527.
8. Wang, X, et al. Enteral nutrition improves clinical outcome and shortens hospital stay after cancer surgery. *J Invest Surg* 2010;23:309–313.

9. Kaunitz. H., et al. Nutritional properties of the triglycerides of medium chain-length. *J Am Oil Chem Soc* 1958;35:10–13.

10. Kiyasu, J.Y., et al. The portal transport of absorbed fatty acids. *J Biol Chem* 1952;199:415–419.

11. Burke, V. and Danks, D.M. Medium-chain triglyceride diet: Its use in treatment of liver disease. *Brit Med J* 1966;2:1050–1051.

12. Kuo, P.T. and Huang, N.N. The effect of medium chain triglyceride upon fat absorption and plasma lipid and depot fat of children with cystic fibrosis of the pancreas. *J Clin Invest* 1965;44:1924–1933.

13. Cancio, M. and Menendez-Corrrada, R. Absorption of medium chain triglycerides in tropical sprue. *Proc Soc Exp Biol* (NY) 1964;117:182–185.

14. Isselbacher, K.J., et al. Congenital beta-lipoprotein deficiency: An hereditary disorder involving a defect in the absorption and transport of lipids. *Medicine* (Baltimore) 1964;43:347–361.

15. Holt, P.R. Dietary treatment of protein loss in intestinal lymphangiectasia. *Pediatrics* 1964;34:629–635.

16. Greenberger, N.J., et al. Use of medium chain triglycerides in malabsorption. *Ann Internal Med* 1967;66:727–734.

17. Zurier, R.B., et al. Use of medium-chain triglyceride in management of patients with massive resection of the small intestine. *New Engl J Med* 1966;274:490–493.

18. Baba, N., et al. Enhanced thermogenesis and diminished deposition of fat in response to overfeeding with diets containing medium chain triglycerides. *Am J Clin Nutr* 1982;35:678–682.

19. St-Onge, M.P. and Jones, P.J. Physiological effects of medium-chain triglycerides: Potential agents in the prevention of obesity. *J Nutr* 2002;132:329–332.

20. Kabara, J.J., et al. Fatty acids and derivatives as antimicrobial agents. *Antimicrobial Agents and Chemotherapy* 1972;2:23–28.

21. Hilmarsson, H., et al. Virucidal effect of lipids on visna virus, a lentivirus related to HIV. *Arch Virol* 2006;151:1217–1224.

22. Kitahara, T., et al. Antimicrobial activity of saturated fatty acids and fatty amines against methicillin-resistant *Staphylococcus aureus*. *Biological & Pharmaceutical Bulletin* 2004;27:1321–1326.

23. Ogbolu, D.O., et al. In vitro antimicrobial properties of coconut oil on Candida species in Ibadan, Nigeria. *J Med Food* 2007;10:384–387.

24. Neal, E.G., et al. A randomized trial of classical and medium-chain triglyceride ketogenic diets in the treatment of childhood epilepsy. *Epilepsia* 2009;50:1109–1117.

25. Eckel, R.H., et al. Dietary substitution of medium-chain triglycerides improves insulin-mediated glucose metabolism in NIDDM subjects. *Diabetes* 1992;41:641–647.

26. Kono, H., et al. Dietary medium-chain triglycerides prevent chemically induced experimental colitis in rats. *Transl Res* 2010;155:131–141.

27. Zakaria, A.A., et al. Hepatoprotective activity of dried- and fermented-processed virgin coconut oil. *Evidence-Based Complementary and Alternative Medicine* 2011;2011:142739.

28. Monserrat, A.J., et al. Protective effect of coconut oil on renal necrosis occurring in rats fed a methyl-deficient diet. *Ren Fail* 1995;17:525–537.

29. Mizushima, T., et al. Prevention of hyperlipidemic acute pancreatitis during pregnancy with medium-chain triglyceride nutritional support. *Int J Pancreatol* 1998;23:187–192.

30. Kono, H., et al. Medium-chain triglycerides enhance secretory IgA expression in rat intestine after administration of endotoxin. *Am J Physiol Gastrointest Liver Physiol* 2004;286:G1081–G1089.

31. Labarthe, F., et al. Medium-chain fatty acids as metabolic therapy in cardiac disease. *Cardiovasc Drugs Ther* 2008;22:97–106.

32. Prior, I.A., et al. Cholesterol, coconuts, and diet of Polynesian atolls: A natural experiment: the Pukapuka and Tokelau island studies. *Am J Clin Nutr* 1981;34:1552–1561.

33. Zakaria, A.A., et al. In vivo antinociceptive and anti-inflammatory activities of dried and fermented processed virgin coconut oil. *Med Princ Pract* 2011;20:231–236.

34. Intahphuak, S., et al. Anti-inflammatory, analgesic, and antipyretic activities of virgin coconut oil. *Pharm Biol* 2010;48:151–157.

35. Kaunitz, H. Nutritional properties of coconut oil. *J Am Oil Chem Soc* 1970;47:462A–466A.

THE COCONUT RESEARCH CENTER, UNDER THE DIRECTION OF DR. BRUCE FIFE, was established to educate the medical profession and the general public about the health and nutritional aspects of coconut and palm products.

William A. Correll   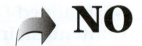 **NO**

FDA Warning Letter to Carrington Farms

David Eben, CEO
Carrington Farms
297 Kinderkamack Road
Suite 101
Oradell, NJ 07649

Re: 431660

Dear Mr. Eben:

This is to advise you that in April 2014, the Food and Drug Administration (FDA) reviewed your product label for Carrington Farms Coconut Oil (54 fl oz). In addition, FDA reviewed labeling on your website at the Internet address http://carringtonfarms.com/ in August 2014 and has determined that you take orders there for the product Carrington Farms Coconut Oil, which both the product label and the website labeling promote for conditions that cause the product to be a "drug" under section 201(g)(1)(B) of the Federal Food, Drug, and Cosmetic Act (the Act) [21 U.S.C. § 321(g)(1)(B)]. The therapeutic claims on your product label and your website labeling establish that the product is a drug because it is intended for use in the cure, mitigation, treatment, or prevention of disease. As explained further below, introducing or delivering this product for introduction into interstate commerce for such uses violates the Act.

Even if your product was not an unapproved new drug, it would be a misbranded food within the meaning of section 403(r)(1) of the Act [21 U.S.C. § 343(r)(1)] as described below.

Unapproved New Drug

Examples of some of the website claims that provide evidence that your product is intended for use as a drug include: Under the webpage titled "Health Benefits":

- "Caprylic acid is considered to have many positive therapeutic qualities—some of which include treating and soothing various infections such as salmonella, ringworm, candidiasis and gastroenteritis . . . Caprylic acid is also excellent for dealing with bacterial infections . . . including certain Streptococcus species and Staphylococcus aureus)."
- "Lauric acid exhibits anti-viral, anti-microbial, and anti-fungal properties."
- "Coconut oil also has been known to: kill bacteria, ease acid reflux . . . lower incidence of hemorrhoids . . . soothes ear aches . . . reduces joint and muscle inflammation."
- "[C]oconut oil may help prevent osteoporosis . . ."
- "Lauric acid [found in coconut oil] has been found to protect your heart by reducing total cholesterol . . ."

Your product is not generally recognized as safe and effective for the above referenced uses and, therefore, the product is a "new drug" under section 201(p) of the Act [21 U.S.C. § 321(p)]. New drugs may not be legally introduced or delivered for introduction into interstate commerce without prior approval from FDA, as described in section 505(a) of the Act [21 U.S.C. § 355(a)]; see also section 301(d) of the Act [21 U.S.C. § 331(d)]. FDA approves a new drug on the basis of scientific data submitted by a drug sponsor to demonstrate that the drug is safe and effective.

Furthermore, your product Carrington Farms Coconut Oil is offered for conditions that are not amenable to self-diagnosis and treatment by individuals who are not medical practitioners; therefore, adequate directions for use cannot be written so that a layperson can use this drug safely for its intended use. Thus, this drug is misbranded within the meaning of section 502(f)(1) of the Act [21 U.S.C. § 352(f)(1)] in that its labeling fails to bear adequate directions for use. The introduction of a misbranded drug into interstate commerce is a violation of section 301(a) of the Act [21 U.S.C. § 331(a)].

Misbranded Food: Nutrient Content Claims

Even if your Carrington Farms Coconut Oil product was not an unapproved drug, it would also be a misbranded food within the meaning of section 403(r)(1)(A) of the Act [21 U.S.C. § 343(r)(1)(A)] because the product label and labeling bear nutrient content claims but do not meet the requirements to make such claims.

Under section 403(r)(1)(A) of the Act [21 U.S.C. § 343(r)(1)(A)], a claim that characterizes the level of a nutrient which is of the type required to be in the labeling of the food must be made in accordance with a regulation promulgated by the Secretary (or, by delegation, FDA) authorizing the use of such a claim. Characterizing the level of a nutrient on food labels and labeling of a product without complying with the specific requirements pertaining to nutrient content claims for that nutrient misbrands the product under section 403(r)(1)(A) of the Act [21 U.S.C. § 343(r)(1)(A)]. Your Carrington Farms Coconut Oil product is misbranded under section 403(r)(1)(A) of the Act because the product label and labeling bear the following nutrient content claims but fail to meet the requirements to make such claims as follows:

1. The label of your Carrington Farms Coconut Oil product bears an implied nutrient content claim, because it bears statements suggesting that because of its nutrient content the product may help consumers maintain healthy dietary practices, and those statements are made in connection with claims or statements about nutrients. The label of your Carrington Farms Coconut Oil product bears the claims "Healthy Foods," "The healthiest oil on earth," "Perfect for healthy . . . cooking," and "Use as a healthy . . . replacement for butter or fat" in connection with the statement "Our unrefined . . . coconut oil is simply pressed and bottled so it retains its original nutrient content . . . No Trans & Hydrogenated Fats." However, this product does not meet the requirements for use of the nutrient content claim "healthy" that are set forth in 21 CFR 101.65(d).

   In accordance with 21 CFR 101.65(d)(2)(i), you may use the term "healthy" as an implied nutrient content claim on the label or in the labeling of a food such as coconut oil provided that the food, among other things, is "low saturated fat" as defined in 21 CFR 101.62(c)(2) (saturated fat content of 1 g or less per Reference Amount Customarily Consumed (RACC) and no more than 15 percent of calories from saturated fat). Furthermore, the product must contain at

least 10 percent of the Daily Value per RACC of one or more of vitamin A, vitamin C, calcium, iron, protein, or fiber.

According to the Nutrition Facts label, this product contains 12 g of saturated fat per tablespoon (14 g) serving of food which is calculated as 83 percent of calories from saturated fat and thus far exceeds the maximum of 1 g of saturated fat per RACC and not more than 15 percent of calories from saturated fat [21 CFR 101.62(c)(2)]. Additionally, according to the Nutrition Facts label this product does not contain at least 10 percent of the Daily Value per RACC of one or more of vitamin A, vitamin C, calcium, iron, protein or fiber. Accordingly, this product does not meet the requirements for the use of the nutrient content claim "healthy" on a food label [21 CFR 101.65(d)(2)].

2. Your website states: "These oils [components of coconut oil] are low in calories."

   Nutrient content claims for calorie content are defined in 21 CFR 101.60. Under 21 CFR 101.60(b)(2), the term "low in calories" may be used on the label or labeling of foods such as coconut oil provided that, among other things, the food does not provide more than 40 calories per RACC and per 50 g. However, according to the Nutrition Facts label, this product contains 130 calories per 14 g serving, which is more than the maximum of 40 calories per RACC and per 50 g allowed under 21 CFR 101.60(b)(2).

3. Your website states: "Coconut oil is rich in antioxidants."

   Nutrient content claims using the term "antioxidant" must comply with the requirements listed in 21 CFR 101.54(g). These requirements state, in part, that for a product to bear such a claim, an RDI must have been established for each of the nutrients that are the subject of the claim [21 CFR 101.54(g)(l)], and these nutrients must have recognized antioxidant activity [21 CFR 101.54(g)(2)]. The level of each nutrient that is the subject of the claim must also be sufficient to qualify for the claim under 21 CFR 101.54(b), (c), or (e) [21 CFR 101.54(g)(3)]. For example, to bear the claim "rich in antioxidant vitamin C," the product must contain 20 percent or more of the RDI for vitamin C under 21 CFR 101.54(b). Such a claim must also include the names of the nutrients that are the subject of the claim as part of the claim or, alternatively, the term "antioxidant" or "antioxidants" may be linked by a symbol (e.g., an asterisk) that refers to the same symbol that appears elsewhere on the same panel of the product label, followed by the name or names of the nutrients with recognized antioxidant activity [21 CPR 101.54(g)(4)]. The antioxidant claim on your website does not indicate the names of the nutrients that are the subject of the claim or link the nutrients with the claim by use of a symbol.

Misbranded Food: Unauthorized Health Claims

Your Carrington Farms Coconut Oil product is also misbranded within the meaning of section 403(r)(l)(B) of the Act because the labeling on your website includes the following unauthorized health claims:

1. "Coconut oil is made up of medium chain fatty acids (MCFA). These fatty acids . . . are known to lower the risk of heart disease and arteriosclerosis."

   There are no health claims authorized by regulation or the Act that provide for claims relating coconut oil or MCFAs to heart disease or arteriosclerosis.

2. "Coconut oil may lower the risk of diabetes, heart disease and improve cholesterol levels. Studies show people who take coconut oil improved their cholesterol profile along with higher HDL levels and higher HDL:LDL ratio."

   Because high blood total- and low density lipoprotein (LDL)-cholesterol levels are associated with increased risk of developing coronary heart disease, the claim that your product "improve(s) cholesterol levels" and "improve[s] [the consumer's] cholesterol profile along with higher HDL levels and higher HDL:LDL ratio" implies that your product is intended for use in the treatment, mitigation, and prevention of coronary heart disease. There are no health claims authorized by regulation or the Act that provide for claims relating coconut oil to coronary heart disease. There are also no health claims authorized by regulation or the Act that provide for claims relating coconut oil to diabetes.

The above violations are not meant to be an all-inclusive list of violations that exist in connection with your products or their labeling. It is your responsibility to ensure that all of your products are in compliance with the Act and its implementing regulations. You should take prompt action to correct the violations cited in this letter and to prevent their reoccurrence. Failure to promptly correct the violations may result in legal action without further notice, such as seizure or injunction.

In addition to the violations cited above, we offer the following comments:

1. The statement for the place of business does not include the street address in accordance with 21 CFR 101.5(d). We note that the street address may be omitted if it is shown in a current city directory or telephone directory.

2. Your Carrington Farms Coconut Oil bears the claim "No Trans & Hydrogenated Fat," and we note that your ingredient statement lists coconut oil and does not include a partially hydrogenated oil as an ingredient in the ingredient list. Under section 403(r)(1)(A) of the Act, a nutrient content claim in food labeling must be made in accordance with a regulation authorizing the use of the claim in order for the food bearing such claim not to be misbranded. Although FDA has not defined the term "no trans-fat" by regulation, we announced in the *Federal Register* dated July 11, 2003 [68 FR 41507 at 41509] that we would likely consider exercising enforcement discretion for a trans-fat nutrient content claim that is demonstrably true, balanced, adequately substantiated, and not misleading.

Scientific evidence suggests that trans-fat acts in a similar manner to saturated fat with respect to raising LDL cholesterol [68 FR 41445 at 41456 (July 11, 2003)]. Higher total and LDL cholesterol levels are associated with increased risk of developing coronary heart disease [68 FR 41445 (July 11, 2003)]. Under 21 CFR 101.13(h), if a food bears a nutrient content claim and also contains more than 13.0 grams of fat, 4.0 grams of saturated fat, 60 milligrams cholesterol, and 480 milligrams of sodium per reference amount customarily consumed (RACC), per labeled serving (or for a food with a RACC of 30 grams or less or 2 tablespoons or less, per 50 grams), then the food must bear a statement disclosing that the nutrient exceeding the specified level is present in the food as follows: "See nutrition information for _____ content" with the blank replaced with the identity of the nutrient exceeding the specified level. Your Carrington Farms Coconut Oil contains 12 g of saturated fat per RACC (1 tbsp. serving) but does not contain the disclosure statement "See nutrition information for saturated fat content."

We intend to consider the exercise of our enforcement discretion for the use of the "No Trans & Hydrogenated Fat" claim on Carrington Farms Coconut Oil provided the claim includes a disclosure statement, in accordance with the requirements in 21 CFR 101.13(h). We will review such claims on a case-by-case basis.

Please respond to this letter within 15 working days from receipt with the actions you plan to take in response to this letter, including an explanation of each step being taken to correct the current violations and prevent similar violations. Include any documentation necessary to show that correction has been achieved. If you cannot complete corrective action within 15 working days, state the reason for the delay and the time within which you will complete the corrections.

You should direct your written reply to Carrie Lawlor, Food and Drug Administration, Center for Food Safety and Applied Nutrition, 5100 Paint Branch Parkway, Office of Compliance (HFS-608), Division of Enforcement, College Park, Maryland 20740-3835. If you have any questions regarding this letter, you may contact Ms. Lawlor via email at carrie.lawlor@fda.hhs.gov.

Sincerely,

/S/
William A. Correll, Jr.
Director
Office of Compliance
Center for Food Safety and Applied Nutrition

William Correll is Director, Office of Compliance at Center for Food Safety and Applied Nutrition of the Food and Drug Administration.

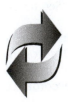

EXPLORING THE ISSUE

Does Coconut Oil Provide Health Benefits?

Critical Thinking and Reflection

1 Using PubMed or a search engine for scientific or academic research, find a peer-reviewed article that describes a study that examines virgin coconut oil (or caprilyc, capric, or lauric acid) and some aspect of health. Write a summary of the article.

2 Visit your local grocery store and compare the Nutrition Facts labels and ingredient lists of the regular coconut oil to virgin or extra virgin coconut oil. Also, compare the prices.

3 Using Index Mundi, compare the coconut oil consumption in the United States to other oils and describe the affect that the 2013 Typhoon Haiyan has had on coconut oil consumption.

4 The "YES" article was written by authors of the "Coconutresearchcenter.org." They included the disclaimer, "This website is for educational purposes only. The information supplied here comes from a variety of sources and authors and not every statement made has been evaluated by the FDA. This information is not intended to diagnose, treat, cure or prevent any disease." Select one of the claims made about coconut oil and find two other articles from reliable sources that either support or refute their claims.

5 The coconut industry is a major source of income for populations in many tropical areas. Using the United Nations Conference on Trade and Development's website, describe which countries produce the greatest amount of coconuts, how coconut trees are grown, and the products that are produced from coconuts.

Is There Common Ground?

Both the Coconut Research Center (CRC) and FDA are concerned about the health and well-being of the people they serve. The problem begins with the differences between whom they serve and the goals of both entities. The CRC was developed to "dispel the myths surrounding coconut and palm products and to present a more accurate and scientific viewpoint." They go on to claim that the health benefits of coconut "are so numerous and so remarkable that this information needs to be available to all." One can assume they serve the coconut oil industry, such as Carrington Farms. Many of the claims that the FDA considers to be unsubstantiated on Carrington's website and their coconut oil labels are similar to claims on the CRC site.

In contrast, the goal of FDA is to "protect consumers and enhance public health by maximizing compliance of FDA regulated products and minimizing risk associated with those products." The coconut oil craze is relatively new, especially in the United States. Even the *Scientific Report of the 2015 Dietary Guidelines Advisory Committee* (*DGAC*) acknowledges that there are many unknowns about virgin coconut oil. In the DGAC report, one area in the "Needs for Future Research" is:

Topic: Examine the effects of saturated fat from different sources, including animal products (e.g.,

butter, lard), plant (e.g., palm vs. coconut oils), and production systems (e.g., refined deodorized bleached vs. virgin coconut oil) on blood lipids and cardiovascular disease risk.

Rationale: Different sources of saturated fat contain different fatty acid profiles and thus, may result in different lipid and metabolic effects. In addition, virgin and refined coconut oils have different effects in animal models, but human data are lacking.

Currently, we do not know about the long-term effects of coconut oil and health. And "virgin coconut oil" may affect the body in a totally different way than refined coconut oil. Based on the FDA letter, "virgin coconut oil" is not mentioned—only "coconut oil." FDA is taking a prudent stance and complying with its mission to protect the public. One might consider CRC as more progressive in its stance.

Additional Resources

Babu AS, Veluswamy SK, Arena R, Guazzi M, Lavie CJ. Virgin coconut oil and its potential cardioprotective effects. *Postgrad Med.* 2014;126(7):76–83.

Fernando WM, Martins IJ, Goozee KG, Brennan CS, Jayasena V, Martins RN. The role of dietary coconut for the prevention and treatment of Alzheimer's disease: Potential mechanisms of action. *Br J Nutr.* 2015;114(1):1–14.

Law KS, Azman N, Omar EA, et al. The effects of virgin coconut oil (VCO) as supplementation on quality of life (QOL) among breast cancer patients. *Lipids Health Dis.* 2014;13:139.

Shilling M, Matt L, Rubin E, et al. Antimicrobial effects of virgin coconut oil and its medium-chain fatty acids on *Clostridium difficile. J Med Food.* 2013;16(12):1079–85.

Internet References . . .

Coconut Oil Research Center

coconutresearchcenter.org

Food and Drug Administration (FDA)

www.fda.gov

Index Mundi

www.indexmundi.com

Organic Facts

www.organicfacts.net/

Republic of the Philippines Department of Agriculture

www.da.gov.ph/

United Nations Conference on Trade and Development

www.unctad.org

Selected, Edited, and with Issue Framing Materials by:
Janet M. Colson, *Middle Tennessee State University*

ISSUE

Should Physicians Use BMI to Assess Overall Health?

YES: Jeremy Singer-Vine, from "Beyond BMI: Why Doctors Won't Stop Using an Outdated Measure for Obesity," *Slate* (2009)

NO: Keith Devlin, from "Do You Believe in Fairies, Unicorns, or the BMI?" *Devlin's Angle* (2009)

Learning Outcomes
After reading this issue, you will be able to: • Outline how and when the BMI formula was developed. • Discuss the mathematical and health-related criticisms of using BMI as an indicator of health status. • Explain why BMI is currently used by physicians and the medical community to assess weight status.

ISSUE SUMMARY

YES: Journalist Jeremy Singer-Vine points out "the circumference around a person's waist provides a much more accurate reading of his or her abdominal fat and risk for disease than BMI." He also acknowledges that waist measurements require slightly more time and training than it takes to record a BMI; however, because BMI is cheap and easy to use, physicians and the medical community will continue using it.

NO: Mathematician Keith Devlin, who is labeled as "overweight" by his physician because his BMI is 25.1, despite his 32 inch waist, considers that BMI is "numerological nonsense." While he applauds the knowledge that physicians have about the human body and health issues, he feels that the mathematics behind the BMI calculations are used irresponsibly and says BMI should not be used in medical practice. He calls for mathematicians to demand responsible use of math.

The mathematical formula to determine BMI was developed almost 200 years ago, but was not widely used to define weight status until the 1980s. Its popularity is credited to Ancel Keys who wrote the "Indices of Relative Weight and Obesity" that was published in the July 1972 issue of *Journal of Chronic Disease*. The results of his landmark study have become one of the most debated topics related to obesity. Based on data from more than 7400 men in five countries, Keys examined which of the height-weight formulas matched up best with each subject's body-fat percentage. It turned out that the best predictor came from the Quetelet Index, developed in 1832. Keys renamed it the "body mass index," and the rest is history.

Before BMI, doctors generally used weight-for-height tables, one for men and one for women, which included ranges of body weights for each inch of height. The tables were originally developed by the Association of Life Insurance Medical Directors of America in 1897 and refined by the Metropolitan Life Insurance Company in 1943. They provide a weight range based on frame size, with desirable weight higher as frame size increases. One of the criticisms with the tables was that a decision had to be made to determine if the person had a small, medium, or large frame. The larger the frame, the more weight a person could weigh, and many people would classify themselves as "large" framed to prevent being in the overweight category.

BMI became an international standard for obesity measurement in the 1980s. The public learned about BMI in the late 1990s, when the government launched an initiative to encourage healthy eating and exercise.

Originally, a BMI of 27.8 and above was used to define "overweight" for men while women with a BMI of 27.3 or higher classified as overweight. In 1998, the National Institutes of Health (NIH) lowered the overweight threshold to 25 to match international guidelines. The move added 30 million Americans who were previously in the "healthy weight" category to the "overweight" category. Today, the NIH advises doctors to include BMI in a complete assessment of a person's overall health. The 2000 NIH report *The Practical Guide: Identification, Evaluation, and Treatment of Overweight and Obesity in Adults* includes the following recommendation for physicians:

> Assessment of a patient should include the evaluation of body mass index (BMI), waist circumference, and overall medical risk. . . . There is evidence to support the use of BMI in risk assessment since it provides a more accurate measure of total body fat compared with the assessment of body weight alone. Neither bioelectric impedance nor height-weight tables provide an advantage over BMI in the clinical management of all adult patients, regardless of gender. Clinical judgment must be employed when evaluating very muscular patients because BMI may overestimate the degree of fatness in these patients. The recommended classifications for BMI [were] adopted by the Expert Panel on the Identification, Evaluation, and Treatment of Overweight and Obesity in Adults and endorsed by leading organizations of health professionals.

Is BMI valuable in assessing health and should it be part of routine health assessments? As you read the following articles, decide why BMI has become the "standard measure" to determine weight status, the pitfalls associated with it, and why physicians continue to use it.

TIMELINE

1832 Belgian's Adolphe Quetelet devises the Quetelet Index.

1897 A standard height and weight table is adopted by the Association of Life Insurance Medical Directors of America.

1942 The Metropolitan Life Insurance Company introduces their standard height-weight tables for men and women.

1972 Ancel Keys publishes "Indices of Relative Weight and Obesity" in the July issue of *Journal of Chronic Disease* and coins the term "body mass index" (BMI) which use Quetelet's Index to assess weight status.

1985 CDC adopts BMI to describe weight status using BMI over 27.8 for men and 27.3 for women to define overweight.

1998 NIH lowers "overweight" BMI threshold from 27.8 to 25 to match international (WHO) guidelines.

YES ↵

Jeremy Singer-Vine

Beyond BMI: Why Doctors Won't Stop Using an Outdated Measure for Obesity

A few extra pounds can extend your life. Or so chirped the press, reporting on a recent study from the journal *Obesity*. The new research, which supports earlier findings that being slightly overweight is associated with living longer, has added to an ongoing controversy over how we measure obesity. At the center of this debate is the body mass index, a simple equation (your weight in kilograms divided by the square of your height in meters) that has in the last decade claimed a near-monopoly on obesity statistics. Some researchers now argue that this flawed and overly reductive measure is skewing the results of research in public health.

For years, critics of the body mass index have griped that it fails to distinguish between lean and fatty mass. (Muscular people are often misclassifed as overweight or obese.) The measure is mum, too, about the distribution of body fat, which makes a big difference when it comes to health risks. And the BMI cutoffs for "underweight," "normal," "overweight," and "obese" have an undeserved air of mathematical authority. So how did we end up with such a lousy statistic?

Belgian polymath Adolphe Quetelet devised the equation in 1832 in his quest to define the "normal man" in terms of everything from his average arm strength to the age at which he marries. This project had nothing to do with obesity-related diseases, nor even with obesity itself. Rather, Quetelet used the equation to describe the standard proportions of the human build—the ratio of weight to height in the average adult. Using data collected from several hundred countrymen, he found that weight varied not in direct proportion to height (such that, say, people 10 percent taller than average were 10 percent heavier, too) but in proportion to the square of height. (People 10 percent taller than average tended to be about 21 percent heavier.)

The new equation had little impact among the medical community until long after Quetelet's death. While doctors had suspected the ill effects of obesity since at least as far

back as the 18th century, their evidence was anecdotal. The first large-scale studies of obesity and health were conducted in the early 20th century, when insurance companies began using comparisons of height and weight among their policy-holders to show that "overweight" people died earlier than those of "ideal" weight. Subsequent actuarial and medical studies found that obese people were also more likely to get diabetes, hypertension, and heart disease.

By the early 1900s, it was well-established that these ailments were the result of having too much adipose tissue—so the studies used functions of height and weight as little more than a proxy for determining how much excess body fat people had. It would have been more accurate for the actuaries to compare longevity data with more direct assessments of body fat—such as caliper-measured skinfold thickness or hydrostatic weighing. But these data were much harder for them to obtain than standard information on height, weight, and sex.

The insurance tables gave us correlations between these physical characteristics and expected lifespan. But medical researchers needed a standard measure of fatness, so they could look at the health outcomes of varying degrees of obesity across an entire population. For decades doctors couldn't agree on the best formula for combining height and weight into a single number—some used weight divided by height; others used weight divided by height cubed. Then, in 1972, physiology professor and obesity researcher Ancel Keys published his "Indices of Relative Weight and Obesity," a landmark study of more than 7,400 men in five countries. Keys examined which of the height-weight formulas matched up best with each subject's body-fat percentage, as measured more directly. It turned out that the best predictor came from Quetelet: weight divided by height squared. Keys renamed this number the *body mass index*.

The new measure caught on among researchers who had previously relied on slower and more expensive measures of body fat or on the broad categories (underweight, ideal weight, and overweight) identified by the insurance companies. The cheap and easy BMI test allowed them to plan and execute ambitious new studies involving hundreds of thousands of participants and to go back through troves of historical height and weight data and estimate levels of obesity in previous decades.

Gradually, though, the popularity of BMI spread from epidemiologists who used it for studies of population health to doctors who wanted a quick way to measure body fat in individual patients. By 1985, the NIH started defining obesity according to body mass index, on the theory that official cutoffs could be used by doctors to warn patients who were at especially high risk for obesity-related illness. At first, the thresholds were established at the 85th percentile of BMI for each sex: 27.8 for men and 27.3 for women. (Those numbers now represent something more like the 50th percentile for Americans.) Then, in 1998, the NIH changed the rules: They consolidated the threshold for men and women, even though the relationship between BMI and body fat is different for each sex, and added another category, "overweight." The new cutoffs—25 for overweight, 30 for obesity—were nice, round numbers that could be easily remembered by doctors and patients.

Keys had never intended for the BMI to be used in this way. His original paper warned against using the body mass index for individual diagnoses, since the equation ignores variables like a patient's gender or age, which affect how BMI relates to health. It's one thing to estimate the average percent body fat for large groups with diverse builds, Keys argued, but quite another to slap a number and label on someone without regard for these factors.

Now Keys' misgivings are gaining traction across the world of medicine: BMI simply doesn't work when it comes to individual measurements. Whether that's a problem worth worrying about is another question. Some researchers say BMI's inaccuracies in individual measurements result in little actual harm, since an attentive doctor can spot outliers and adjust her diagnosis accordingly. But this begs the question: If a doctor's eye is better than BMI at determining a patient's healthy weight, then why use BMI for individuals at all?

No matter how attentive they might be, health professionals have increasingly used body mass index to justify lifestyle recommendations for their patients. And online BMI calculators—there's even one hosted by the NIH—invite people to diagnose themselves without any medical supervision whatsoever. Faulty readings could promote a negative self-image among healthy people and lead them to pursue unnecessary diets. Or the opposite problem: People with a little too much body fat might be lulled into a false sense of complacency by a misleading BMI.

A recent critique (PDF) of the body mass index in the journal *Circulation* suggests that BMI's imprecision and publicity-friendly cutoffs may distort even the large epidemiological studies. (There's no definitive count of how many people are misclassified by BMI, but several studies have suggested that the error rate is significant for people of certain ages and ethnicities.) It's impossible to know which studies have been affected and in what direction they might have been skewed.

Our continuing reliance on BMI is especially grating given there's a very reasonable alternative. It turns out that the circumference around a person's waist provides a much more accurate reading of his or her abdominal fat and risk for disease than BMI. And wrapping a tape measure around your gut is no more expensive than hopping on a scale and standing in front of a ruler. That's why the American Society for Nutrition, the American Diabetes Association, and other prominent medical groups have lately promoted waist circumference measurements as a supplement to, or replacement for, the body mass index.

Yet few doctors have made the switch. The waist measurements require slightly more time and training than it takes to record a BMI reading, and they don't come with any official cutoffs that can be used to make easy assessments. The sensitivity of doctors to these slight inconveniences signals just how difficult it will be to unseat Quetelet's equation. The body mass index is cheap and easy, and it has the incumbent advantage. In short, BMI is here to stay—despite, but also because of, its flaws.

JEREMY SINGER-VINE is a journalist and computer programmer with the New York City–based *Slate* and writes the "Research Report" for the *Wall Street Journal*. He also develops multimedia projects and edits *Slate's* environmental coverage.

Keith Devlin   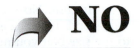 **NO**

Do You Believe in Fairies, Unicorns, or the BMI?

... [T]he Centers for Disease Control and Prevention classify people as overweight on a number called the body mass index, or BMI]. Overweight, according to this CDC endorsed metric, are athletes and movie stars Kobe Bryant, George Clooney, Matt Damon, Johnny Depp, Brad Pitt, Will Smith, and Denzel Washington. Tom Cruise scored even worse, being classified as downright obese, as was Arnold Shwarzenegger when he was a world champion body-builder. With definitions like that, no wonder Americans think of themselves as having an overweightness epidemic. (Using the CDC's BMI measure, 66 percent of adults in the United States are considered overweight or obese.)

Yes, it's that time of year again, when I go for my annual physical. I know the routine. My body mass index regularly comes out at around 25.1, putting me just into the "overweight category," and the doctor sends me a fact sheet telling me I need to lose weight, exercise more, and watch my diet. Notwithstanding the fact that the person *he has just examined* has a waist of 32 inches, rides a bicycle in the California mountains between 120 and 160 miles a week, competes regularly in competitive bicycle events up to 120 miles, does regular upper-body work, has a resting pulse of 59 beats per minute, blood pressure generally below 120/80, healthy cholesterol levels, and eats so much broccoli I would not be surprised to wake up one morning to find it sprouting out of my ears. . . . No, I'm not a "fitness junkie." And I am certainly not a professional athlete. I'm just a fairly ordinary guy who was lucky to be born with good genes and who likes being outdoors on my bike when the weather is nice, and I have a competitive streak that makes me want to race every now and then. A not atypical Californian academic, in fact.)

Why do we have this annual BMI charade? Why would otherwise well-educated medical professionals ignore the evidence of their own eyes? Because the BMI is one of those all-powerful magic entities: a *number*. And not just any number, but one that is generated by a *mathematical formula*. So it has to be taken seriously, right?

Sadly, despite that fact that completion of a calculus course is a necessary prerequisite for entry into medical school, the medical profession often seems no less susceptible than the general population to a misplaced faith in anything that looks mathematical, and at times displays unbelievable naivety when it comes to numbers.

(Actually, my own physician is smarter than that. I chose him because he is every bit as compulsive an outdoorsy, activities person as I am, and he seems to know that the BMI routine we go through is meaningless, though the system apparently requires that he play along and send me the "You need to lose weight and exercise more" letter, despite our having spent a substantial part of the consultation discussing our respective outdoors activities.)

So what is the BMI? A quick web search on "BMI" or "body mass index" will return hundreds of sites, many of which offer calculators to determine your BMI. All you do is feed in your height and your weight, and out comes that magic number. Many of the sites also give you a helpful guide so you can interpret the results. For instance, the CDC website gives these ranges:

below 18.5 = Underweight

18.5 to 24.9 = Ideal

25.0 to 29.9 = Overweight

30.0 and above = Obese

(Tom Cruise, with a height of 5'7" and weight of 201 lbs, has a body mass index of 31.5, while the younger Schwarzenegger, at just over six feet tall and about 235 pounds, had a BMI over 31. The figures I quote for athletes and movie stars are from data available on the web, and I believe they are accurate, or were when the information was entered.)

Some sites even tell you how this mystical number is calculated:

$$BMI = \text{weight in pounds} / (\text{height in inches} \times \text{height in inches}) \times 703$$

Hmmm. No mention of waist-size here? Or rump? That's odd. Isn't the amount of body fat you carry related to the size belt you need to wear or how baggy is the seat of the jeans the belt holds up?

And what about the stuff inside the body? One thing all those "overweight" and "obese" athletes and movie stars have in common is that they have very little fat and a lot of muscle, and possibly also stronger, healthier bones. Now, a quick web-search reveals that mean density figures for these three body component materials are: fat 0.9 gm/ml, muscle 1.06 gm/ml, and bone 1.85. In other words, the less fat you have, and the more your body weight is made up of muscle and bone, the greater the numerator in that formula, and the higher your BMI. In other words, if you are a fit, healthy individual with little body fat but strong bones and lots of muscle, the CDC (and other medical authorities) will classify you as overweight. Note the absurdity of the whole approach. If I actually did take my physician's BMI-triggered, form-letter advice and exercise more, I would put on even more muscle and lose even more of what little body fat I have, and my BMI would increase! With a medical profession like that, who needs high cholesterol as an enemy?

Admittedly, those same authorities also say that a male waistline of 40 inches and a female waistline of 35 inches are where "overweight" begins. But this of course is totally inconsistent with their claim that the BMI is a reliable indicator of excess body fat. In contrast, it is consistent with my observation that it is the density of the stuff inside the body that is key, not the body weight. If you ignore that wide variation in densities, then of course you will end up classifying people with 32 inch waists as overweight. Yet this blatant inconsistency does not seem to cause anyone to pause and ask if there is not something just a little odd going on here. Isn't it time to inject some science into this part of medical practice?

Time to take a look at that BMI formula and ask where it came from. I've already noted that it ignores waistline, rump-size, and the different densities of fat, muscle, and bone. Next question: Why does it mysteriously *square* the height? What possible *scientific* reason could there be to square someone's height for heaven's sake? (Multiplying height by girth at least has some rationale, as it would give an indication of total body volume, but it would put girth into the denominator in the formula, which is not what you want.) But height squared? Beats me.

Then there is that mysterious number 703. Most websites simply state it as if it were some physical constant. A few make the helpful remark that it is a "conversion factor." But I could not find a single source that explains what exactly it is converting. It did not take long to figure

it out, however. The origins of the BMI, of which more later, goes back to a Belgian mathematician. The original formula would thus have been in metric units, say

$$BMI = \text{weight in kilograms}/(\text{height in meters} \times \text{height in meters})$$

To give an equivalent formula in lbs and inches, you need to solve the following equation for C

$$1\text{lb}/(1\text{in} \times 1\text{in}) \times C = 0.4536\text{kg}/(0.0254\text{m} \times 0.0254\text{m})$$

which gives C = 703 (to the nearest whole number).

Well that at least explains the 703. Sort of. But given that the formula is self-evidently just a kludge, why not round it to 700. Stating it as 703 gives an air of accuracy the formula cannot possibly merit, and suggests that the folks who promote this piece of numerological nonsense either have no real understanding of numbers or they want to blind us by what they think we will accept as science.

Another question: Why is the original metric formula expressed in terms of kilograms and meters? Why not grams and centimeters? Or some other units? Well, given the scientific absurdity of dividing someone's weight by the square of their height it really doesn't matter what the units are. I suspect the ones chosen were so that the resulting number comes out between 1 and 100, and thus looks reassuringly like a percentage. I'm beginning to suspect my "blind-us-with-science" conspiracy theory may be right after all.

So which clown first dreamt up this formula and why? Well, it was actually no clown at all, but one of the smartest mathematicians in history: the Belgian polymath Lambert Adolphe Jacques Quetelet (1796–1874). Quetelet received a doctorate in mathematics from the University of Ghent in 1819, and went on to do world class work in mathematics, astronomy, statistics, and sociology. Indeed, he was one of the founders of both these last two disciplines, being arguably the first person to use statistical methods to draw conclusions about societies.

It is to Quetelet that we can trace back that important figure in twentieth century society, the "average man." (You know, the one with 2.4 children.) He (Quetelet, not the average man) realized that the most efficient way to organize society, allocate resources, etc. was to count and measure the population, using statistical methods to determine the (appropriate) "averages." He looked for mathematical formulas that would correlate, *numerically,* with those "average citizens."

(Elementary) statistics being the highly simplistic (but extremely powerful) tool[,] it is generally not difficult to find simple formulas that correlate pretty well with society's averages. You just play around with a few variables until you find a formula that fits. If you can provide a scientific rationale for the formula, so much the better, and you are justified in having more confidence in your ability to use the formula predictively. But it is generally enough that your formula is empirically representative. *Provided* that all you are doing is trying to draw conclusions about society as a whole . . . Quetelet knew what he was doing. Many since then, including, it appears, the CDC, do not.

The absurdity of using statistical formulas to make *any* claim about a single individual is made clear by the old joke about the man who had his head in the refrigerator and his feet in the fire: on average he felt fine!

Yet the CDC says, on its website,

"BMI is a reliable indicator of body fatness for people."

Nonsense. It is off-the-charts unreliable for me and for millions of people like me. True, a few sentences later, the CDC—doubtless at the insistence of their lawyers—says

"However, BMI is not a diagnostic tool."

You're telling me! Come on guys, either the BMI is, as you claim, "a reliable indicator of body fatness," in which case you can so use it or, as you also admit, it cannot be used to diagnose excess body fat. Which is it to be?

The CDC's answer becomes clear as we read on. Lest we note the disclaimer that the BMI cannot be used to diagnose excess body fat and demand a more reliable procedure, they immediately go on to mask their legal get-out by claiming,

Calculating BMI is one of the best methods for population assessment of overweight and obesity. Because calculation requires only height and weight, it is inexpensive and easy to use for clinicians and for the general public. The use of BMI allows people to compare their own weight status to that of the general population.

I'll say it again. This statement is completely false; there are several *much* better methods—some of which the CDC actually lists on its website! The only part of this second statement that I see as having any validity is the very telling admission that the BMI method is inexpensive and easy to use.

There is another problem with the manner in which the CDC and other medical authorities explain the BMI. Notice that the interpretive ranges into the categories

underweight, ideal, etc. are given to one decimal place, with equal signs. This suggests a level of precision in the formula that cannot possibly be warranted. (Some sites give two decimal places.) It would at least be more honest to give the ranges like this:

below 19 you are likely to be underweight

between 19 and 25 is the range generally viewed as ideal

between 25 and 30 suggests you may be overweight

if you are above 30 you are likely to be obese

This would not make the formula any less a piece of numerological junk, but at least would indicate that the ranges are just rough guidelines. The only possible reason for giving the ranges in the precise way the CDC does is to try to mislead patients that there is something scientific going on here. It's a classic example of "lying with numbers."

So here is the beef (lean, of course). The BMI was formulated, *by a mathematician, not a medical physician,* to provide a simple, easy-to-apply mathematical formula to give a broad, society-level measure of weight issues. It has absolutely no scientific or medical basis. It is based purely on a crude statistical analysis. It measures a general society trend, it does not predict. Since the majority of people today (and in Quetelet's time) lead fairly sedentary lives, and are not particularly active, the formula tacitly assumes low muscle mass and high relative fat content. It applies moderately well when applied to such people because it was formulated by focusing on them! Duh!

But this is not science—it's not even good statistics—and as a result it should not be accepted medical practice, to be regularly flouted as some magical mumbo jumbo and used as a basis for giving advice to patients. (For heavens sake, even seven times Tour de France winner Lance Armstrong's own Livestrong website provides a BMI calculator, despite the fact that the boss himself, when he first became a world champion cyclist—before chemotherapy for cancer took 20 lbs off him—found himself classified as "overweight" by the wretched formula.)

As you might expect, once a piece of numerological nonsense is held up for proper scrutiny, it doesn't take long before the whole house of cards comes tumbling down. The surprising thing about the BMI is that it has survived for so long (as a diagnostic for individual patients). As I indicated earlier, I suspect that much of the appeal is that it is a single number, easy to calculate, given an air of scientific authority by a *mathematical formula,* and (just as my earlier quote from the CDC makes clear) it is easier and quicker to base a diagnosis on a number than on properly examining a patient. But at that point you have stopped doing medicine and are just doing kindergarten arithmetic.

The good news is, at last there is hope of some sanity entering the story. The science (the real science) is finally coming. For instance, a study of 33,000 American adults, published recently in the *American Journal of Public Health* (Vol 96, No. 1, January 2006, 173–178), showed that male life expectancy is greatest for BMIs of about 26—overweight under the CDC's rule, and equivalent to 24 lb extra for the typical man. For women, the study found an optimum BMI of about 23.5, about 7 lbs heavier than the CDC's standard.

The paper's author, Dr Jerome Gronniger, a government scientist, concluded that, "I found that the current definitions of obesity and overweight are imprecise predictors of mortality risk."

"Imprecise predictors"? Gronniger was clearly using "scientific understatement." It was, after all, a scientific publication. Dr David Haslam, the clinical director of Britain's National Obesity Forum was more blatant in a statement he made to the Daily Telegraph newspaper: "It's now widely accepted that the BMI is *useless* for assessing the healthy weight of individuals." (My italics.) [In the UK, it's almost impossible to be sued, and there is no massive lobby of medical insurance companies looking for ways to avoid paying for your medical treatment, so commentators tend to be more forthcoming.]

Of course, any mathematician surely knew what Haslam now confirms the moment he or she took their first look at Quetelet's formula. It screams "junk math."

Numbers are one of the most powerful tools we have to understand our world and to improve our lives. But like all powerful tools, when used irresponsibly, they can do more harm than good. Medical professionals have enormous knowledge and experience that we all benefit from. I do regularly go for my annual physical, and for the most part I listen to my physician's advice. He knows a lot more than I do about the human body and health issues. I trust him—for the most part. But when the BMI comes up, we are definitely into territory where my expertise trumps his, and I can recognize a piece of numerological nonsense when I see it, and as a result I ignore that part of the proceedings. But if trained medical practitioners, backed up by august professional organizations such as a the CDC, are still so over-awed by such rubbish (mathematics does that to people, I see it all the time) that they continue to preach it as if it were gospel, then how can a patient with less mathematical sophistication hope to resist this annual incantation.

Since the entire sorry saga of the BMI was started by a mathematician—one of us—I think the onus is on us, as the world's experts on the formulation and application of mathematical formulas, to start to eradicate this nonsense and demand the responsible use of our product.

Heavens, next thing we know, some authority will be claiming that the golden ratio is the aspect ratio of the rectangle most pleasing to the human eye. Where will it all end?

After all that, I think I need a good long bike ride over the mountains to bring my blood pressure down.

KEITH DEVLIN is senior researcher for the Center for the Study of Language and Information and was founder and currently executive director of H-STAR Institute at Stanford. He received his PhD in Mathematics from University of Bristol, U.K.

EXPLORING THE ISSUE

Should Physicians Use BMI to Assess Overall Health?

Critical Thinking and Reflection

1. Describe how the BMI formula was developed.
2. List the strengths and weaknesses of using BMI to assess the health status of an adult.
3. You have been asked to conduct a study to determine the prevalence of overweight and obesity of students at your university. Ideally, you need to include at least 1000 students in your study. Outline the steps you would take to gather and assess the weight status and the methods you would use.
4. Compare the probable health status of a man whose BMI is 31 and has a waist circumference of 35.5 inches to a non-pregnant woman whose BMI is 27 and waist circumference is 36 inches.
5. What is your opinion on use of BMI for weight assessment by physicians and in other health care practices? Write a letter to NIH explaining your position on the topic; include specific suggestions to either change the method or strengthen the existing one.

Is There Common Ground?

Both authors point out that BMI is not an accurate method to label a person as being underweight, normal weight, or obese. However, because use of BMI is cheap and easy to use, both agree that physicians and the medical community will continue to use it and are even encouraged to determine the BMI on routine health check-ups. Frequently, insurance companies require the BMI of individuals when completing eligibility applications.

Both authors agree that the medical community needs a better way to assess health based on body size. Waist circumference is a better indicator, but requires more time to assess. More recently, use of the waist-to-height ratio, or even waist-to-neck ratio, is becoming commonplace and may replace use of the waist circumference alone.

Additional Resources

Akin I, Nienaber CA. "Obesity paradox" in coronary artery disease. *World J Cardiol*. 2015; 7(10):603–8.

Carmienke S, Freytag MH, Piston T, et al. General and abdominal obesity parameters and their combination in relation to mortality: A systematic review and meta-regression analysis. *Ear J Clan Nutria*. 2013;67(6):573–85.

Chang Y, Guo X, Li T, Li S, Guo J, Sun Y. A body shape index and body roundness index: Two new body indices to identify left ventricular hypertrophy among rural populations in northeast China. *Heart Lung Circ*. 2015. doi: +10.1016/j.hlc.2015.08.009.

Dhana K, Kavousi M, Ikram MA, Tiemeier HW, Hofman A, Franco OH. Body shape index in comparison with other anthropometric measures in prediction of total and cause-specific mortality. *J Epidemiol Community Health*. 2015. doi: +10.1136/jech-2014-205257.

Sahakyan KR, Somers VK, Rodriguez-Escudero JP, et al. Normal-weight central obesity: Implications for total and cardiovascular mortality. *Ann Intern Med*. 2015.doi: +10.7326/M14-2525

Tanamas SK, Lean ME, Combet E, Vlassopoulos A, Zimmet PZ, Peeters A. Changing guards: Time to move beyond Body Mass Index for population monitoring of excess adiposity. *QJM*. 2015. doi: http://dx.doi.org/10.1093/qjmed/hcv201.

Internet References . . .

Centers for Disease Control and Prevention

www.cdc.gov

National Heart, Lung, and Blood Institute

www.nhlbi.nih.gov

Penn State Hershey PRO Wellness Center

http://prowellness.vmhost.psu.edu

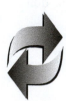

Unit 3

UNIT

Our Food Supply

*W*hat we eat depends largely on foods that are available. Therefore, the food industry has a tremendous influence on the nation's nutritional status. The leading food manufacturers employ food and nutrition experts to formulate new products and recipes—and most have a marketing team to persuade the public to eat their company's products. The issues in this unit focus on foods that are available and the modifications that the food industry has made to our food supply.

Debate begins with the way foods are grown, starting with farming practices. Advances in agriculture allow farmers to use seeds that are genetically modified, soil enhanced with fertilizer, and industrial strength pesticides. Debate focuses on the unknown, as these practices are relatively new. Many ask, "What effect will they have in the long-term?" And the concerns are not only over the health status of humans, but for animals, other plants, and the environment. Other apprehensions center around new food products—new foods hit the market every week. The leading food manufacturers employ food and nutrition experts to formulate new items and recipes—and most have a marketing team to persuade the public to eat their company's products. Are these new products beneficial or detrimental to our health?

The opinions expressed in these selections are from a variety of perspectives. Some are based on opinions of the food industry and researchers who have decades of research experience related to our food supply. Others selections are written by advocacy groups and journalists. As you read the selections, think critically about who has written the article and their motives behind their positions.

Selected, Edited, and with Issue Framing Material by:
Janet M. Colson, *Middle Tennessee State University*

ISSUE

Should All Trans Fat Be Banned in Processed Foods?

YES: Food and Drug Administration, from "Final Determination Regarding Partially Hydrogenated Oils," from www.federalregister.gov/articles/2015/06/17/2015-14883/final-determination-regarding-partially-hydrogenated-oils (2015)

NO: The Grocery Manufacturers Association, from "A Petition to the Food and Drug Administration (FDA) about Partially Hydrogenated Vegetable Oils (PHOs)," https://cspinet.org/new/201508051.html (2015)

Learning Outcomes

After reading this issue, you will be able to:

- Describe why and when FDA removed partially hydrogenated oils (PHOs) from the "generally recognized as safe" (GRAS) list.
- Outline FDA's responses to the public's comments about PHOs and their rationale to remove them from GRAS status.
- Explain the justification that the Grocery Manufacturers Association uses to request to continue adding PHOs to processed foods.
- Identify the amounts of PHOs that the Grocery Manufacturers Association is requesting to be allowed in processed foods.

ISSUE SUMMARY

YES: In June 2015, the Food and Drug Administration issued the final determination that partially hydrogenated oils (PHOs) are no longer on the GRAS list because they are not "generally considered as safe." In effect, this means that *trans* fats are banned from foods because PHOs are the main source of *trans* fat. The FDA announced that PHOs must be removed from processed foods by June 2018.

NO: The Grocery Manufacturers Association filed a detailed petition outlining the safety of PHOs and requesting that low levels of PHOs be allowed in certain processed foods.

More than a century ago, Procter & Gamble introduced Americans to the first vegetable oil that looks and acts like lard and butter. Through the chemical process of adding hydrogen to cottonseed oil, the liquid oil took on the properties of a solid fat, similar to lard. Liquid oils are fluid because they are composed mainly of unsaturated fatty acids. The addition of hydrogens to unsaturated fatty acids causes them to become saturated, resulting in a very solid fat. Fatty acids for which all fatty acids are saturated with hydrogen are "fully hydrogenated oils," whereas fatty acids that contain some fatty acids that are hydrogenated are known as "partially hydrogenated oils." Partial hydrogenation results in a chemical change in the structure of the fatty acid changing it from a bent *"cis"* configuration to a straight *"trans"* shape. *Cis* oils are fluid whereas *trans* are solid, and look and act like saturated fats found in lard and butter. Therefore, partially hydrogenated oils are also known as *"trans* fats."

Procter & Gamble called their product "Crisco" because it was made from "crystalized cottonseed oil." The newly developed product was also called "shortening" because of its ability to "shorten" the strands of gluten in baked products making biscuits and pastries tender. Crisco and other partially hydrogenated oils also have a longer shelf life than liquid oils and are much cheaper than butter or lard, so it soon became a favorite with home makers and the food industry.

In the early part of the 1900s, when women still made pie crusts and biscuits from scratch and home-cooked meals were the norm, Crisco shortening became a staple in American homes. As we switched from home-cooking to eating processed and fast foods, the food industry reaped the benefits of a cheap way to make tasty confectioneries with a long shelf life and the use of shortening became a standard way to fry fast foods.

The love affair for shortening hit some bumpy roads in the 1990s when groups such as the Center for Science in the Public Interest (CSPI) began to spread the word that the *trans* fats in foods that contain partially hydrogenated oils are worse on the heart than foods that contain cholesterol or saturated fat. In fact, CSPI began urging the FDA to require food labels to include *trans* fat in 1993 and filed a formal petition one year later requesting that Nutrition Facts labels include *trans* fat content. Five years later, the FDA complied with the CSPI request and proposed that labels list *trans* fat content. In 2003 the FDA finalized the rule requiring food manufacturers to list *trans* fat content on food labels by 2006. As with most FDA food label definitions, "*trans*-fat free" means the product contains less than 0.5 g/serving. (So there is still some *trans* fat in the foods labeled "zero *trans*-fat.")

In 2004, CSPI filed petition to totally "revoke the authority for industry to use partially hydrogenated vegetable oils in foods." Five years later, biochemist Fred Kummerow filed a similar petition to the FDA requesting that they "ban partially hydrogenated fat from the American diet." In 2013, almost 10 years after the original CSPI petition, the FDA announced its preliminary determination that partially hydrogenated oil is no longer "generally recognized as safe." So removal from the GRAS list means that American food manufacturers cannot use any partially hydrogenated oils in their foods.

The selections for this issue pick up in 2015 and include FDA's "Final Determination Regarding Partially Hydrogenated Oils" as the YES selection. The NO selection consists of excerpts from the 19-page letter by the Grocery Manufacturers Association to the FDA petitioning them to allow some partially hydrogenated oil in processed food.

TIMELINE

1902 The first patent for hydrogenated vegetable oils is filed in Germany.

1911 Procter & Gamble introduces Crisco shortening made with partially hydrogenated oil.

1939–45 During both World Wars, butter is rationed so the public switches to *trans* fat-containing margarines made from vegetables oils.

1957 Ancel Keys publishes first report linking saturated fats to heart disease (*Lancet*, 1957) and the American Heart Association (AHA) recommends replacing animal fats with margarine and shortening made from partially hydrogenated vegetable oils.

1985 The Center for Science in the Public Interest and *The New York Times* (November 14) report that many fast food restaurants use beef tallow to fry foods. Media attention prods restaurant chains to switch to hydrogenated vegetable oils, which are high in *trans* fats. FDA concludes that *trans* fats are probably similar to saturated fats in their cholesterol-raising properties, but that more research is needed.

1990 Netherlands scientist Martijn Katan and colleagues publish report in the August *New England Journal of Medicine* showing a diet high in *trans* fats increases LDL cholesterol as much as saturated fats.

1992 *Trans* fat-free margarines are introduced in the United States.

1993 In May, the results of the Nurses' Health Study are published in *Lancet*; the authors find ties between *trans* fats and coronary artery disease. The Center for Science in the Public Interest (CSPI) requests the FDA to take steps to add *trans* fat content to nutrition labels. After inviting comments, the FDA concludes that research does not support this requirement.

1994 CSPI formally petitions FDA to require *trans* fat to be listed on food labels. After inviting comments, the FDA concludes that research does not support this requirement.

1994 In May, Harvard's Alberto Ascherio and Walter Willett write a commentary in the *American Journal of Public Health* that describes how *trans* fats are more damaging to heart health than saturated fats and are likely responsible for at least 30,000 premature U.S. deaths per year. They call for a "regulated phase-out or strict limitation" of *trans* fats and request *trans* fat labeling requirements on all foods, including fast foods.

1996 CSPI calls on restaurants and food manufacturers to disclose *trans* fat levels and switch to liquid vegetable oils.

1999 FDA proposes rules requiring that the amount of *trans* fat be listed on nutrition labels and advises consumers to cut their intake as much as possible.

2004 CSPI petitions FDA to remove *trans* fat from the list of ingredients that are "generally recognized as safe" (GRAS list).

2005 *Dietary Guidelines for Americans* includes "Limit intake of fats and oils high in saturated and/or *trans* fatty acids."

2005 Tiburon, California, is the first U.S. city to ban *trans* fat.

2006 FDA requires food labels to include the grams of *trans* fat.

2006 The AHA recommends that less than 1 percent of calories be from *trans* fats.

2010 California bans *trans* fat in restaurants.

2011 The *Dietary Guidelines for Americans 2010* includes "Keep *trans* fatty acids as low as possible."

2013 FDA announces the "preliminary determination" that *trans* fats are no longer on the GRAS list.

2015 The FDA files the final determination that *trans* fats are no longer GRAS and will not be allowed in foods after June 18, 2018.

YES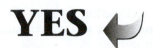

Final Determination Regarding Partially Hydrogenated Oils

I. Background

In accordance with the process set out in § 170.38(b)(1), we issued a notice on November 8, 2013, announcing our tentative determination that, based on currently available scientific information, PHOs are no longer GRAS under any condition of use in human food and therefore are food additives subject to section 409 of the Federal Food, Drug, and Cosmetic Act.

FDA's evaluation of the GRAS status of PHOs centers on the *trans* fatty acid (TFA, also referred to as "*trans* fat") component of these oils. Although we primarily use the word "oil" when discussing PHOs in this document, partially hydrogenated fats (such as partially hydrogenated lard), are included within the definition of PHOs (discussed in section II) and therefore within the scope of this order, and references to "oil" in this document should be read in most cases to include fats. PHOs are the primary dietary source of industrially-produced *trans* fatty acids. As explained in the tentative determination, all refined edible oils contain some *trans* fat as an unintentional byproduct of their manufacturing process; however, unlike other edible oils, *trans* fats are an integral component of PHOs and are purposely produced in these oils to affect the properties of the oils and the characteristics of the food to which they are added. In addition, the *trans* fat content of PHOs is significantly greater than the amount in other edible oils. Non-hydrogenated refined oils may contain *trans* fatty acids as a result of high-temperature processing, at levels typically below 2 percent. Low levels (below 2 percent) may also be found in fully hydrogenated oils (FHOs) due to incomplete hydrogenation. Small amounts (typically around 3 percent) may be found in the fat component of dairy and meat products from ruminant animals.

FDA's tentative determination identified the significant human health risks associated with the consumption of *trans* fat. The tentative determination was based on evidence including results from a number of controlled feeding studies on *trans* fatty acid consumption in humans, findings from long-term prospective epidemiological studies, and the opinions of expert panels. The latter included the 2005 recommendation of the Institute of Medicine (IOM) to limit *trans* fat consumption as much as possible while consuming a nutritionally adequate diet, recognizing that *trans* fat occurs naturally in meat and dairy products from ruminant animals and that naturally-occurring *trans* fat is unavoidable in ordinary, non-vegan diets without significant dietary adjustments that may introduce undesirable effects. In addition, in the tentative determination FDA cited a peer reviewed, published estimate of deaths and coronary events that would be prevented annually in the United States from elimination of remaining uses of PHOs from the food supply. Given all this evidence, we tentatively determined that there is no longer a consensus among qualified experts that PHOs, the primary dietary source of IP-TFA, are safe for human consumption, either directly or as ingredients in other food products.

PHOs have a long history of use as food ingredients. The two most common PHOs currently used by the food industry, partially hydrogenated soybean oil and partially hydrogenated cottonseed oil, are not listed as GRAS or as approved food additives in FDA's regulations. However, these and other commonly used PHOs (*e.g.,* partially hydrogenated coconut oil and partially hydrogenated palm oil) have been considered GRAS by the food industry based on a history of use prior to 1958. By contrast, the partially hydrogenated versions of low erucic acid rapeseed oil (21 CFR 184.1555) and menhaden oil have been affirmed by regulation as GRAS for use in food. Partially hydrogenated LEAR oil was affirmed as GRAS for use in food through scientific procedures. Partially hydrogenated menhaden oil was affirmed as GRAS for use in food on the basis that the oil is chemically and biologically comparable to commonly used partially hydrogenated vegetable oils such as corn and soybean oils. FDA believes that partially hydrogenated LEAR and menhaden oils are not currently widely used by the food industry. We plan to amend these regulations in a future rulemaking.

In the November 2013 notice, FDA requested additional data and scientific information related to our tentative determination and, in particular, requested comment on several questions. Interested persons were originally given until January 7, 2014, to comment on the notice. However, in response to several requests, we extended the comment period to March 8, 2014 (December 31, 2013).

We received over 6000 comments in response to the November 2013 notice announcing our tentative determination, including over 4500 form letters. In addition to submissions from individuals, we received comments from industry and trade associations, consumer and advocacy groups, health professional groups, and state/local governments. Most comments generally supported the tentative determination or supported aspects of it. FDA also received numerous comments stating that although they agreed with FDA's efforts to further reduce *trans* fat in the food supply, they disagreed with our tentative determination regarding the GRAS status of PHOs. Of the comments that objected to the tentative determination, many disagreed with FDA's scientific analysis and offered alternative approaches to address *trans* fat in the food supply. Some comments addressed issues outside the scope of the tentative determination (such as disruptions to trade, taxation of foods, and requests for bans on other substances) and were not considered. We reviewed all comments that were submitted to the docket before arriving at the decision outlined in this order.

We have arranged comments and our responses by topic throughout the remainder of this document. To make it easier to identify the comments and our responses, the word "Comment," in parentheses, appears before the comment's description and the word "Response," in parentheses, appears before FDA's response. . . .

The major provisions of this order are:

- PHOs are not GRAS for any use in human food.
- Any interested party may seek food additive approval for one or more specific uses of PHOs with data demonstrating a reasonable certainty of no harm of the proposed use(s).
- For the purposes of this declaratory order, FDA is defining PHOs as those fats and oils that have been hydrogenated, but not to complete or near complete saturation, and with an iodine value (IV) greater than 4.
- FDA is establishing a compliance date of June 18, 2018.

II. Definitions and Scope, and Related Comments with FDA Responses

(Comment 1) Some comments requested that we define PHOs and clearly delineate them from FHOs. The comments suggested various parameters for defining these fats and oils, including setting a specification for *trans* fat content (*e.g.*, a percentage) or using iodine value (IV; also interchangeably called iodine number).

(Response) FDA agrees with the comments that we should define PHOs to differentiate them from FHOs, which are outside the scope of this order. When a fat or oil is hydrogenated, the degree of hydrogenation can be tailored to obtain the desired properties for the application. FHOs are produced by allowing the hydrogenation process to proceed to complete or near complete saturation to obtain a more solid fat. In practice, the reaction does not proceed to 100 percent completion, even when producing FHOs, and some degree of unsaturation unavoidably remains in the final fat or oil. Non-hydrogenated refined fats and oils generally contain *trans* fatty acids as an unavoidable impurity as a result of high-temperature processing, at levels typically below 2 percent. The IV of a fat or oil is not a direct measure of the TFA content, but is a measure of the degree of unsaturation. Thus, in a fat or oil that has been hydrogenated, a low degree of unsaturation (*i.e.*, a low IV number) will correlate to a low level of TFA. FHOs with an IV of 4 or less generally contain *trans* fat at levels similar to non-hydrogenated refined fats and oils (less than 2 percent). By contrast, when the hydrogenation process is arrested before near complete saturation, *trans* fat content is typically higher, and IV is typically greater than 4.

Based on data for FHOs that are currently available on the market, which are indicative of modern hydrogenation technology, we define FHOs for the purposes of this order as fats and oils that have been hydrogenated to complete or near complete saturation, and with an IV of 4 or less, as determined by a method that is suitable for this analysis. FHOs are outside the scope of this order. For the purposes of this order, we define PHOs as fats and oils that have been hydrogenated, but not to complete or near complete saturation, and with an IV greater than 4 as determined by a method that is suitable for this analysis. . . .

(Comment 2) We received several comments requesting clarification on the scope of FDA's tentative determination, including whether it applies only to PHOs used in human food; whether it applies to ingredients that contain only naturally occurring *trans* fat, such as those ingredients derived from ruminant sources; and whether it applies to conjugated linoleic acid. We also received a citizen petition (discussed in section V) raising questions related to partially hydrogenated methyl ester of rosin.

(Response) FDA wishes to clarify that this order applies only to PHOs used in human food, not animal feed, and applies to PHOs used as a food ingredient, which includes those uses sometimes considered processing aids or food contact substances (*e.g.*, pan-release agents). By contrast, the use of PHOs as raw materials used to synthesize other ingredients is outside the scope of this order. We do not have specific information on the intake of industrially-produced *trans* fat from this source. . . .

This order does not apply to ingredients that contain only naturally occurring *trans* fat, such as those ingredients derived from ruminant sources.

This order does not apply to the use of conjugated linoleic acid (CLA) as a food ingredient. CLA does not fit the definition of PHO. CLAs are a class of fatty acid isomers derived from linoleic acid and do not contain non-conjugated double bonds in a *trans* configuration nor are CLAs triglyceride molecules. On the other hand, PHOs are primarily mixtures of triglycerides, produced by partial hydrogenation and include at least one nonconjugated double bond(s) in a *trans* configuration. . . .

This order also does not apply to the use of partially hydrogenated methyl ester of rosin. . . . Partially hydrogenated methyl ester of rosin is composed of resin acids that are chemically and structurally distinct from fatty acids found in PHOs. Resin acids are terpene-derived aromatic compounds that do not have long chain fatty acid components with *cis/trans* double bonds.

III. Discussion of Legal Issues, and Related Comments with FDA Responses

A. GRAS

Section 409 of the FD&C Act provides that a food additive is unsafe unless it is used in accordance with conditions set forth in that section. "Food additive" is defined . . . as any substance the intended use of which results or may reasonably be expected to result in its becoming a component or otherwise affecting the characteristics of any food, if such substance is not GRAS or otherwise excluded from the definition. Certain other substances that may become components of food are also excluded from the statutory definition of food additive, including pesticide chemicals and their residues, new animal drugs, color additives, and dietary ingredients in dietary supplements.

A substance is GRAS if it is generally recognized, among experts qualified by scientific training and experience to evaluate its safety, as having been adequately shown through scientific procedures (or, in the case of a substance used in food prior to January 1, 1958, through either scientific procedures or experience based on common use in food) to be safe under the conditions of its intended use. However, history of use prior to 1958 is not sufficient to support continued GRAS status if new evidence demonstrates that there is no longer a consensus that an ingredient is safe. . . .

FDA has defined safe as "a reasonable certainty in the minds of competent scientists that the substance is not harmful under the intended conditions of use," and general recognition of safety must be based only on the views of qualified experts. To establish general recognition of safety, there must be a consensus of expert opinion regarding the safety of the use of the substance. . .

Importantly, the GRAS status of a specific use of a particular substance in food may change as knowledge changes. For example, as new scientific data and information develop about a substance or the understanding of the consequences of consumption of a substance evolves, expert opinion regarding the safety of a substance for a particular use may change such that there is no longer a consensus that the specific use is safe. The fact that the status of the use of a substance under section 201(s) of the FD&C Act may evolve over time is the underlying basis for FDA's regulation at § 170.38, which provides, in part, that we may, on our own initiative, propose to determine that a substance is not GRAS. . . .

As noted in section III.A, under section 201(s) of the FD&C Act, a substance that is GRAS for a particular use in food is not a food additive, and may lawfully be utilized for that use without FDA review or approval. Currently, a GRAS determination may be made when the manufacturer or user of a food substance evaluates the safety of the substance and the views of qualified experts and determines that the use of the substance is GRAS. This approach is commonly referred to as "GRAS self-determination" or "independent GRAS determination."

Other substances that are GRAS may be identified in FDA regulations in one of two ways. Following the passage of the 1958 Food Additives Amendment, we established in our regulations a list of food substances that, when used as indicated, are considered GRAS. We made clear that this was not a comprehensive list. This list [is] commonly referred to as the "GRAS list." Thereafter, in 1972, we established the GRAS affirmation process through which we affirmed, through notice and comment rule making, the GRAS status of particular uses of certain substances in food. . . . (As a general matter, we no longer affirm the GRAS status of substances through notice-and-comment rulemaking. In April 1997, we proposed to replace the voluntary GRAS affirmation petition process with a voluntary GRAS notification program, which would not involve rulemaking. At the time of the proposal, we initiated a pilot of the GRAS notification program, which continues to function. A firm may voluntarily submit information on a GRAS self-determination to FDA for review through the GRAS notification program, but is not required to do so.) . . .

(Comment 3) Some comments stated that FDA must show a "severe conflict" among experts about the safety of a substance in order to determine that PHOs are not GRAS.

(Response) FDA disagrees that "severe conflict" is the relevant standard. . . . We have considered all available information and determined that there is no longer a consensus among qualified experts that PHOs are safe for human consumption. To the extent there is disagreement among qualified experts about the safety of PHOs for human consumption, this genuine dispute regarding safety precludes a finding of GRAS.

(Comment 4) Some comments focused on the idea that it may be possible to establish a threshold below which PHOs may be safely used in the food supply. One comment argued that there is no consensus among experts that PHOs are unsafe below some low threshold level of use.

(Response) As discussed later, FDA does not agree that such a threshold has been identified based on the available science. Importantly, even if such a threshold could be identified, this alone would not meet the requirement of "general recognition" for uses below the threshold without there also being consensus among qualified experts that uses below the threshold are safe. . . . We acknowledge that scientific knowledge advances and evolves over time. We encourage submission of scientific evidence as part of food additive petitions under section 409 of the FD&C Act for one or more specific uses of PHOs for which industry or other interested individuals believe that safe conditions of use may be prescribed. We are establishing a compliance date of June 18, 2018 for this order to allow time for such petitions and their review.

(Comment 5) One comment stated that FDA must demonstrate that each and every PHO, and every use of PHOs, is not safe.

(Response) FDA disagrees. FDA need not demonstrate that PHOs are unsafe to determine that they are not GRAS, only that there is a lack of consensus among qualified experts regarding their safety. In addition, our consideration of PHOs as a class is justified because the available, relevant scientific evidence demonstrates an increased risk of coronary heart disease (CHD) attributable to *trans* fat PHOs are the primary dietary source of IP-TFA; and there is a lack of consensus among qualified experts that PHOs are safe for use in food at any level.

(Comment 6) Some comments stated that, by determining that the use of PHOs are not GRAS because they contain a nutrient that increases risk of CHD, FDA would be calling into question the regulatory status of other food sources of *trans* fat.

(Response) FDA disagrees. As noted in section II, this order does not apply to ingredients that contain naturally occurring *trans* fat (such as those ingredients derived from ruminant sources), fully hydrogenated oils, or edible oils that contain IP-TFA as an impurity. FDA has considered the available information and concluded that there is a lack of consensus among qualified experts that PHOs, as the primary dietary source of IP-TFA, are safe for use in human food. . . .

(Comment 8) Some comments stated that the expert panels we cited in the tentative determination (*i.e.*, the Institute of Medicine/National Academy of Sciences (IOM/NAS), American Heart Association, American Dietetic Association, World Health Organization, Dietary Guidelines Advisory Committee, and the FDA Food Advisory Committee Nutrition Subcommittee) were not experts qualified by scientific training and experience to evaluate the safety of substances in food. The comments also stated that these expert panels were not convened for the purposes of evaluating the safety of PHOs and did not make determinations regarding the GRAS status of PHOs. Therefore, the comments argued that the conclusions of these panels do not demonstrate a lack of consensus among qualified experts that PHOs are GRAS.

(Response) FDA disagrees with these comments. The expert panels we cited were composed of scientists qualified by relevant training and experience to review literature on *trans* fat consumption, because of their nationally recognized and established expertise in the area of food and nutrition. For example, the Food and Nutrition Board at IOM/NAS is a recognized national resource for recommendations on health issues, and the Dietary Guidelines Advisory Committee members are nationally recognized experts in nutrition and health. . . .

B. Procedural Requirements

Under section 5(d) of the Administrative Procedure Act (APA), an agency, "in its sound discretion, may issue a declaratory order to terminate a controversy or remove uncertainty." The APA defines "order" as "the whole or a part of a final disposition, whether affirmative, negative, injunctive, or declaratory in form, of an agency in a matter other than rulemaking but including licensing." The APA defines "adjudication" as "agency process for the formulation of an order."

FDA's regulations, consistent with the APA, define "order" to mean "the final agency disposition, other than the issuance of a regulation, in a proceeding concerning any matter. . . ." Our regulations also define "proceeding and administrative proceeding" to mean "any undertaking to issue, amend, or revoke a regulation or order, or to take or not to take any other form of administrative action, under the laws administered by the Food and Drug Administration." Moreover, our regulations establish that the Commissioner may initiate an administrative proceeding to issue, amend, or revoke an order.

FDA's regulations also set forth a process by which we, on our own initiative or on the petition of an interested person, may determine that a substance is not GRAS. Specifically, FDA may initiate this process by issuing a notice in the Federal Register proposing to determine that a substance is not GRAS and is a food additive subject to section 409 of the FD&C Act. The notice must allow a period of 60 days for comment. If, after review of comments, FDA determines that there is a lack of convincing evidence that a substance is GRAS or is otherwise exempt from the definition of a food additive in section 201(s) of the FD&C Act, FDA will publish a notice thereof in the Federal Register. Such a notice "shall provide for the use of the additive in food or food contact surfaces as follows: (1) It may promulgate a food additive regulation governing use of the additive[;] (2) It may promulgate an interim food additive regulation governing use of the additive[;] (3) It may require discontinuance of the use of the additive[;] (4) It may adopt any combination of the above three approaches for different uses or levels of use of the additive." . . .

IV. Discussion of Scientific Issues, and Related Comments with FDA Responses

A. Intake Assessment

In the November 2013 notice, we discussed dietary intake of *trans* fat from PHOs, estimated in 2010 and updated in 2012. The intake assessment was done for four reasons: (1) To determine the impact of the 2003 labeling rule and subsequent reformulations; (2) to assist in our review of the citizen petitions, which are discussed in section V;

(3) to consider strategies for further *trans* fat reduction, if warranted; and (4) to better understand the current uses of PHOs and identify products that still contain high levels of *trans* fat. Our determination regarding the GRAS status of PHOs relies on an analysis of whether PHOs meet the GRAS standard based on available scientific evidence; the intake assessment was not the basis for this determination.

In 2012, we estimated the mean *trans* fat intake from the use of PHOs to be 1.0 grams per person per day (g/p/d; 0.5 percent of energy based on a 2,000 calorie diet) for the U.S. population aged 2 years or more. We also estimated intake for high-level consumers (represented by intake at the 90th percentile), as well as a "high-intake" scenario that assumed consumers consistently chose products with the highest *trans* fat levels. We received a number of comments on our intake assessment, including comments on assumptions, methodology, and recommendations for future studies. . . .

(Comment 17) Many comments stated that a substantial number of products have been reformulated since the 2012 intake assessment and that we should revise our intake assessment for *trans* fat before issuing our final determination on the GRAS status of PHOs.

(Response) FDA agrees that reformulation efforts by industry are continuing. However, the 2012 intake assessment was intended to be a snapshot in time and was based on products containing PHOs that were in the market at that time, and was done for the reasons described previously in this section. Given the evidence FDA has reviewed and our determination that PHOs are not GRAS for any use in human food, an updated intake assessment for *trans* fats from PHOs is not needed at this time. Our determination that PHOs are not GRAS for use in human food does not rely on the intake assessment.

. . .

(Comment 20) One comment urged FDA to reevaluate the intake of *trans* fat using the most recent National Health and Nutrition Examination Survey (NHANES) data. The comment suggested that the intake of *trans* fat would be lower if the more recent NHANES data were used because the mandatory labeling rule for *trans* fat became effective on January 1, 2006.

(Response) While the 2003–2006 NHANES food consumption data were used in the 2010 and 2012 intake assessments, the levels of *trans* fat in the food products were determined based on products that were available in the market from 2009 to 2012, therefore capturing *trans* fat reductions due to product reformulation as a result of the regulation in § 101.9(c)(2)(ii) (effective in 2006) requiring declaration of the *trans* fat content of food in the nutrition label. . . .

(Comment 25) Two comments stated that intake should be evaluated based on the presumption that all products with PHOs as an ingredient contain *trans* fat at a specified level (*e.g.*, 0.2 g/serving or per reference amount customarily consumed). These comments suggested that such an assessment could provide support for an alternative approach such as setting an allowable level of *trans* fat in foods.

(Response) Because we have concluded that PHOs are no longer GRAS, evaluating intake for alternative approaches, such as setting an allowable level of *trans* fat in foods, is not planned at this time.

B. Safety

In the Federal Register of November 17, 1999, we issued a proposed rule entitled "Food Labeling: *Trans* Fatty Acids in Nutrition Labeling, Nutrient Content Claims, and Health Claims." The proposed rule would require that *trans* fat content be provided in nutrition labeling, and concluded that dietary *trans* fats have adverse effects on blood cholesterol measures that are predictive of CHD risk, specifically low-density lipoprotein cholesterol (LDL-C) levels. In the Federal Register of July 11, 2003, we issued a final rule (the July 2003 final rule) amending the labeling regulations to require declaration of *trans* fat content of food in the nutrition label of conventional foods and dietary supplements. In the July 2003 final rule, we cited authoritative reports that recommended limiting intake of *trans* fat to reduce CHD risk.

In the November 2013 notice containing our tentative determination that PHOs are no longer GRAS for any use in human food, we summarized findings reported in the literature since 2003, when we had last reviewed the adverse effects of dietary *trans* fat in support of the July 2003 final rule. We noted that since 2003, both controlled feeding trials and prospective observational studies published on *trans* fat consumption have consistently confirmed the adverse health effects of *trans* fat consumption on risk factor biomarkers (*e.g.*, serum lipoproteins including LDL-C) and increased risk of CHD. . . .

Since publication of the November 2013 notice, we re-reviewed key literature and expert panel reports published since the 1990s on the relationship between *trans* fat consumption and CHD risk. Our review focused on the two main lines of scientific evidence linking *trans* fat intakes and CHD: (1) The effect of *trans* fat intake on blood lipids in controlled feeding trials, a type of randomized clinical trial; and (2) observational (epidemiological) studies of *trans* fat intake and CHD risk in populations. Additionally, we reviewed the conclusions of recent U.S. and international expert panels on the health effects of *trans* fat. As summarized in our review memorandum, the scientific evidence, including combined analyses of multiple studies (meta-analyses), supports a progressive and linear cause and effect relationship between *trans* fatty acid intake and adverse effects on blood lipids that predict CHD risk, including LDL-C, high-density lipoprotein cholesterol (HDL-C) and ratios such as total cholesterol (total-C)/HDL-C and LDL-C/HDL-C. . . .

In controlled feeding trials, a type of randomized clinical trial, *trans* fatty acid intake increased LDL-C ("bad" cholesterol), decreased HDL-C ("good" cholesterol) and increased ratios of total-C/HDL-C and LDL-C/HDL-C compared with the same amount of energy intake (calories) from *cis*-unsaturated fatty acids. Increases in LDL-C, total-C/HDL-C and LDL-C/HDL-C and decreases in HDL-C are adverse changes with respect to CHD risk. These adverse effects of *trans* fat intake on blood lipids are based on controlled feeding trials. . . .

Epidemiology is the study of the distribution and causes of disease in human populations. Analytic epidemiology studies are those designed to test hypotheses regarding whether or not a particular exposure is associated with causing or preventing a specific disease outcome. In prospective observational (cohort) studies, subjects are classified according to presence or absence of a particular factor (such as usual dietary intake of *trans* fat) and followed for a period of time to identify disease outcomes (such as heart attack or death from CHD). Strengths of the prospective observational study design are that the time sequence of exposure and disease is clearly shown; exposures are identified at the outset of the study; and measurement of exposure is not affected by later disease status. Results of four major prospective studies, some with one or more updates during the follow up period, consistently show higher *trans* fat intake associated with increased CHD risk. . . .

As described in our review memorandum, international and U.S. expert panels, using additional scientific evidence available since 2002, have continued to recognize the positive linear trend between LDL-C and *trans* fat intake and the consistent association of *trans* fat intake and CHD risk in prospective observational studies. The panels have concluded that *trans* fats are not essential nutrients in the diet, and have recommended that consumption be kept as low as possible. . . .

Since publication of the November 2013 notice, we also conducted a systematic search of the peer-reviewed literature published since 2008 and summarized the findings. The major human health endpoints evaluated for associations with *trans* fat intake reported in the literature included CHD, all-cause mortality, cardiovascular disease and stroke. Other human health endpoints addressed in our search included various types of cancer, metabolic syndrome and diabetes, and adverse effects on fertility, pregnancy outcome, cognitive function, and mental health. . . .

We have also analyzed the comments we received regarding the scientific basis for our tentative determination in the November 2013 notice. Comments regarding the safety of PHOs that were opposed to our tentative determination were generally related to one of four subject areas: (1) Dose-response relationship of *trans* fat intake and adverse health effects in human studies and whether there is a threshold below which intake of *trans* fats is generally recognized as safe; (2) reliance on expert panel reports and recommendations; (3) health benefits and clinical significance of replacements for PHOs; and (4) alternative approaches. Comments regarding the safety of PHOs that were in support of our determination raised concerns about other adverse health effects besides effects on LDL-C, such as adverse effects on other risk factors for CHD (e.g., HDL-C, total-C/HDL-C ratio, LDL-C/HDL-C ratio, and other lipid and non-lipid biomarkers), inflammatory effects, harm to subpopulations, and increased diabetes risk. . . .

(Comment 30) Several comments cited a 2011 publication by FDA authors as evidence of PHO safety and evidence that a threshold can be determined below which there is general recognition of safety. The comments argued that these authors reviewed data from clinical trials to assess the relationship between *trans* fat intake and LDL-C and total-C and that their regression analysis showed no association between *trans* fat consumption and either LDL-C or total-C levels. Also, the comments stated that the authors do not "force" the regression line through zero unlike in the Ascherio et al. 1999 paper, relied upon by FDA in the tentative determination.

(Response) FDA disagrees. We note that the authors of this paper stated that their regression analysis of TFA intake and LDL-C "supports the IOM's conclusion that any intake level of *trans* fat above 0 percent of energy increased LDL cholesterol concentration." This paper did not identify a threshold level at which LDL-C began to increase. The analysis in the paper was limited to validated surrogate endpoint biomarkers of CHD, total cholesterol and LDL-C, and did not consider other CHD risk factor biomarkers such as HDL-C, or total-C/HDL-C or LDL-C/HDL-C ratios. The paper focused on methodology for attempting to identify a tolerable upper intake level for *trans* fat. The appropriateness of fitting the intercept through zero in a regression analysis depends on the meaning of the data, the research question to be answered, and the particular study design, and is discussed further in our response to Comment 28.

. . .

(Comment 33) Some comments stated that FDA should convene an expert panel to specifically address whether evidence exists to indicate the effect of TFA on LDL-C is linear at low intakes (below 3% energy). Other comments stated that there is consensus among qualified experts that TFA intake should be less than 1% of energy, and cited expert panel reviews as evidence. Similar comments stated that PHOs are safe at current intake levels, and TFA intake is already below levels recommended by nutrition experts.

(Response) We decline to convene another expert panel in light of the substantial evidence available on the adverse effects of consuming *trans* fat. FDA notes that a 2013 National Institutes of Health, National Heart, Lung, and Blood Institute (NIH/NHLBI) expert panel conducted a systematic evidence review and concluded with moderate confidence that, for every 1 percent of energy from TFA replaced by mono- or polyunsaturated fatty acids (MUFA or PUFA), LDL-C decreases by an estimated 1.5 milligrams per deciliter (mg/dL) and 2.0 mg/dL, respectively. The panel also concluded that replacement of TFA with saturated fatty acids (SFA), MUFA, or PUFA increases HDL-C by an estimated 0.5, 0.4 and 0.5 mg/dL, respectively. This panel's conclusions were not limited to a specific TFA dose range and did not indicate any threshold TFA intake. . . .

We also disagree that, based on generally available information, there is a consensus among qualified experts that *trans* fats are safe at some level, and we note that recommendations from expert panels either: (1) Do not state a recommended level; or (2) recommend consideration of further reduction in IP-TFA intake, below current levels. Since 2002, many expert panels have considered the adverse effects associated with *trans* fat consumption. . . .

(Comment 34) Several comments questioned whether further reductions in TFA intake will be clinically significant and subsequently affect public health.

(Response) Since publication of the November 2013 notice, we have quantitatively analyzed the public health significance of removing PHOs from the food supply, and the results show that removing PHOs from human food would have an expected positive impact on public health. We note that further reductions in IP-TFA intake below current levels may result in small reductions in LDL-C and small improvements in other biomarkers that may not seem clinically significant for an individual; however, when considered across the U.S. population, small reductions in CHD risk would be expected to prevent large numbers of heart attacks and deaths, as illustrated in FDA estimates. . . .

(Comment 36) Several comments proposed that we should limit the percentage of *trans* fat in finished foods or oils, or set a threshold in foods for the maximum grams (g) of *trans* fat per serving. Some comments suggested various specification levels ranging from 0.2 to 0.5 g *trans* fat per serving or as a percentage of total fat in foods or oils. Another comment urged FDA to establish a reasonable level for *trans* fat in food to specifically account for minor uses of PHOs as processing aids.

Some comments urged us to declare that certain uses of PHOs in foods are GRAS, or to issue interim food additive regulations for specific low level uses. Examples of such uses provided by comments included emulsifiers, encapsulates for flavor agents and color additives, pan release agents, anti-caking agents, gum bases, and use in frostings, fillings, and coatings. The use of PHOs in chewing gum was specifically noted in some comments as deserving special consideration due to the claim that there is no meaningful PHO intake from this use. Several comments suggested we issue interim food additive regulations that would allow certain uses of PHOs in food, pending completion of studies evaluating the health effects of low level consumption of *trans* fat that reflect current intake levels. Furthermore, one comment advised that if we decide to treat certain low-level uses of PHOs as food additives, then the GRAS status for these uses should not be revoked until a food additive approval is issued.

In contrast, we also received numerous comments opposed to establishing limits of *trans* fat in foods. Most of these comments noted that scientific evidence has shown that no amount of *trans* fat in food is safe and therefore, supported our tentative determination. One comment noted that *trans* fat threshold limits in food would be too difficult to monitor and enforce, and therefore, should not be established.

(Response) Regarding the proposals for alternate approaches suggesting a threshold for *trans* fat in food or oils or suggesting that FDA declare some uses of PHOs as GRAS, no comments provided evidence that any uses of PHOs meet the GRAS standard, or evidence that would establish a safe threshold exposure level. Further, although the intake from such minor uses may be low, adequate data (*e.g.*, specific conditions of use, use level, *trans* fat content of the PHOs used) were not provided so that intake from these uses could be estimated. Therefore we are not setting a threshold for *trans* fat. If industry or other interested individuals believe that safe conditions of use for PHOs can be demonstrated, it or they may submit a food additive petition or food contact notification to FDA for review. . . .

(Comment 37) Several comments suggested various changes to our labeling regulations to encourage industry to reformulate products to contain less *trans* fat and help consumers reduce *trans* fat intake. In addition, one comment stated that a 0 g *trans* fat declaration should not be allowed on a label if a PHO is in the ingredient list. Some comments indicated that a statement recommending that consumers limit their intake of *trans* fat should be added to the Nutrition Facts Panel. A few comments suggested we set a Daily Value for *trans* fat and consider establishing disclosure or disqualifying levels of *trans* fat for nutrient content and health claims. Many comments noted that the risk of developing CHD is dependent on many factors, and therefore, the association between intake of macronutrients, such as PHOs, and adverse health outcomes is best addressed through nutrition labeling and consumer education.

(Response) FDA disagrees that labeling is the best approach to address the use of PHOs because FDA has determined that PHOs are not GRAS for any use in human food and therefore are food additives subject to the requirement of premarket approval under section 409 of the FD&C Act. Although we recognize that the requirement to label *trans* fat content led to significant reduction in *trans* fat levels in products, further changes to labeling are outside the scope of this determination, which relates to ingredient safety.

(Comment 38) Some comments suggested that we should work with industry to encourage voluntary reductions in PHO use and to foster the development of innovative hydrogenation technologies that produce PHOs containing low levels of *trans* fat.

(Response) FDA disagrees that a voluntary program is the best way to remove PHOs from the food supply, given our conclusion on the GRAS status of PHOs. FDA has determined that PHOs are not GRAS for any use in human food. FDA agrees, however, that we should work with the food industry to review new regulatory submissions or data as new technologies and/or ingredients are developed that may serve as alternatives to PHOs, and we will continue to do so.

V. Citizen Petitions

As discussed in the tentative determination, we received two citizen petitions regarding the safety of PHOs. In 2004, the Center for Science in the Public Interest (CSPI) submitted a citizen petition requesting that we revoke the GRAS status of PHOs, and consequently declare that PHOs are food additives. The petition also asked us to revoke the safe conditions of use for partially hydrogenated products that are currently considered food additives, to prohibit the use of partially hydrogenated vegetable oils that are prior sanctioned, and to initiate a program to encourage manufacturers and restaurants to switch to more healthy oils. The CSPI citizen petition excluded *trans* fat that occurs naturally in meat from ruminant animals and dairy fats, and that forms during the production of non-hydrogenated oils. It also did not include FHOs, which contain negligible amounts of *trans* fat, and PHOs that may be produced by new technologies that result in negligible amounts of *trans* fat in the final product. The CSPI citizen petition stated that *trans* fat promotes CHD by increasing LDL-C and also by lowering HDL-C, and therefore has greater adverse effects on serum lipids (and possibly CHD) than saturated fats. The CSPI citizen petition also stated that, beyond its adverse effects on serum lipids, *trans* fat may promote heart disease in additional ways. Based on these findings, CSPI asserted that PHOs can no longer be considered GRAS.

In 2009, Dr. Fred Kummerow submitted a citizen petition requesting that we ban partially hydrogenated fat from the American diet. The Kummerow citizen petition cited studies linking intake of IP-TFA to the prevalence of CHD in the United States. The Kummerow citizen petition also asserted that *trans* fat may be passed to infants via breast milk and that the daily intake of *trans* fat related to the health of children has been ignored since children do not exhibit overt heart disease. The Kummerow citizen petition further stated that inflammation in the arteries is believed to be a risk factor in CHD and studies have shown that *trans* fatty acids elicit an inflammatory response.

This order constitutes a response, in part, to the citizen petitions. As discussed above in section III.C, we plan to amend the regulations regarding LEAR and menhaden PHOs in a future action, and we will consider taking future action regarding related regulations. As discussed in

section III.B, we intend to address any claims of prior sanction for specific uses of PHO in a future action.

. . .

VI. Compliance Date and Related Comments with FDA Responses

We received numerous comments about the time needed to reformulate products to remove PHOs should FDA make a final determination that PHOs are not GRAS. We also received comments about challenges to reformulation, specific product types that will be difficult to reformulate, and effects on small businesses.

(Comment 39) The comments recommended compliance dates ranging from immediate to over 10 years. Several comments stated that fried foods should have less time (*i.e.*, 6 months) to phase out the use of PHOs. One comment stated that if the use of low levels of PHOs were to remain permissible by virtue of being GRAS or through food additive approval, then the estimated time to reformulate would be 5 years; however, if FDA does not authorize low level uses of PHOs, the timeline would need to be 10 years. In general, the food industry urged FDA to provide sufficient time for all companies to secure a supply of alternatives and transition to new formulations. Some comments stated that FDA should coordinate the compliance date with updates to the Nutrition Facts Panel.

Some comments stated that domestically grown oilseed crops must be planted about 18 months prior to their expected usage in order for the crop to be grown, harvested, stored, crushed, oil extracted, processed, refined, delivered, and used in foods. One comment stated that the oil industry will need a minimum of 3 years to fully commercialize the various oils capable of replacing PHOs in food. A number of comments stated that it could take several additional years to reformulate after the development of the new oils.

Several comments expressed concern about adequate availability of alternative oils, especially palm oil. One comment stated that the food industry would prefer to replace PHOs with domestically produced vegetable oils (*e.g.*, high-oleic soybean oil) rather than palm oil, but time is needed to commercialize these options. Some comments stated that sudden demand for palm oil would pose challenges for obtaining sustainably-sourced palm oil, as the current market would likely not be able to meet the demand.

Other comments indicated that the time needed for removal of PHOs is dependent on the product category.

A number of comments indicated that the baking industry will have difficulty replacing the solid shortenings used in bakery products. Other comments indicated difficulties in the categories of cakes and frostings, fillings for candies, chewing gum, snack bars, and as a component of what the comments termed minor use ingredients, such as for use in coatings, anti-caking agents, encapsulates, emulsifiers, release agents, flavors, and colors.

. . .

A number of comments noted challenges faced by small businesses, such as access to alternative oils, inability to compete for supply, fewer resources to commit to research and development, and effect of ingredient costs on growth of the business. Some comments noted that small businesses represent a relatively small contribution to overall IP-TFA intake. One comment recommended that we allow small businesses an additional 2 years beyond the rest of industry. Another comment stated that small businesses would need at least 5 years due to their limitations in research and development expertise, inability to command supply of scarce ingredients, and economic pressures of labeling changes. . . .

(Response) Based on our experience and on the changes we have already seen in the market, we believe that 3 years is sufficient time for submission and review and, if applicable requirements are met, approval of food additive petitions for uses of PHOs for which industry or other interested individuals believe that safe conditions of use may be prescribed. For this reason, we are establishing a compliance date for this order of June 18, 2018. We recognize that the use of PHOs in the food supply is already declining and expect this to continue even prior to the compliance date. Regarding the use of "low levels" of PHOs, no comments provided a basis upon which we can currently conclude that any use of PHO is GRAS. We recognize the challenges faced by small businesses, however, considering our determination that PHOs are not GRAS

for any use in human food, we conclude that providing 3 years for submission and review of food additive petitions and/or food contact notifications is reasonable, and will have the additional benefit of allowing small businesses time to address these challenges. We understand the difficulties faced by small businesses due to limited research and development resources and potential challenges to gain timely access to suitable alternatives.

The compliance date will have the additional benefit of minimizing market disruptions by providing industry sufficient time to identify suitable replacement ingredients for PHOs, to exhaust existing product inventories, and to reformulate and modify labeling of affected products. Three years also provides time for the growing, harvesting, and processing of new varieties of edible oilseeds to meet the expected demands for alternative oil products and to address the supply chain issues associated with transition to new oils. . . .

VII. Conclusion and Order

As discussed in this document, for a substance to be GRAS, there must be consensus among qualified experts based on generally available information that the substance is safe under the intended conditions of use. In accordance with the process set forth in FDA's regulations in § 170.38, FDA has determined that there is no longer a consensus that PHOs, the primary source of industrially-produced *trans* fat, are generally recognized as safe for use in human food, based on current scientific evidence . . . regarding the health risks associated with consumption of *trans* fat. FDA considers this order a partial response to the citizen petitions from CSPI and Dr. Kummerow.

FOOD AND DRUG ADMINISTRATION is the agency of the United States Department of Health and Human Services and is responsible for regulating food, dietary supplements, drugs, biological medical products, blood products, medical devices, radiation-emitting devices, veterinary products, and cosmetics in the United States.

The Grocery Manufacturers Association   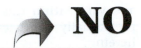 **NO**

A Petition to the Food and Drug Administration (FDA) about Partially Hydrogenated Vegetable Oils (PHOs)

Executive

The Grocery Manufacturers Association (GMA) submits this petition to the Food and Drug Administration (FDA) which demonstrates that partially hydrogenated vegetable oils (PHOs) meet the "reasonable certainty of no harm" safety standard required for food additives and generally recognized as safe (GRAS) ingredients. GMA continues to believe PHOs are GRAS on the basis of common use in foods; nonetheless, GMA is committed to working cooperatively with FDA and submits this food additive petition in the interest of furthering the science and understanding regarding PHOs. This petition details the safety of partially hydrogenated vegetable oils (PHOs) manufactured from the following vegetable oils: soy cottonseed, coconut, canola, palm, palm kernel and sunflower oils, or blends of these oils, under the identified conditions of use.

As described in more detail in the sections below, the uses of PHOs satisfy the reasonable certainty of no harm standard for the following reasons:

- Recent intervention studies, meta-analyses and a mode of action (MOA) study support a 1.5 %en/day threshold level below which TFA does not have a significant effect on changes in LDL-C.
- The 90th percentile exposure of TFAs from the petitioned PHO uses combined with the intrinsic ruminant *trans* fatty acids (rTFAs) is 1.33 %en/day, a level of TFA exposure below the 1.5 %en/day threshold.
- The non-threshold linear model relied upon in the previous assessment by FDA did not consider recent intervention studies, meta-analyses and a mode of action study that support a 1.5 %en/day threshold level below which TFAs do not have a significant effect on change in LDL-C.

- Nonetheless, application of a linear dose model similar to that used by FDA in the past, and which FDA asked GMA specifically to consider, demonstrates that the petitioned PHO uses do not increase hypothetical CHD risk.

Triglycerides are the main components of vegetable oils, comprised predominantly of fatty acids present in the form of esters of glycerol. Mixtures of triglycerides composed of both saturated and unsaturated fatty acids are present in vegetable oils. Chemical hydrogenation is the process by which hydrogen atoms are added to unsaturated sites on the carbon chains of fatty acids, in the presence of catalysts, thereby reducing the number of double bonds. "Partial hydrogenation" describes an incomplete saturation of the double bonds, in which some double bonds remain but may shift to a different position along the carbon chain and alter their configuration from *cis* to *trans*. The *trans* arrangement of hydrogen atoms results in a relatively straight configuration of the fatty acids and increases the melting point, shelf life, and flavor stability of the partially hydrogenated oil.

The *trans* fat components of partially hydrogenated vegetable oils mainly contain the *trans* isomers of oleic acid, the major one being C18:1 *trans*-9 or elaidic acid and C18:1 *trans*-10. Partially hydrogenated vegetable oils also contain smaller amounts of C18:1 *trans*-8, and C18:1 *trans*-11 or vaccenic acid, lesser amounts of C18:2 *trans* and C18:3 *trans*, and very minor levels, generally reported at less than one percent, of *trans* isomers of alpha-linolenic acid may arise during deep-fat frying.

The *trans* fatty acid (TFA) content of PHOs can vary from approximately 5 to 60 percent of the oil, depending on how the oil is manufactured. The average TFA content will depend upon the product type and vary within this range. The general specifications for partially hydrogenated vegetable oils are provided herein. . . .

Partially hydrogenated vegetable oils have been used for decades in numerous food applications. PHOs are used in the production of foods, food ingredients, processing aids and incidental additives to improve the oxidative stability and/or melting and crystallization properties of food grade oils and fats, and combinations thereof. The data and information compiled by FDA demonstrate that since 2003, *trans* fat intake exposure from PHOs has been reduced by approximately 80 percent. This food additive petition includes uses of PHOs: (i) as an anti-caking, anti-dusting and free flow agent, (ii) as a dough strengthener, (iii) as an emulsifier, (iv) as a formulation aid, e.g., serving as a carrier, binder, film former, tableting aid, (v) as a humectant, (vi) as a lubricant and release agent, either alone or in combination with other components, (vii) as a processing aid or component thereof, (viii) as a solvent and vehicle for fat soluble ingredients including coloring agents, flavors, flavor enhancers and vitamins, (ix) as a stabilizer or thickener, (x) as a surface-active agent, (xi) as a surface-finishing agent or (xii) as a texturizer (tenderness and moisture retention in gluten-containing foods).

PHOs are also used as (xiii) a heat transfer medium (i.e., in deep frying, heat energy is transferred from the heat source to the food in the PHO).

The food additive petition would cover the following uses of PHOs:

(i) PHO, or a blend of PHOs, as a carrier or component thereof for flavors and flavorings, and as a diluent or component thereof for color additives intended for food use, provided the PHOs in the carrier or diluent contribute no more than 300 parts per million (300 mg/kg) TFA to the finished food as consumed.

(ii) PHO, or a blend of PHOs, as an incidental additive, including as a processing aid, or component thereof, provided the PHOs in the incidental additive contribute no more than 50 parts per million (50 mg/kg) TFA to the finished food as consumed.

(iii) PHO, or a blend of PHOs, in the below-listed foods when the standards of identity established under section 401of the Act do not preclude such use:

Limitation—PHO(s) contribute no more than	Food Categories
0.01 g TFA/100 g	• Protein drinks, such as instant breakfast drinks, meal supplement drinks, meal replacement drinks, etc.
0.02 g TFA/100 g	• Tea bags and tea powder mixes
0.05 g TFA/100 g	• Breakfast cereals, ready-to-eat • Chewing gums • Processed meat products, such as emulsified or formed products like bologna, hot dogs (frankfurter), meat loafs, sausage, or meatballs, etc.
0.06 g TFA/100 g	• Artichoke hearts, marinated • Pancakes waffles, frozen
0.07 g TFA/100 g	• Meat alternatives, such as meatless bacon, breakfast links, chicken, fish sticks, frankfurters/hot dogs, luncheon meat and meatballs, vegetarian meat loaf or patties, etc.
0.08 g TFA/100 g	• Frozen entrees or side dishes, such as vegetables for steaming, Salisbury steak, sirloin with gravy, Swedish meatballs, fried chicken, chicken and noodles, chicken with rice and vegetables, turkey dinner, fish dinner, spaghetti and meatballs, lasagna, scrambled eggs with sausage and hash brown, French fries, etc.
0.10 g TFA/100 g	• Pie fillings
0.12 g TFA/100 g	• Candies, caramel
0.13 g TFA/100 g	• Pudding, dry mix
0.15 g TFA/100 g	• Pizza, frozen
0.16 g TFA/100 g	• Potatoes and potato meal and side dishes, shelf-stable, including mashed potatoes, scalloped potatoes, au gratin potatoes, potatoes with cheese, julienne potatoes, hashbrown potatoes, potato casseroles, etc.
0.17 g TFA/100 g	• Soups, canned, including meal starter sauces

Limitation—PHO(s) contribute no more than	Food Categories
0.19 g TFA/100 g	• Cream-based or cheese-based frozen entrees or side dishes, such as vegetables in cheese or cream sauces, chicken divan, chicken or turkey a la king, chicken in cream sauce with noodles and vegetables, fish in lemon-butter sauce, enchilada with chicken, macaroni and cheese, pasta with vegetable and cheese sauce, etc. • Tortillas and taco shells, flour, soft
0.20 g TFA/100 g	• Hot cocoa mix, liquid • Ice cream sauces, ready to eat • Pinto beans, canned • Pudding, ready to eat
0.21 g TFA/100 g	• Frozen dairy-containing desserts (non–ice cream) and novelties, including frozen custards, gelatos, frozen yogurts and sherbets • Ice cream products, including tubs, cups, bars, sticks, sandwiches or cones. • Pizza rolls, frozen
0.24 g TFA/100 g	• Cakes and cupcakes, ready-to-eat, with or without filling or icing
0.25 g TFA/100 g	• Breakfast or dessert pastry-type foods, such as fritters, strudels, Danishes, doughnuts, tarts, turnovers, etc.
0.28 g TFA/100 g	• Seasoning, dry mixes
0.30 g TFA/100 g	• Cheese cake dry mix
0.35 g TFA/100 g	• Bread or dough products, refrigerated or frozen, such as hand-held sandwiches (i.e., meat or breakfast turnover), cinnamon rolls, dinner rolls, biscuits, pizza crust, bread sticks, etc.
0.40 g TFA/100 g	• Candies, soft chocolate with nut inclusions
0.42 g TFA/100 g	• Rice cake type products, including rice cakes, rice crackers, puffed rice cakes, popcorn cakes, etc.
0.43 g TFA/100 g	• Pies and cobblers, frozen • Salad dressings
0.47 g TFA/100 g	• Cookies, including ready-to-eat cookies, bars and brownies, ready-to-bake cookies, ice cream cones (cone only), etc.
0.50 g TFA/100 g	• Pasta or rice dish dry mixes, such as macaroni or noodles with cheese mixes, flavored pasta mixes, rice pilaf mixes, flavored rice and/or pasta mixtures, Spanish rice mixes, etc. • Savory snacks, such as crackers, crispbread, corn or cornmeal based salty snacks (i.e., corn/tortilla chips and cheese puffs), multigrain chips, pretzels, potato chips, vegetable chips, etc.
0.55 g TFA/100 g	• Cake, muffin and quick bread mixes, including frozen or refrigerated muffin batters, etc.
0.60 g TFA/100 g	• Hot cereal mixes, such as oatmeal, etc.
0.70 g TFA/100 g	• Nutrition or granola bars, such as breakfast bars, snack bars, protein bars, fiber bars, etc.
0.73 g TFA/100 g	• Soup and bouillon, dry mixes and pastes
0.74 g TFA/100 g	• Stuffing, dry mix
0.84 g TFA/100 g	• Candies, hard
0.86 g TFA/100 g	• Sauces, cheese, ready-to-eat
0.87 g TFA/100 g	• Pancake, waffle and biscuit mixes
0.88 g TFA/100 g	• Dough mix for pizza crust
0.90 g TFA/100 g	• Frostings and fillings, including whipped toppings and icings, confectionery toppings, etc.
1.0 g TFA/100 g	• Sugar used as doughnuts coating • Margarine sticks, including light margarine, unsalted margarine and lactose-free margarine sticks • Popcorn, sweet or savory, including ready-to-eat, microwave, etc. • Wafer-containing, chocolate-covered confections
1.04 g TFA/100 g	• Cookie, bar and brownie mixes
1.06 g TFA/100 g	• Sauces and gravies, dry mixes

Limitation—PHO(s) contribute no more than	Food Categories
1.07 g TFA/100 g	• Cream substitutes, such as frozen, liquid or powdered non- dairy creamers, etc.
1.13 g TFA/100 g	• Cultured dips, ready-to-eat
1.28 g TFA/100 g	• Pie crust mixes
1.70 g TFA/100 g	• Breading in meat and poultry products, including breading mixes and breadcrumbs
1.75 g TFA/100 g	• Pie crusts, frozen
1.91 g TFA/100 g	• Candies, soft fruit snack
3.0 g TFA/100 g	• Shortening

TFA in PHOs is determined by the method entitled "Fatty Acid Composition by Capillary GC for Nutritional Labeling," AOCS Ce 1h–05 (09). Compliance with the proposed TFA limits in foods may be calculated based on the TFA content of the PHO and the amount of PHO called for in the food product recipe. Validated analytical methods may be another option for confirming compliance with the TFA limits (e.g., AOCS Ce 1j-07).

History Of Use and Regulatory Status

Partially hydrogenated oils have a long history of use in the United States (U.S.) food supply as ingredients in food. PHOs are formed from the partial hydrogenation of vegetable oils and are semi-solid fats at room temperature. This process was developed in the 1930s and has been used commercially for over seventy years. PHOs were originally used to replace butter and lard which are high in saturated fat; today, they are used to improve flavors, increase shelf-life and provide flavor stability of foods. The presence of PHOs in foods increased during the 1980s to replace tropical oils because of their low saturated fat levels. PHOs have no formal regulatory definition. The two most common PHOs marketed today are partially hydrogenated soybean oil and partially hydrogenated cottonseed oil. PHOs have been determined to be Generally Recognized as Safe (GRAS) at levels consistent with Good Manufacturing Practices (GMP) based on historical use in food prior to the 1958 Food Additives Amendment to the FD&C Act. The Select Committee on GRAS Substances (SCOGS) confirmed the GRAS status of soybean PHO in 1976 and two additional PHOs were affirmed as GRAS by FDA in the mid- and late 1980s, i.e., low erucic acid rapeseed (LEAR) oil per 21 CFR 184.1555(c)(2) and menhaden oil per 21 CFR 184.1472(b). FDA based its GRAS affirmations of the LEAR and menhaden PHOs on the fact that those PHOs are comparable, chemically and biologically, to commonly used PHOs such as corn and soybean PHOs.

FDA issued a final rule on July 11, 2003 (68 FR 41434) requiring declaration of the TFA content in the nutrition label of conventional foods and dietary supplements effective January 1, 2006. As a result, many food manufacturers voluntarily reformulated products to reduce the levels of *trans* fat in food products. At the time of the 2003 labeling proposed rule, the daily mean intake of TFAs from PHOs among adults 20 years of age and older was 4.6 g/day (2 %en/day) and total TFA from both animal and PHO sources was 5.8 g/day (2.6 %en/day) (68 FR 41434). In a later assessment by the FDA using updated food composition data from 2009 and 2010 and food consumption data from 2003-2006, intakes of TFAs from PHOs among the US population was found to have dropped by almost 80%, down to 1.3 g/day (0.59 %en/day) when TFA data weighted by market share and representative of the TFA levels in foods available in the markets were used.

In 2004 and 2009, two citizen petitions were submitted to the FDA requesting the revocation of the GRAS status of PHOs. On November 8, 2013, the FDA issued a tentative determination that PHOs used in processed food are not GRAS and requested comments, scientific data, and information. (78 FR 67169, Docket No. FDA-2013-N-1317). In response to FDA's request, GMA submitted comments addressing scientific, legal, and policy considerations relevant to FDA's Tentative Determination, including a review of scientific and other factors demonstrating continued GRAS status of PHOs under current conditions of use.[1]

Estimated Daily Intake

Estimated daily intakes (EDI) of TFAs from the following sources were computed: a) Intrinsic (background), b) Petitioned PHO Uses, c) Cumulative (Intrinsic + Petitioned PHO Uses).

Food consumption data were obtained from the 2007–10 What We Eat in America (WWEIA) dietary component of the National Health and Nutrition

Examination Surveys (NHANES). Consumption data in the WWEIA NHANES are reported on an "as consumed basis." Several databases were used to map the foods reported consumed in WWEIA, NHANES to their respective ingredients, or to identify nutrients and weights of typical portions, etc. including the Food Intakes Converted to Retail Commodities Database (FICRCD), the Food Patterns Equivalent Database (FPED), the Food Commodity Intake Database (FCID), and the Food and Nutrient Database for Dietary Studies (FNDDS).

The USDA National Nutrient Database for Standard Reference (SR) (Standard Reference, Release 27) (SR27) was the source of the intrinsic TFA concentrations used in the assessment of TFA intakes from intrinsic sources. The distributions of TFA levels from intrinsic sources derived from SR27 for those food groups with at least 25 observations were reviewed and Crystal Ball® (Release 11.1.2.0.00) was used to determine the best fitting parametric distribution. Stochastic modeling was used to estimate TFA intakes from intrinsic sources. **The mean TFA intake from intrinsic sources for the US 2+ y is 1.04 g/day (95% CI: 0.94–1.15) or 0.46 %en/day (95% CI: 0.41–0.50).** TFA intakes from beef and dairy products constitute almost 75% of the total TFA intake from intrinsic sources.

For the assessment of TFA intakes from the petitioned uses of PHOs in the above-listed food categories (see above and Table 4 within this petition), food codes reported consumed in NHANES 2007–10 were reviewed and mapped to the listed food categories. Several of the listed food categories are for dry mixes with proposed maximum TFA limits for the foods "as sold" and not as consumed. In these cases percent recipe adjustments were applied to derive the TFA level in the foods as consumed. Deterministic modeling was used to estimate TFA intakes from petitioned PHO uses. Each food category was assigned a maximum TFA level contributed by the petitioned use of PHOs in that food category and a deterministic assessment was used to estimate the population mean and 90th percentile using the Food Analysis and Residue Evaluation Program (FARE) TM. **The mean TFA intake from petitioned uses of PHOs in the select food categories for the U.S. population 2 years (y) and older (U.S. 2+ y) is 0.77 g/day (95% CI: 0.75–0.79) or 0.34 %en/day (95% CI: 0.33–0.35).**

TFA intakes from petitioned PHO uses as flavor carriers, color additive diluents and incidental additives (including processing aids) were derived using a *per capita* intake approach. Specifically, the maximum TFA level of 300 ppm for flavor carriers and color additive diluents, and maximum level of 50 ppm for incidental additives, including processing aids, were applied to a 3 kg diet, and assuming 38% of the diet is from processed foods.

The TFA intake from PHO uses as flavor carriers and color additive diluents is estimated to be 0.34 g/day or 0.15 %en/day. The TFA intake from incidental additive (including processing aid) uses of PHOs is estimated to be 0.057 g/day or 0.026 %en/day.

Stochastic modeling was used to estimate combined TFA intakes from intrinsic sources and petitioned PHO uses in the select food categories. The mean *per capita* intake estimates from flavor carrier and color additive diluent uses and from incidental (including processing aid) uses are added to the total deterministically. **The mean cumulative EDI of TFAs from all sources (intrinsic + petitioned uses of PHOs) for the US 2+ y is 2.21 g/day (95% CI: 2.10–2.33) or 0.98 %en/day (95% CI: 0.93–1.02). The 90th percentile cumulative EDI from all sources (intrinsic + petitioned uses of PHOs) for the US 2+ y is 3.49 g/day (95% CI: 3.26–3.73) or 1.33 %en/day (95% CI: 1.24–1.43).**

Safety Information

TFA, Blood Lipid Metabolism, and Coronary Heart Disease (CHD) Risks

Similar to all other triglycerides consumed in the diet, PHOs have effects on various lipoproteins and other physiological biomarkers related to blood lipid metabolism. Lipid metabolism is not an adverse effect in and of itself. As discussed in detail below, while high levels of TFA intake contributed by PHOs in the diet are associated with changes of low density lipoprotein cholesterol (LDL-C), there are numerous other dietary constituents (e.g., saturated fatty acids) that also have the potential to impact biomarkers of lipid metabolism, including LDL-C. High density lipoprotein – cholesterol (HDL-C) has in some studies, but not others, been shown to be decreased by high levels of TFA intake.

In addition to LDL-C and HDL-C, several biological markers of CHD risk have been examined to determine whether associations with TFA intake exist, including Lp(a), apo-B, apo-A1, C-reactive protein (CRP), serum triglycerides (TG), and serum cholesterol ratios (i.e., LDL-C:HDL-C and TC:HDL-C). However, the use of lipoprotein ratios (i.e., LDL-C:HDL- CTC:HDL-C, apoB:apoA1) can be difficult to interpret for magnitude of effect. In addition, the effect of TFA intake on these alternative measures is not consistently reported in the scientific literature and therefore, many recent reviews have not been able to conduct meta-analyses to quantify overall summary effect sizes for these biomarkers for use in a safety assessment.

No Effects of Low Levels of TFA (<1.5 %en/day) on LDL-C

There is no evidence from randomized, controlled intervention studies on adverse effects attributable to increased risk of CHD at the petitioned low levels of consumption of PHO (i.e., 90% percentile cumulative intake from naturally-occurring TFA and industrially-produced TFA at 1.33 %en/day). In fact, a recent randomized, controlled intervention study showed no statistically significant difference in impact on LDL-C levels between the test group which consumed 1.47 %en/day TFA and the control group which consumed 0.399 %en/day TFA.

The Association between Levels of TFA and LDL-C

An association between TFA intake and increased CHD risk has been observed in US prospective cohorts groups consuming high levels of TFA. Intake of TFA in the individual cohorts ranged from 0.44 %en/day to ~5 %en/day at the upper quintile. Two initial studies examining intakes from the Nurses Health Study (NHS) cohort found significant increase in risk for CHD but this relationship was only statistically significant at levels of TFA intake of 3.2 %en/day compared to 1.3 %en/day and 2.9 %en/day. In a 20 year follow-up study of this population (NHS) increased risk for CHD was significantly associated with the third and fifth quintile of TFA consumption (i.e., 1.9 %en/day and 2.8 %en/day) but not with the second and fourth quintile (i.e., 1.6 %en/day and 2.2 %en/day) when compared to the lowest quintile of TFA intake of 1.3 %en/day in models adjusted for dietary fat intake, fiber, and fruits and vegetables. While CHD risk was not significantly associated with each increasing quintile of intake, there was a significant trend (p for trend = 0.01). In the Health Professional Follow-up Study (HPFS) the lowest TFA intake level that was associated with an increased risk of myocardial infarction was 4.3 g/day (1.6 %en/day) when compared to 1.5 g/day, but this relationship was no longer significant after adjustment for fiber intake. In the Zutphen Elderly Study there was no significant effect of TFA intake on CHD risk in the middle tertile of TFA intake (median TFA intake = 3.87 %en/day) compared to the lowest tertile (median TFA intake = 2.36 %en/day). The Alpha-Tocopheral Beta-Carotene Cancer Prevention Study found no significant relationship between risk for major coronary event and total TFA (including all TFA isomers) but this relationship did reach significance with intake of 5.6 g/d (2.0 %en/day) and risk of coronary death. The results from these studies, while not able to demonstrate causality, provide supporting evidence that although a relationship between increased CHD risk and high levels of TFA intake exists, this observed relationship has not been established at low levels of intake below 1.3 %en/day (i.e., the reference group).

Non-Threshold Model

Quantitative estimates of the effect of TFAs in the diet on LDL-C and HDL-C included several meta-analyses of randomized controlled feeding trials in humans. These analyses include a comprehensive review of the dietary intervention trials conducted between the years 1982–2011. Four analyses included LDL-C as a measured endpoint while [one] analysis examined the relationship between change in TFA intake and change in calculated ratio of LDL-C to HDL-C.

All of these analyses relied upon application of a dose-dependent linear regression method. With the exception of Trumbo 2011, all analyses made an *a priori* decision to arbitrarily set the intercept at zero, regardless of whether this is biologically plausible for lipoprotein endpoints.

It is important to note that the Ascherio et al. (1999) study was the first regression analysis to assume the linear dose response between TFA intakes and blood lipids. Moreover, Ascherio et al. (1999) included only one study that evaluated TFAs at a dose below 3% (0.36 %en/day change in TFA intakes) and the remainder of the test diets ranged from >3 %en/day to 11 %en/day.

Therefore, this linear dose model draws a straight line to zero relying on a single non-significant finding in the low dose region of the dose response. This approach assumes that there is no threshold for TFA intake below which there is no meaningful effect on LDL-C levels.[2]

Recent Intervention Trials, Meta-Analyses and a Mode of Action Study Support a 1.5 %en/day Threshold

These early analyses included very few intervention diets with TFA intakes in the low dose range (i.e., with the majority at 4 %en/day to 7 %en/day and as high as 11 %en/day). Subsequent to the Brouwer et al (2010) regression-analysis, several dietary intervention trials have investigated the effect of TFA on LDL-C in the lower dose region of the response curve with null findings indicating a linear dose response model through zero may not be the most appropriate fit for the data.

Researchers on behalf of the Food Standards Australia New Zealand (FSANZ) recently published an updated meta-analysis of randomized controlled trials with TC,

LDL-C or HDL-C as an outcome and feeding duration >3 weeks. The FSANZ meta- analysis was based on 10 data points from 8 trials that included both sources of TFAs (i.e., ruminant and industrial) and reported no significant effect on LDL-C from a 1 %en/day TFA intake in exchange for mono-unsaturated fatty acids (MUFAs) (0.0145 mmol/L; 95%CI,-0.0375, 0.0664 mmol/L). The TFA intakes in these later trials provides LDL-C responses in the lower TFA dose range (<2 %en/day), allowing a focus on the lower end of the dose response curve where previous trials and meta-analyses were lacking data. These new findings support the existence for a threshold TFA intake below which there is no meaningful effect on LDL-C levels. However, the determination of whether a threshold exists would be based on an examination of the proposed mode of action for TFA, which consists of two receptor-mediated events (i.e., increased very low density lipoprotein (VLDL) synthesis and decreased LDL clearance) that are non-linear biological processes. Therefore, the relationship between exposure and response would be expected to have a threshold as indicated by the underlying biology.

To address this critical research gap, a group of researchers recently modeled the effect of change in TFA intake on change in LDL using a meta-regression approach to improve the accuracy of estimating the relationship between exposure and response by considering the variance in individual studies and weighting the results appropriately. This work was focused at the low end of the dose response with TFA intake. They concluded that TFA intakes within the range of 1.5 %en/day results in "a negligible increase in the TFA-associated change in LDL-C." The slight increases in LDL-C that occur within this range of TFA intake are consistent with accepted measurement variability of LDL-C (i.e., 5%).

Haber et al. (2015) also presented a description of the mode of action (MOA) to aid the interpolation and/or extrapolation of the effect of TFAs on blood lipids in the low dose region of the response curve. The MOA for the raising of LDL-C levels from TFA intake results from two key events that are both functions of non-linear biological processes: 1) increased LDL production and 2) decreased LDL clearance. The shape of the dose response curve between TFA intake and LDL-C is hypothesized to be non-linear due to feedback loops and homeostatic controls that regulate blood lipid levels and underlie the two key events.

Other Health Outcomes

A review of published guidance documents on the level of evidence regarding the association between TFA intake and other health outcomes by national and international scientific expert panels within food safety and public health authorities was conducted. Based on the published guidance documents from the scientific expert panels described above, the conclusions consistently reported limited, inconsistent, and/or weak evidence for any effects of TFA on other health outcomes including diabetes, cancer, and obesity.

Ruminant v. Industrial Sources of TFA

The differentiation of the effect between industrially produced PHOs and natural, or ruminant, sources of TFA in the diet has only been evaluated in a small number of studies with inconsistent findings. Several researchers conclude that null results in the meta-analyses measuring the association between ruminant TFAs (rTFAs) and LDL-C are most likely in part due to a lack of statistical power to detect a significant effect due to the small number of studies. Further, the naturally low intakes of TFA from ruminant sources in the diet make it difficult to estimate effects that are typically measured of industrial TFAs (iTFAs) in clinical trials. The majority of rTFA trials reported intakes <2 %en/day while the iTFA trials are typically in the 5–7 %en/day range and as high as 11–12 %en/day. A cross-over study by Motard-Belanger et al. (2008) showed that when a high intake of iTFA (10.2 g/2500 kcal or 3.7 %en) was compared to a moderate intake of rTFA (4.2 g/ 2500 kcal or 1.5 %en/day), there was a significantly higher LDL-C level among the iTFA diet. However, when a high rTFA was achieved (10.2 g/2500 kcal diet or 3.7 %en/day), LDL-C levels were significantly higher compared to a low TFA diet from any source (0.8 %en/day). This study suggests that when comparable levels of rTFA and iTFA are achieved, the effects on LDL-C are also comparable. Several national and international organizations have evaluated the importance of the source of the TFA on risk of CHD for purposes of dietary recommendations. EFSA summarized results of two human intervention studies and concluded that the available evidence indicates that rTFA and iTFA have similar adverse effects on blood lipids. In the WHO FAO's third Expert Consultation on Fats and Fatty Acids in Human Nutrition, it was concluded that there is evidence to indicate that TFA from natural sources have similar effects on the TC:HDL-C ratio to those from industrial sources. In the WHO Scientific Update on TFA, it was stated that "despite the inherent differences in chemical structure, limited evidence indicates that industrial and ruminant TFAs may have similar effects on serum lipoproteins when ruminant TFA are consumed in sufficient quantities (much higher than seen with usual dietary intakes) in experimental studies."

Safety Evaluation

While several blood lipid and lipoprotein measurements have been evaluated as surrogate biomarkers for the relationship between dietary fat intakes and risk of CHD, LDL-C has an established biological plausibility and has been the focus of dietary guidelines and recommendations. In particular, an association between TFA intake, LDL-Cs and an individual's risk of CHD was recognized by the IOM/ NAS in the 2005 Dietary Reference Intakes (DRIs) for macronutrients and relied upon in the FDA's Final Rule on "Food Labeling: *Trans* Fatty Acids in Nutrition Labeling, Nutrient Content Claims, and Health Claims" (68 Federal Register (FR) 133:41434–41456). Although HDL-C has been found to be independently associated with CHD risk, its causal association is not as well established. The IOM's review of the evidence on biomarkers for disease risk states that LDL-C is a known, independent risk factor for CHD with decades of consistent data supporting this conclusion, but noted that the value of HDL-C as a biomarker for CHD is less clear with controlled intervention studies showing inconsistent results and providing little evidence that an increase in HDL-C confers any predicted benefit. While recognizing the complex pathway between TFA intake and CHD risk and that any one biomarker will not be the only contributor to the pathway, given the IOM's review on the CHD predictive value of HDL-C and the robust and measured relationship between LDL-C levels and CHD risks from intervention studies (summarized herein), the associated changes of LDL-C with TFA intake and increased CHD risk is the focus of the dose response assessment and safety evaluation in this petition.

Non-Threshold Linear Dose Response Models

As discussed above, non-threshold linear model relied upon by FDA in its Tentative Determination did not consider the more recent studies, analyses and an MOA study supporting a threshold TFA intake level on LDL-C. Nonetheless, to accommodate consideration of the linear regressions reported in previous nutritional and epidemiological assessments of clinical association, and at the direct request of FDA, a linear dose response model was developed to quantify the change in risk of CHD associated with an incremental increase in dietary intake of TFAs. This model assumes that any TFA intake greater than 0 %en/day is associated with an increase in LDL-C levels that are in turn associated with CHD risk. However, as previously reviewed in the above section, the fundamental limitation of this linear approach is that it is not consistent with the mechanistic data describing the key events in the pathway between diet intake and LDL-C

concentrations, which are non-linear. The implementation of the dose-response model to quantify the change in risk of CHD that could result from a given increase in TFA intake (e.g. 1 %en/day) requires estimates for two model parameters: 1) the change in LDL-C associated with changes in TFA intake and 2) the associated risk of CHD events with a change in LDL-C.

To ensure that the totality of the evidence is captured, both intervention and observational studies were considered in the dose response model. Two linear dose response models were implemented based on the available data to capture the range of the magnitude of change in LDL-C associated with a unit change in TFA intake (e.g., 1 %en) and the change in CHD risk associated with a unit change in LDL-C. Replacement of TFA with MUFA in the diet was assumed in the modeling. Although this is not reflective of functional replacement scenarios, it was chosen to represent the most conservative case.

The two dose response models were combined with the estimated daily intake of TFA from background (intrinsic) sources, PHO uses, and total (intrinsic sources + PHO uses), which are below the TFA intake level of 1.5 %en/day that Haber et al. (2015) identified as the threshold level below which TFAs do not have a significant effect on changes in LDL-C (see below), to estimate hypothetical CHD risks and 95% CI. Hypothetical risk estimates were derived for mean and 90th percentile TFA intakes from intrinsic sources, PHO uses, and from total combined. To characterize the uncertainty surrounding the magnitude and variability in the estimates of changes in LDL-C and hypothetical CHD risks depending on the source of the safety data (i.e., intervention or observational studies), as well as variability and uncertainty associated with the EDI, hypothetical CHD risk estimates were stochastically derived using Crystal Ball® (Release 11.1.2.0.00), a spreadsheet application for predictive modeling and simulation. The mean, 2.5th, and 97.5th percentiles of the 1000 simulated risk values represent the mean risk and associated 95% CI corresponding to the mean TFA intake. A similar approach was used for estimating the hypothetical risk and 95% CI corresponding to the 90th percentile TFA intake.

The predicted percent increase in hypothetical CHD Risks and 95% CI associated with the estimated daily intake of TFA from intrinsic sources, PHO uses and total combined (intrinsic sources + PHO) uses overlap. In all cases, whether at the mean or 90th percentile TFA intake, or linear dose response models 1or 2, the lower bound difference in hypothetical CHD risk estimates between background TFA intake from intrinsic source and TFA intake from PHO uses or TFA intake from both sources (intrinsic + PHO uses) is 0% (non-significant differences). Therefore, the hypothetical CHD risks associated with background TFA intake from intrinsic sources are not statistically significantly different from hypothetical CHD risks associated with TFA intake from petitioned PHO uses or risks associated with total TFA intake (intrinsic + PHO uses), irrespective of which linear dose response models are applied. This is true at both the mean and 90th percentile TFA intake estimates.

1.5 %en/day Threshold Level

Recently, there have been several dietary intervention trials that investigated the effect of TFA intakes on LDL-C in the lower dose region of the response curve with null findings. The recent FSANZ meta-analysis that was based on 10 data points from 8 trials that included both sources of TFAs (i.e., ruminant and industrial) reported no significant effect on LDL-C from a 1 %en/day TFA intake in exchange for MUFAs (0.0145 mmol/L; 95% CI, −0.0375, 0.0664 mmol/L). The TFA intakes in these later trials provide LDL-C information in the lower TFA dose range (<2 %en), allowing a focus on the lower end of the dose response curve where previous trials and meta-analyses were lacking data. These new findings support a threshold level that must be exceeded for TFA intake to have a significant effect on changes in LDL-C.

In order to assess the available clinical data and define the relationship of TFA and LDL-C, Haber et al. (2015) completed a comprehensive MOA evaluation for the effects of TFA on LDL- C, as well as a meta-regression analysis of this effect. These critical assessments clearly show that the prevailing reliance on the linear non-threshold relationship to describe the relationship of TFA and LDL-C is not biologically correct. The meta-regression analysis of 16 published controlled dietary intervention studies with 34 data points that measured the association between TFA intake and LDL-C levels concluded that the best fitting model was non-linear. Haber et al. identified a threshold level of 1.5 %en/day TFA below which TFA intake does not have a significant effect on change in LDL-C.

The cumulative EDI for TFA from all sources (intrinsic + PHO uses) is 0.98 %en/day and 1.3 %en/day at mean and the 90th percentile, respectively for the U.S. 2 + y. The highest cumulative TFA intake is among boys 13-19y, which is 1.4 %en/day at the 90th percentile. These cumulative EDIs are below the threshold level of 1.5 %en/day.

The MOA for the raising of LDL-C levels from TFA intake further supports a threshold level for TFA. Potential effects from TFA can result from two key events that are both functions of non-linear biological processes: 1) increased LDL production and 2) decreased LDL clearance. The shape of the dose response curve between TFA intake and LDL-C is hypothesized to be non-linear due to feedback loops and homeostatic controls that regulate blood lipid levels and underlie the two key events.

Thus, based on a comprehensive review of all available data, a non-linear model provides the best fit model and demonstrates a threshold of effect. Regardless of the approach used, all available data reviewed support the safety of PHO added to the diet under the conditions of intended use described in this petition.

Safety Conclusion

Safety assessments of dietary macro constituents such as PHOs are complex and require consideration of the totality of the relevant evidence, including chemistry, metabolism, nutrition, and toxicological factors. The body's biological response to diet, genetic, and lifestyle factors is dynamic, fluid, and constantly changing through regeneration and repair as part of normal processes of metabolism, utilization, and elimination. Numerous dietary constituents, including saturated and unsaturated fatty acids, fiber, and other food components, have a demonstrated effect on surrogate biomarkers of CHD, and are recognized confounders.

The progression to CHD is a complex pathway and research on this pathway has resulted in hundreds of variables that are statistically associated with CHD outcomes. Of these numerous risk factors, the evidence consistently supports that the majority of CHD events can be explained by a smaller group of factors including dyslipidemia, blood pressure, smoking, and diabetes which are often clustered within individuals. However, even within this smaller group of factors, the pathway is complex and mediated or effected by an individual's characteristics, including genetics and the environment, with some individuals with clearly identified risk factors such as high blood pressure or dyslipidemia never experiencing CHD events. Alternatively, to further add to the complexity of the causal pathway to CHD, relatively normal levels of established risk factors within an individual can interact beyond a simple additive relationship and predict events at a multiplicative rate. As such, removal of a single dietary factor, such as PHOs (and associated TFAs), may not result in meaningful risk reduction.

As recognized by the IOM (2005), "... *trans* fatty acids are unavoidable in ordinary, nonvegan diets, [and] consuming 0 percent of energy [from *trans fats*] would require significant changes in patterns of dietary intake . . . Such adjustments may introduce undesirable effects (e.g., elimination of commercially prepared foods, dairy products, and meats that contain *trans* fatty acids may result in inadequate intakes of protein and certain micronutrients) and unknown and unquantifiable health risks."

In defining the safety standard for a food additive, FDA has long recognized that "[i]t is impossible . . . to establish with complete certainty the absolute harmlessness of the use of any substance." A food additive is therefore deemed safe if "there is a reasonable certainty in the minds of competent scientists that the substance is not harmful under the intended conditions of use." See 21 CFR § 170.3(i). As described further below, the petitioned uses of PHOs under the intended condition of use as described herein satisfy the reasonable certainty of no harm standard.

The PHOs that are the subject of this petition have a long history of safe use in the food supply and meet appropriate food grade specifications and heavy metals limits.

The estimated mean daily intake of TFAs from the PHOs, under the conditions of use in or on foods as described in this petition, among the US 2+ y and adults 20+ y is 1.17 g/day (0.52 %en/day) and 1.18 g/day (0.52 %en/day), respectively. These estimated intakes assume that all foods in a given category will contain TFAs at the maximum proposed limits, and do not account the fact that some products could contain lower TFA levels, thus the true TFA intake estimates from PHOs could be even lower.

Relative to the mean daily intake of TFAs from intrinsic sources (i.e., meat, milk, dairy and other products), which is 1.042 g/day (0.46 %en/day) among the US 2+ y, the estimated mean daily intake of TFAs from the petitioned uses of PHOs in or on foods as an incidental additive, including as a processing aid, is 0.06 g/day (0.03 %en/day), which is approximately 15 times lower than and within the decimal range of the background TFA intake from intrinsic sources.

Relative to the mean daily intake of TFAs from intrinsic sources, the estimated mean daily intake of TFAs from the petitioned use of PHOs in or on foods as flavor carrier and color additive diluent (0.34 g/day or 0.15 %en/day) is approximately 1/3 of the background TFA intake from intrinsic sources. The estimated mean daily intake of TFAs from the petitioned use of PHOs in or on specified foods in the select categories (0.77 g/day or 0.34 %en/day) is lower than the background TFA intake from intrinsic sources.

For expediency, and to respond most directly to questions FDA has raised about TFAs and LDL- C, this Petition examines the safety of the TFA intake resulting from the petitioned PHO uses from several different perspectives. First, the Petition summarizes systematic/evidence-based reviews and meta-analyses in which possible quantitative relationships between TFAs, blood lipids, and CHD were estimated. Then, to address numerous limitations with analyses that assume a linear dose response relationship, and to consider more recent trials and predictive models investigating the effects of lower intakes of TFA, the Petition reviews support for a threshold TFA intake level below which TFA has no significant effect on change in LDL-C levels. Finally, in response to a direct request from FDA, the Petition applies non-threshold linear dose response models to model hypothetical CHD risk from TFA intake under the conditions of intended use described in the petition.

Until recently, most of the published analyses on the relationship between TFA intake, LDL-C and CHD risks based on feeding trials of TFA from PHOs at high doses assumed a non-threshold linear dose-response relationship, arbitrarily forced through zero in the absence of data at the low levels. Based on this assumption and to capture the evidence and associated uncertainty in the magnitude of effect, both intervention and observational studies are included in the parameterization of two dose response modes. Since there is no evidence of differential effects between ruminant TFA and TFA from PHOs, these dose response models were applied to TFA intake from both intrinsic and PHO uses. Applying these dose response models to the TFA intake from intrinsic sources, TFA intake from PHO uses, as well as total TFA from combined intrinsic and PHO uses, the predicted percent increase in hypothetical CHD Risks and 95% CI associated with TFA intake from intrinsic sources, TFA intake from PHO uses and total TFAs from combined intrinsic and PHO uses overlap, irrespective of the linear dose response models. In all cases, whether at the mean or 90th percentile TFA intake, or linear dose response models 1or 2, the lower bound difference in hypothetical CHD risk estimates between background TFA intake from intrinsic source and TFA intake from PHO uses or TFA intake from both sources (intrinsic + PHO uses) is 0% (non-significant differences). Therefore, the hypothetical CHD risks associated with background TFA intake from intrinsic sources are not statistically significantly different from hypothetical CHD risks associated with TFA intake from petitioned PHO uses or risks associated with cumulative TFA intake (intrinsic + PHO uses). This is true at both the mean and 90th percentile intake estimates. In other words, the additional TFA intake from the petitioned uses of PHOs does not alter existing hypothetical CHD risk that is assumed through linear modeling.

Early analyses included very few intervention diets with TFA intakes in the low dose range; several dietary intervention trials have investigated the effect of TFA on LDL-C in the lower dose region of the response curve with null findings indicating a linear dose response model through zero may not be the most appropriate fit for the data. Indeed, the recent analysis by Haber et al. (2015) identified a TFA intake threshold of 1.5 %en/day below which TFA does not significantly affect change in LDL- C. The cumulative EDI for TFA from all sources (intrinsic + PHO uses) is 0.98 %en/day and 1.3 %en/day at the mean and 90th percentile, respectively for the US 2+ y. The highest cumulative TFA intake is found among boys 13–19 y, which is 1.4 %en/day at the 90th percentile. These cumulative EDIs are below the TFA threshold intake level of 1.5 %en/day, below which TFA has no significant effect on change in LDL-C. Therefore, there can be no inference of any increase in hypothetical CHD risk via the LDL-C mediated pathway as the result of the proposed uses of PHOs.

There is a reasonable certainty of no harm because the 90th percentile exposure of TFAs from the uses of PHOs covered by this petition combined with the rTFAs is 1.33 %en/day; a level of use lower than the 1.5 %en/day threshold supported by the Haber et al. analysis (2015) . . . which TFAs do not have a significant effect on change in LDL-C. Further, even using the non-threshold linear model, PHO uses covered by this petition would not increase hypothetical CHD risk beyond that which is inherent in the human diet due to consumption of meat, milk, dairy and other products. To the extent that humans continue to consume meat for protein, milk/dairy for calcium, etc., there will always be TFA in the diet. Accordingly, there is a reasonable certainty of no harm from the additional exposure of the petitioned uses of PHOs because the incremental intake of TFA from the petitioned PHO uses does not alter existing hypothetical CHD risk.

Notes

1. GMA continues to view all past and current uses of PHOs as GRAS for the reasons set forth in our comments. The submission of this Petition does not constitute evidence that GMA has changed its position that past and current uses of PHOs are GRAS.
2. Issues and concerns presented by the use of regression analyses to support a "zero tolerance" standard for food ingredients have been comprehensively reviewed by GMA and others and are not further examined here. For completeness, this Petition evaluates PHO safety from several perspectives, including the non-threshold linear approach relied upon in the Tentative Determination and a threshold approach supported by biological plausibility.

THE GROCERY MANUFACTURER ASSOCIATION is an international association that represents the makers of foods, beverage, and merchandise.

EXPLORING THE ISSUE

Should All Trans Fat Be Banned in Processed Foods?

Critical Thinking and Reflection

1. Describe what partially hydrogenated oils (PHOs) are and how they are made.
2. Look over the Nutrition Facts panels and ingredients lists of the following: a can of shortening, a jar of peanut butter, stick margarine and tub (soft) margarine. Compare the fat content and ingredient lists of the items.
3. Modify and prepare a recipe that calls for shortening by using cold coconut oil to replace the shortening. Describe how it compares to the product made with shortening.
4. Compare the *trans* fat regulations of countries around the world.

Is There Common Ground?

Both the FDA and the Grocery Manufacturers Association (GMA) are concerned about the health and well-being of the nation and want to ensure that the food supply is safe and causes no adverse health effects. Both are very cordial in their correspondence and very knowledgeable in their approach. Both are interested in furthering the science and understanding regarding PHOs.

FDA acknowledges that "scientific knowledge advances and evolves over time." And it "encourage[s] submission of scientific evidence as part of food additive petitions under section 409 of the FD&C Act for one or more specific uses of PHOs for which industry or other interested individuals believe that safe conditions of use may be prescribed." It also has given the industry three additional years to allow time for such petitions. So will the FDA agree with the GMA request and allow some foods to contain relatively trace amounts of added PHOs or will it decide that "ban" means to totally ban *trans* fat from foods?

Additional Resources

Ascherio A, Katan MB, Zock PL, Stampfer MJ, Willett WC. *Trans* fatty acids and coronary heart disease. *N Engl J Med* 1999;340:1994–8.

Gebauer SK, Destaillats F, Dionisi F, Krauss RM, Baer DJ. Vaccenic acid and *trans* fatty acid isomers from partially hydrogenated oil both adversely affect LDL cholesterol: A double-blind, randomized controlled trial. *Am J Clin Nutr.* 2015;102:1339–46.

Restrepo BJ, Rieger M. Denmark's policy on artificial *trans* fat and cardiovascular disease. *Am J Prev Med* 2015, August.

Stender S. In equal amounts, the major ruminant *trans* fatty acid is as bad for LDL cholesterol as industrially produced trans fatty acids, but the latter are easier to remove from foods. *Am J Clin Nutr.* 2015; doi: 10.3945/ajcn.115.123646.

Stender S, Astrup A, Dyerberg J. Tracing artificial *trans* fat in popular foods in Europe: A market basket investigation. *BMJ* Open 2014;4: e005218.

Stender S, Dyerberg J, Bysted A, Leth T, Astrup A. A *trans* world journey. *Atheroscler* (Suppl) 2006;7:47–52.

Willett WC, Stampfer MJ, Manson JE, Colditz GA, Speizer FE, Rosner BA, Sampson LA, Hennekens CH. Intake of *trans* fatty acids and risk of coronary heart disease among women. *Lancet* 1993;341:581–5.

Internet References . . .

Food and Drug Administration (FDA)

www.fda.gov

The Grocery Manufacturer Association

www.gmaonline.org

Health.gov

health.gov

Selected, Edited, and with Issue Framing Materials by:
Janet M. Colson, *Middle Tennessee State University*

ISSUE

Are Organic Foods Better Than Conventional Foods?

YES: Ed Hamer and Mark Anslow, from "10 Reasons Why Organic Can Feed the World" *The Ecologist* (2008)

NO: Mark Bittman, from "Eating Food That's Better for You, Organic or Not?" *The New York Times* (2009)

Learning Outcomes
After reading this issue, you will be able to: • List the factors that make organic foods superior to conventionally grown foods.   • Outline the benefits that eating an organic, locally grown plant-based diet will have on the environment and our health.   • Describe the trends in organic food consumption by Americans and people of the United Kingdom.

ISSUE SUMMARY

YES: Ed Hamer and Mark Anslow indicate that organically produced foods use less energy, water, and pesticides and produce less pollution while producing foods that taste better and contain more nutrients.

NO: Mark Bittman says that eating organically offers no guarantee of eating well, healthfully, sanely, even ethically. He points out that people may feel better about eating an organic Oreo than a conventional Oreo, and sides with Marion Nestle who says "Organic junk food is still junk food."

For centuries, organic farming was all that existed. During the first few decades of the 1900s, farmers began to use fertilizers, pesticides, and herbicides to increase crop production. Then, use of antibiotics, vaccinations, and hormones to improve the quality of livestock and other farm animals became widespread throughout the world. And handpicking was replaced with large machines. The organic movement, as we know it today, began when a few environmentally conscious people objected to this "industrialized agriculture."

One of the first people to speak out against the new way of farming was British botanist Sir Albert Howard, who is often thought of as the father of organic farming. He wrote several books about farming practices in India where he used compost as a natural fertilizer and promoted that compost is superior to modern fertilizers. In the United States, Jerome Irving Rodale published the magazine *Organic Farming and Gardening* that focuses on how to grow food without using chemicals. The magazine, which began publication in 1942, is one of the most highly read gardening magazines.

In 1962, environmentalist Rachel Carson's book *Silent Spring* was published. Her book is credited with further increasing awareness of organics. She describes how the insecticide dichlorodiphenyltrichloroethane (DDT) destroys not only malaria-spreading mosquitoes, but also birds and other wildlife. She was concerned that chemicals were being used with "little or no advance investigation of their effect on soil, water, wildlife, and man himself." Her book was instrumental in the formation of the Environmental Protection Agency (EPA) and the ban of DDT in 1972.

Another factor that stimulated awareness of organics was the hippy movement of the 1960s. Hippies rebelled against the established ways of life, opting for a more natural lifestyle. Females burned their bras, stopped wearing makeup, and were among the first to return to breast-feeding. Men let their hair grow long and quit shaving. They formed communes where they lived off the land. Part of their return to nature included organic gardening. By the early 1970s, people who preached "organic and natural" were considered by most of mainstream America to be hippies.

Farmers of California led the nation in organic agriculture and founded the California Certified Organic Farmers (CCOF) association in 1973. The organization is still considered a leader in organic certification in North America. California was first to pass its "Organic Food Act" in 1979. Members of CCOF were instrumental with the passage of the Federal Organic Foods Production Act of 1990.

Even after the federal act was passed, there was still no way that a person could look at food in a local grocery store and know the product was organic or not. Therefore, in 2004, the United States Department of Agriculture (USDA) and the Food and Drug Administration (FDA) developed the USDA-certified labeling. Organic-related definitions allowed on food labels are listed below.

- **100 percent organic.** Products that are completely organic or made of all organic ingredients.
- **Organic.** Products that are at least 95 percent organic.
- **Made with organic ingredients.** These are products that contain at least 70 percent organic ingredients. The organic seal can't be used on these packages.
- **All-natural, free-range, or hormone-free.** These descriptions *do not* mean the food is organic.

More and more of us are grabbing organic foods. According to Ed Hamer and Mark Anslow, organic foods can feed the world, if we farm and eat differently. They say organically produced foods are more nutritious than conventionally grown foods and are earth friendly. Mark Bittman disagrees and insists that eating organically offers "no guarantee of eating well, healthfully, sanely, even ethically." After you read their articles, decide if organic foods are better than conventionally grown ones.

Distinctions Between Conventional and Organic Farming

Conventional Farming	Organic Farming
Apply chemical fertilizers to promote plant growth.	Apply natural fertilizers, such as manure or compost, to feed soil and plants.
Spray insecticides to reduce pests and disease.	Use beneficial insects and birds, mating disruption or traps to reduce pests and disease.
Use chemical herbicides to manage weeds.	Rotate crops, till, hand weed, or mulch to manage weeds.
Give animals antibiotics, growth hormones, and medications to prevent disease and spur growth.	Give animals organic feed and allow them access to the outdoors. Use preventive measures—such as rotational grazing, a balanced diet, and clean housing—to help minimize disease.

Source: http://usda-fda.com/Articles/Organic.htm.

TIMELINE

Early 1900s   Industrialized agriculture begins.
1942   J.I. Rodale publishes *Organic Farming and Gardening*.
1962   Rachel Carson's book *Silent Spring* is published.
1972   DDT banned in the United States.
1973   California Certified Organic Farmers (CCOF) is formed.
1979   California Organic Food Act is passed.
1990   Federal Organic Foods Production Act is passed.
2002   USDA and FDA begin organic foods labeling.

YES ↵

Ed Hamer and Mark Anslow

10 Reasons Why Organic Can Feed the World

Can organic farming feed the world? Ed Hamer and Mark Anslow say yes, but we must eat and farm differently.

1. Yield

Switching to organic farming would have different effects according to where in the world you live and how you currently farm.

Studies show that the less industrialised world stands to benefit the most. In southern Brazil, maize and wheat yields doubled on farms that changed to green manures and nitrogen-fixing leguminous vegetables instead of chemical fertilisers. In Mexico, coffee-growers who chose to move to fully organic production methods saw increases of 50 per cent in the weight of beans they harvested. In fact, in an analysis of more than 286 organic conversions in 57 countries, the average yield increase was found to be an impressive 64 per cent.

The situation is more complex in the industrialised world, where farms are large, intensive facilities, and opinions are divided on how organic yields would compare.

Research by the University of Essex in 1999 found that, although yields on US farms that converted to organic initially dropped by between 10 and 15 per cent, they soon recovered, and the farms became more productive than their all-chemical counterparts. In the UK, however, a study by the Elm Farm Research Centre predicted that a national transition to all-organic farming would see cereal, rapeseed and sugar beet yields fall by between 30 and 60 percent. Even the Soil Association admits that, on average in the UK, organic yields are 30 per cent lower than non-organic.

So can we hope to feed ourselves organically in the British Isles and Northern Europe? An analysis by former *Ecologist* editor Simon Fairlie in *The Land* journal suggests that we can, but only if we are prepared to rethink our diet and farming practices.

In Fairlie's scenario, each of the UK's 60 million citizens could have organic cereals, potatoes, sugar, vegetables and fruit, fish, pork, chicken and beef, as well as wool and flax for clothes and biomass crops for heating. To achieve this we'd each have to cut down to around 230 g of beef (½ lb), compared to an average of 630 g (1½ lb) today, 252 g of pork/bacon, 210 g of chicken and just under 4 kg (9 lb) of dairy produce each week—considerably more than the country enjoyed in 1945. We would probably need to supplement our diet with home-grown vegetables, save our food scraps as livestock feed and reform the sewage system to use our waste as an organic fertiliser.

2. Energy

Currently, we use around 10 calories of fossil energy to produce one calorie of food energy. In a fuel-scarce future, which experts think could arrive as early as 2012, such numbers simply won't stack up.

Studies by the Department for Environment, Food and Rural affairs over the past three years have shown that, on average, organically grown crops use 25 per cent less energy than their chemical cousins. Certain crops achieve even better reductions, including organic leeks (58 per cent less energy) and broccoli (49 per cent less energy).

When these savings are combined with stringent energy conservation and local distribution and consumption (such as organic box schemes), energy-use dwindles to a fraction of that needed for an intensive, centralised food system. A study by the University of Surrey shows that food from Tolhurst Organic Produce, a smallholding in Berkshire, which supplies 400 households with vegetable boxes, uses 90 per cent less energy than if non-organic produce had been delivered and bought in a supermarket.

Far from being simply 'energy-lite', however, organic farms have the potential to become self-sufficient in energy—or even to become energy exporters. The 'Dream

From *The Ecologist*, March 1, 2008, pp. 43–46. Copyright © 2008 by The Ecologist. Reprinted by permission.

Farm' model, first proposed by Mauritius-born agroscientist George Chan, sees farms feeding manure and waste from livestock and crops into biodigesters, which convert it into a methane-rich gas to be used for creating heat and electricity. The residue from these biodigesters is a crumbly, nutrient-rich fertiliser, which can be spread on soil to increase crop yields or further digested by algae and used as a fish or animal feed.

3. Greenhouse Gas Emission and Climate Change

Despite organic farming's low-energy methods, it is not in reducing demand for power that the techniques stand to make the biggest savings in greenhouse gas emissions.

The production of ammonium nitrate fertiliser, which is indispensable to conventional farming, produces vast quantities of nitrous oxide—a greenhouse gas with a global warming potential some 320 times greater than that of CO_2. In fact, the production of one tonne of ammonium nitrate creates 6.7 tonnes of greenhouse gases ($CO_2{}^e$), and was responsible for around 10 percent of all industrial greenhouse gas emissions in Europe in 2003.

The techniques used in organic agriculture to enhance soil fertility in turn encourage crops to develop deeper roots, which increase the amount of organic matter in the soil, locking up carbon underground and keeping it out of the atmosphere.

The opposite happens in conventional farming: high quantities of artificially supplied nutrients encourage quick growth and shallow roots. A study published in 1995 in the journal *Ecological Applications* found that levels of carbon in the soils of organic farms in California were as much as 28 per cent higher as a result. And research by the Rodale Institute shows that if the US were to convert all its corn and soybean fields to organic methods, the amount of carbon that could be stored in the soil would equal 73 per cent of the country's Kyoto targets for CO_2 reduction.

Organic farming might also go some way towards salvaging the reputation of the cow, demonised in 2007 as a major source of methane at both ends of its digestive tract. There's no doubt that this is a problem: estimates put global methane emissions from ruminant livestock at around 80 million tonnes a year, equivalent to around two billion tonnes of CO_2, or close to the annual CO_2 output of Russia and the UK combined. But by changing the pasturage on which animals graze to legumes such as clover or birdsfoot trefoil (often grown anyway by organic farmers to improve soil nitrogen content), scientists at the Institute of Grassland and Environmental Research believe that methane emissions could be cut dramatically. Because the leguminous foliage is more digestible, bacteria in the cow's gut are less able to turn the fodder into methane. Cows also seem naturally to prefer eating birdsfoot trefoil to ordinary grass.

4. Water Use

Agriculture is officially the most thirsty industry on the planet, consuming a staggering 72 per cent of all global freshwater at a time when the UN says 80 per cent of our water supplies are being overexploited.

This hasn't always been the case. Traditionally, agricultural crops were restricted to those areas best suited to their physiology, with drought-tolerant species grown in the tropics and water-demanding crops in temperate regions.

Global trade throughout the second half of the last century led to a worldwide production of grains dominated by a handful of high-yielding cereal crops, notably wheat, maize and rice. These thirsty cereals—the 'big three'—now account for more than half of the world's plant-based calories and 85 per cent of total grain production.

Organic agriculture is different. Due to its emphasis on healthy soil structure, organic farming avoids many of the problems associated with compaction, erosion, salinisation and soil degradation, which are prevalent in intensive systems. Organic manures and green mulches are applied even before the crop is sown, leading to a process known as 'mineralisation'—literally the fixing of minerals in the soil. Mineralised organic matter, conspicuously absent from synthetic fertilisers, is one of the essential ingredients required physically and chemically to hold water on the land.

Organic management also uses crop rotations, undersowing and mixed cropping to provide the soil with near-continuous cover. By contrast, conventional farm soils may be left uncovered for extended periods prior to sowing, and again following the harvest, leaving essential organic matter fully exposed to erosion by rain, wind and sunlight.

In the US, a 25-year Rodale Institute experiment on climatic extremes found that, due to improved soil structure, organic systems consistently achieve higher yields during periods both of drought and flooding.

5. Localisation

The globalisation of our food supply, which gives us Peruvian apples in June and Spanish lettuces in February, has seen our food reduced to a commodity in an increasingly volatile global marketplace.

Although year-round availability makes for good marketing in the eyes of the biggest retailers, the costs to the environment are immense.

Friends of the Earth estimates that the average meal in the UK travels 1,000 miles from plot to plate. In 2005, Defra released a comprehensive report on food miles in the UK, which valued the direct environmental, social and economic costs of food transport in Britain at £9 billion each year. In addition, food transport accounted for more than 30 billion vehicle kilometres, 25 percent of all HGV journeys and 19 million tonnes of carbon dioxide emissions in 2002 alone.

The organic movement was born out of a commitment to provide local food for local people, and so it is logical that organic marketing encourages localisation through veg boxes, farm shops and stalls. Between 2005 and 2006, organic sales made through direct marketing outlets such as these increased by 53 per cent, from £95 to £146 million, more than double the sales growth experienced by the major supermarkets. As we enter an age of unprecedented food insecurity, it is essential that our consumption reflects not only what is desirable, but also what is ultimately sustainable. While the 'organic' label itself may inevitably be hijacked, 'organic and local' represents a solution with which the global players can simply never compete.

6. Pesticides

It is a shocking testimony to the power of the agrochemical industry that in the 45 years since Rachel Carson published her pesticide warning *Silent Spring*, the number of commercially available synthetic pesticides has risen from 22 to more than 450.

According to the World Health Organization there are an estimated 20,000 accidental deaths worldwide each year from pesticide exposure and poisoning. More than 31 million kilograms of pesticide were applied to UK crops alone in 2005, 0.5 kilograms for every person in the country. A spiralling dependence on pesticides throughout recent decades has resulted in a catalogue of repercussions, including pest resistance, disease susceptibility, loss of natural biological controls and reduced nutrient-cycling.

Organic farmers, on the other hand, believe that a healthy plant grown in a healthy soil will ultimately be more resistant to pest damage. Organic systems encourage a variety of natural methods to enhance soil and plant health, in turn reducing incidences of pests, weeds and disease.

First and foremost, because organic plants grow comparatively slower than conventional varieties they have thicker cell walls, which provide a tougher natural barrier to pests. Rotations or 'break-crops', which are central to organic production, also provide a physical obstacle to pest and disease lifecycles by removing crops from a given plot for extended periods. Organic systems also rely heavily on a rich agro-ecosystem in which many agricultural pests can be controlled by their natural predators.

Inevitably, however, there are times when pestilence attacks are especially prolonged or virulent, and here permitted pesticides may be used. The use of organic pesticides is heavily regulated and the International Federation of Organic Agriculture Movements (IFOAM) requires specific criteria to be met before pesticide applications can be justified.

There are in fact only four active ingredients permitted for use on organic crops: copper fungicides, restricted largely to potatoes and occasionally orchards; sulphur, used to control additional elements of fungal diseases; Rotenone, a naturally occurring plant extract; and soft soap, derived from potassium soap and used to control aphids. Herbicides are entirely prohibited.

7. Ecosystem Impact

Farmland accounts for 70 per cent of UK land mass, making it the single most influential enterprise affecting our wildlife. Incentives offered for intensification under the Common Agricultural Policy are largely responsible for negative ecosystem impacts over recent years. Since 1962, farmland bird numbers have declined by an average of 30 per cent. During the same period more than 192,000 kilometres of hedgerows have been removed, while 45 per cent of our ancient woodland has been converted to cropland.

By contrast, organic farms actively encourage biodiversity in order to maintain soil fertility and aid natural pest control. Mixed farming systems ensure that a diversity of food and nesting sites [is] available throughout the year, compared with conventional farms where autumn sow crops leave little winter vegetation available.

Organic production systems are designed to respect the balance observed in our natural ecosystems. It is widely accepted that controlling or suppressing one element of wildlife, even if it is a pest, will have unpredictable impacts on the rest of the food chain. Instead, organic producers regard a healthy ecosystem as essential to a healthy farm, rather than a barrier to production.

In 2005, a report by English Nature and the RSPB on the impacts of organic farming on biodiversity reviewed more than 70 independent studies of flora, invertebrates, birds and mammals within organic and conventional farming systems. It concluded that biodiversity is enhanced at every level of the food chain under organic management practices, from soil micro-biota right through to farmland birds and the largest mammals.

8. Nutritional Benefits

While an all-organic farming system might mean we'd have to make do with slightly less food than we're used to, research shows that we can rest assured it would be better for us. In 2001, a study in the *Journal of Complementary Medicine* found that organic crops contained higher levels of 21 essential nutrients than their conventionally grown counterparts, including iron, magnesium, phosphorus and vitamin C. The organic crops also contained lower levels of nitrates, which can be toxic to the body.

Other studies have found significantly higher levels of vitamins—as well as polyphenols and antioxidants—in organic fruit and veg, both of which are thought to play a role in cancer-prevention within the body.

Scientists have also been able to work out why organic farming produces more nutritious food. Avoiding chemical fertilizer reduces nitrates levels in the food; better quality soil increases the availability of trace minerals, and reduced levels of pesticides mean that the plants' own immune systems grow stronger, producing higher levels of antioxidants. Slower rates of growth also mean that organic food frequently contains higher levels of dry mass, meaning that fruit and vegetables are less pumped up with water and so contain more nutrients by weight than intensively grown crops do.

Milk from organically fed cows has been found to contain higher levels of nutrients in six separate studies, including omega-3 fatty acids, vitamin E, and beta-carotene, all of which can help prevent cancer. One experiment discovered that levels of omega-3 in organic milk were on average 68 per cent higher than in non-organic alternatives.

But as well as giving us more of what we do need, organic food can help to give us less of what we don't. In 2000, the UN Food and Agriculture Organization (FAO) found that organically produced food had 'lower levels of pesticide and veterinary drug residues' than non-organic did. Although organic farmers are allowed to use antibiotics when absolutely necessary to treat disease, the routine use of the drugs in animal feed—common on intensive livestock farms—is forbidden. This means a shift to organic livestock farming could help tackle problems such as the emergence of antibiotic-resistant bacteria.

9. Seed-Saving

Seeds are not simply a source of food; they are living testimony to more than 10,000 years of agricultural domestication. Tragically, however, they are a resource that has suffered unprecedented neglect. The UN FAO estimates that 75 per cent of the genetic diversity of agricultural crops has been lost over the past 100 years.

Traditionally, farming communities have saved seeds year on year, both in order to save costs and to trade with their neighbours. As a result, seed varieties evolved in response to local climatic and seasonal conditions, leading to a wide variety of fruiting times, seed size, appearance and flavour. More importantly, this meant a constant updating process for the seed's genetic resistance to changing climatic conditions, new pests and diseases.

By contrast, modern intensive agriculture depends on relatively few crops—only about 150 species are cultivated on any significant scale worldwide. This is the inheritance of the Green Revolution, which in the late 1950s perfected varieties Filial 1, or F1 seed technology, which produced hybrid seeds with specifically desirable genetic qualities. These new high-yield seeds were widely adopted, but because the genetic makeup of hybrid F1 seeds becomes diluted following the first harvest, the manufacturers ensured that farmers return for more seed year on year.

With its emphasis on diversity, organic farming is somewhat cushioned from exploitation on this scale, but even Syngenta, the world's third-largest biotech company, now offers organic seed lines. Although seed-saving is not a prerequisite for organic production, the holistic nature of organics lends itself well to conserving seed.

In support of this, the Heritage Seed Library, in Warwickshire, is a collection of more than 800 open-pollinated organic varieties, which have been carefully preserved by gardeners across the country.

Although their seeds are not yet commercially available, the Library is at the forefront of addressing the alarming erosion of our agricultural diversity.

Seed-saving and the development of local varieties must become a key component of organic farming, giving crops the potential to evolve in response to what could be rapidly changing climatic conditions. This will help agriculture keeps pace with climate change in the field, rather than in the laboratory.

10. Job Creation

There is no doubt British farming is currently in crisis. With an average of 37 farmers leaving the land every day, there are now more prisoners behind bars in the UK than there are farmers in the fields.

Although it has been slow, the decline in the rural labour force is a predictable consequence of the industrialisation of agriculture. A mere one per cent of the UK workforce is now employed in land-related enterprises, compared with 35 per cent at the turn of the last century.

The implications of this decline are serious. A skilled agricultural workforce will be essential in order to maintain food security in the coming transition towards a new model of post-fossil fuel farming. Many of these skills have already been eroded through mechanisation and a move towards more specialised and intensive production systems.

Organic farming is an exception to these trends. By its nature, organic production relies on labour-intensive management practices. Smaller, more diverse farming systems require a level of husbandry that is simply uneconomical at any other scale. Organic crops and livestock also demand specialist knowledge and regular monitoring in the absence of agrochemical controls.

According to a 2006 report by the University of Essex, organic farming in the UK provides 32 per cent more jobs per farm than comparable non-organic farms. Interestingly, the report also concluded that the higher employment observed could not be replicated in non-organic farming through initiatives such as local marketing.

Instead, the majority (81 per cent) of total employment on organic farms was created by the organic production system itself. The report estimates that 93,000 new jobs would be created if all farming in the UK were to convert to organic.

Organic farming also accounts for more younger employees than any other sector in the industry. The average age of conventional UK farmers is now 56, yet organic farms increasingly attract a younger more enthusiastic workforce, people who view organics as the future of food production. It is for this next generation of farmers that Organic Futures, a campaign group set up by the Soil Association in 2007, is striving to provide a platform.

ED HAMER is a freelance journalist specializing in agricultural globalization issues in the United Kingdom.

MARK ANSLOW is editor of the *Ecologist* magazine, one of the world's leading environmental publications.

Mark Bittman 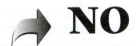 **NO**

Eating Food That's Better for You, Organic or Not

In the six-and-one-half years since the federal government began certifying food as "organic," Americans have taken to the idea with considerable enthusiasm. Sales have at least doubled, and three-quarters of the nation's grocery stores now carry at least some organic food. A Harris poll in October 2007 found that about 30 percent of Americans buy organic food at least on occasion, and most think it is safer, better for the environment and healthier.

"People believe it must be better for you if it's organic," says Phil Howard, an assistant professor of community, food and agriculture at Michigan State University.

So I discovered on a recent book tour around the United States and Canada.

No matter how carefully I avoided using the word "organic" when I spoke to groups of food enthusiasts about how to eat better, someone in the audience would inevitably ask, "What if I can't afford to buy organic food?" It seems to have become the magic cure-all, synonymous with eating well, healthfully, sanely, even ethically.

But eating "organic" offers no guarantee of any of that. And the truth is that most Americans eat so badly—we get 7 percent of our calories from soft drinks, more than we do from vegetables; the top food group by caloric intake is "sweets"; and one-third of nation's adults are now obese—that the organic question is a secondary one. It's not unimportant, but it's not the primary issue in the way Americans eat.

To eat well, says Michael Pollan, the author of "In Defense of Food," means avoiding "edible food-like substances" and sticking to real ingredients, increasingly from the plant kingdom. (Americans each consume an average of nearly two pounds a day of animal products.) There's plenty of evidence that both a person's health—as well as the environment's—will improve with a simple shift in eating habits away from animal products and highly processed foods to plant products and what might be called

"real food." (With all due respect to people in the "food movement," the food need not be "slow," either.)

From these changes, Americans would reduce the amount of land, water and chemicals used to produce the food we eat, as well as the incidence of lifestyle diseases linked to unhealthy diets, and greenhouse gases from industrial meat production. All without legislation.

And the food would not necessarily have to be organic, which, under the United States Department of Agriculture's definition, means it is generally free of synthetic substances; contains no antibiotics and hormones; has not been irradiated or fertilized with sewage sludge; was raised without the use of most conventional pesticides; and contains no genetically modified ingredients.

Those requirements, which must be met in order for food to be labeled "U.S.D.A. Organic," are fine, of course. But they still fall short of the lofty dreams of early organic farmers and consumers who gave the word "organic" its allure—of returning natural nutrients and substance to the soil in the same proportion used by the growing process (there is no requirement that this be done); of raising animals humanely in accordance with nature (animals must be given access to the outdoors, but for how long and under what conditions is not spelled out); and of producing the most nutritious food possible (the evidence is mixed on whether organic food is more nutritious) in the most ecologically conscious way.

The government's organic program, says Joan Shaffer, a spokeswoman for the Agriculture Department, "is a marketing program that sets standards for what can be certified as organic. Neither the enabling legislation nor the regulations address food safety or nutrition."

People don't understand that, nor do they realize "organic" doesn't mean "local." "It doesn't matter if it's from the farm down the road or from Chile," Ms. Shaffer said. "As long as it meets the standards it's organic."

Hence, the organic status of salmon flown in from Chile, or of frozen vegetables grown in China and sold in the United States—no matter the size of the carbon footprint left behind by getting from there to here.

Today, most farmers who practice truly sustainable farming, or what you might call "organic in spirit," operate on small scale, some so small they can't afford the requirements to be certified organic by the government. Others say that certification isn't meaningful enough to bother. These farmers argue that, "When you buy organic you don't just buy a product, you buy a way of life that is committed to not exploiting the planet," says Ed Maltby, executive director of the Northeast Organic Dairy Producers Alliance.

But the organic food business is now big business, and getting bigger. Professor Howard estimates that major corporations now are responsible for at least 25 percent of all organic manufacturing and marketing (40 percent if you count only processed organic foods). Much of the nation's organic food is as much a part of industrial food production as midwinter grapes, and becoming more so. In 2006, sales of organic foods and beverages totaled about $16.7 billion, according to the most recent figures from Organic Trade Association.

Still, those sales amounted to slightly less than 3 percent of overall food and beverage sales. For all the hoo-ha, organic food is not making much of an impact on the way Americans eat, though, as Mark Kastel, co-founder of The Cornucopia Institute, puts it: "There are generic benefits from doing organics. It protects the land from the ravages of conventional agriculture," and safeguards farm workers from being exposed to pesticides.

But the questions remain over how we eat in general. It may feel better to eat an organic Oreo than a conventional Oreo, but, says Marion Nestle, a professor at New York University's department of nutrition, food studies and public health, "Organic junk food is still junk food."

Last [year], Michelle Obama began digging up a patch of the South Lawn of the White House to plant an organic vegetable garden to provide food for the first family and, more important, to educate children about healthy, locally grown fruits and vegetables at a time when obesity and diabetes have become national concerns.

But Mrs. Obama also emphasized that there were many changes Americans can make if they don't have the time or space for an organic garden.

"You can begin in your own cupboard," she said, "by eliminating processed food, trying to cook a meal a little more often, trying to incorporate more fruits and vegetables."

Popularizing such choices may not be as marketable as creating a logo that says "organic." But when Americans have had their fill of "value-added" and overprocessed food, perhaps they can begin producing and consuming more food that treats animals and the land as if they mattered. Some of that food will be organic, and hooray for that. Meanwhile, they should remember that the word itself is not synonymous with "safe," "healthy," "fair" or even necessarily "good."

MARK BITTMAN is a food journalist and author. He writes a weekly column for *The New York Times* dining section called *The Minimalist*. He has authored over 10 books on food and cooking.

EXPLORING THE ISSUE

Are Organic Foods Better Than Conventional Foods?

Critical Thinking and Reflection

1. Define what is meant by "organic and local."
2. Describe how both the articles compare the way organic foods are grown today to the way the early organic farmers originally intended them to be grown.
3. List the benefits that organic foods provide to people, the environment, and society.
4. Ed Hamer and Mark Anslow say that organic farming can feed the world if we "farm and eat differently." Explain what they mean by this.
5. Design a program that will ensure all people in your city have access to affordable organic foods.

Is There Common Ground?

Both Hamer and Anslow are U.K.-based journalists and look at the influence that conventional farming has on the global environment. They begin by acknowledging that the yield from organic foods will vary depending on current farming practices of the country. They point out that less fossil energy, water, and pesticides are used by organic practices and that organic results in less greenhouse emissions. And organic practices are kinder to wildlife. They cite several studies that claim organic foods and beverages provide more nutrients than conventionally grown foods.

In contrast, Mark Bittman says that eating organically "offers no guarantee" that the foods are healthier or even grown more ethically. He points out that "most Americans eat so badly . . . that the organic question is secondary." Bittman agrees with Michael Pollan's recommendation that we should avoid "edible food-like substances" and eat real foods with the least processing as possible. He also agrees that eating more from the plant kingdom and less animal products is better. Changes like this would reduce the amount of land, water, and chemicals used. Bittman says the foods don't necessarily need to meet the USDA definition of "organic" to improve health.

Bittman criticizes current practices of organic food production and points out that the current practices are not what the original organic crusaders wanted. Currently, major food corporations are responsible for 25 percent of all organic food manufacturing and marketing. This makes it difficult for small local organic farms to thrive. There are differences between "locally grown" and "organic." He criticizes the carbon footprints that organic foods leave behind that are flown to America

from around the world and says they defeat the purpose of the organic movement. He concludes by applauding the garden Michelle Obama planted on the lawn of the White House. The garden educates Americans about the benefits of fresh fruits and vegetables and encourages less reliance on overly processed foods. He concludes that we all need to eat better, some of the foods may not meet the definition of "organic," but we can all strive to eat foods that are less processed and grown in a manner that is easier on the environment.

Additional Resources

Johansson E, Hussain A, Kuktaite R, Andersson SC, Olsson ME. Contribution of organically grown crops to human health. *Int J Environ Res Public Health.* 2014;11(4):3870–93.

Niggli U. Sustainability of organic food production: Challenges and innovations. *Proc Nutr Soc.* 2015;74(1):83–8.

Smith-spangler C, Brandeau ML, Hunter GE, et al. Are organic foods safer or healthier than conventional alternatives?: A systematic review. *Ann Intern Med.* 2012;157(5):348–66.

Strassner C, Cavoski I, Di cagno R, et al. How the organic food system supports sustainable diets and translates these into practice. *Front Nutr.* 2015;2:19.

Vallverdú-queralt A, Lamuela-raventós RM. Foodomics: A new tool to differentiate between organic and conventional foods. *Electrophoresis.* 2015. doi:+10.1002/elps.201500348.

Internet References . . .

Organic Consumers

www.organicconsumers.org

Organic Foods Research Foundation

www.ofrf.org/organic-faqs

United States Department of Agriculture

www.usda.gov

Selected, Edited, and with Issue Framing Material by:
Janet M. Colson, *Middle Tennessee State University*

ISSUE

Does the World Need Genetically Modified Foods?

YES: William Saletan, from "Unhealthy Fixation: The War against Genetically Modified Organisms Is Full of Fearmongering, Errors, and Fraud. Labeling Them Will Not Make You Safer," *Slate* (2015)

NO: Claire Robinson, from "Lessons in Critical Thinking and William Saletan—Part 1," GMWatch.org (2015)

Learning Outcomes
After reading this issue, you will be able to:
• Discuss how genetic modification (GM) makes certain plants disease resistant. • List the main types of GM that are currently used. • Identify the benefits that GM provides to our food supply and the possible hazards that could occur if we continue to use GM seeds.

ISSUE SUMMARY

YES: William Saletan defends biotechnology used in genetically modifying foods and believes they bring many advantages and help ensure a safe food supply. He says the case AGAINST genetic modification is full of errors, fallacies, misconceptions, misrepresentations, and lies.

NO: *GMWatch* editor Claire Robinson, and co-author of the free online book *GM Myths and Truths,* points out the fallacies of Saletan's defense of GM foods in her rebuttal to his article. She grades his "critical thinking in which Saletan gets a big "F" for "Fail."

If you eat any processed foods, chances are you have eaten genetically modified (GM) ones without even knowing it. Most people have heard of the term, but may not know exactly what "genetically modified" means. The World Health Organization (WHO) defines it as "organisms in which the genetic material (DNA) has been altered in a way that does not occur naturally." Other names for GM are "genetic engineering," "modern biotechnology," "gene technology," "gene splicing," and "bioengineered." The term genetically modified organism (GMO) simply refers to any organism whose genetic material has been altered using genetic engineering techniques.

Scientists have been working on GM techniques for many years in an effort to improve and extend the world's food supply. Some GM involves improving the vitamin, omega-3 fatty acid, or other nutrient content of crops or animals. Others try to speed up the growth or improve the taste or appearance of a food. Some commonly used GMs are designed to make crops tolerant to herbicides, whereas others make the product resistant to insects.

The most common herbicide used in developed countries is Roundup, which contains the potentially toxic chemical glyphosate. The Environmental Protection Agency (EPA) currently considers it safe, whereas the WHO and the United Nations classify glyphosate as a "probable carcinogen." Many environmentalists, such as Claire Robinson, are concerned about long-term exposure to glyphosates, although most conventional farmers use it to kill the weeds and grasses around their crops, as do home gardeners. Use of Roundup eliminates, or at least reduces, the amount of weeds in the garden. The only problem is that Roundup is so strong that it kills the plant.

A seed that is modified to become "Roundup Ready" means a farmer can plant the GM seeds and spray Roundup in the field, on both weeds and plants. Because the plants are tolerant of Roundup, they do not die but the weeds do. To date, "Roundup Ready" is the most common GM procedure used. It is used in soy, corn, sorghum, canola, alfalfa, and cotton.

The USDA Economic Research Services tracks the GM crops, specifically the herbicide-tolerant (HT), such as "Roundup Ready," and the insect-resistant crops that contain the gene from the soil bacterium Bt *(Bacillus thuringiensis)*. The Bt bacteria produce a protein that is toxic to specific insects; if the plant contains the Bt gene, insects cannot attack the plant, and the plant is protected over its entire life.

The vast majority of soybeans, cotton, and corn grown in the United States are from GM seeds. Based on the USDA 2015 survey data:

HT soybeans went from 17 percent of U.S. soybean acreage in 1997 to 68 percent in 2001 and 94 percent in 2014 and in 2015. Plantings of HT cotton expanded from about 10 percent of U.S. acreage in 1997 to 56 percent in 2001, 91 percent in 2014, but declined to 89 percent in 2015. The adoption of HT corn, which had been slower in previous years, has accelerated, reaching 89 percent of U.S. corn acreage in 2014 and in 2015.

Bt-resistant crops have been available since 1996. Plantings of Bt corn grew from about 8 percent of U.S. corn acreage in 1997 to 19 percent in 2000 and 2001, before climbing to 29 percent in 2003 and 81 percent in 2015. The increases in acreage share in recent years may be largely due to the commercial introduction of new Bt corn varieties resistant to the corn rootworm and the corn earworm, in addition to the European corn borer, which was previously the only pest targeted by Bt corn. Plantings of Bt cotton also expanded rapidly, from 15 percent of U.S. cotton acreage in 1997 to 37 percent in 2001 and 84 percent in 2014 and in 2015.

As related to Roundup Ready crops, people are concerned about two things. First, what effect does the Roundup residue that remains on the plant—and the food we eat—have on our bodies? The second is related to the actual genetic changes in the DNA. Is it safe for humans? GM foods have only been around since the 1990s, and the long-term effects they could have on health and the environment are not known. Some laboratory studies have reported problems with fertility, abnormalities in offspring, and kidney problems in laboratory studies using GM foods.

GM crops are a global concern. The European Network of Scientists for Social and Environmental Responsibility (ENSSER) published its position statement, "No scientific consensus on GMO safety." Over 300 experts (scientists, physicians, academics, and experts from disciplines relevant to the scientific, legal, and social and safety assessment aspects of GMO) signed the statement. Part of their position includes:

. . . we strongly reject claims by GM seed developers and some scientists, commentators, and journalists that there is a "scientific consensus" on GMO safety and that the debate on this topic is "over."

We feel compelled to issue this statement because the claimed consensus on GMO safety does not exist. The claim that it does exist is misleading and misrepresents the currently available scientific evidence and the broad diversity of opinion among scientists on this issue. Moreover, the claim encourages a climate of complacency that could lead to a lack of regulatory and scientific rigour and appropriate caution, potentially endangering the health of humans, animals, and the environment.

Science and society do not proceed on the basis of a constructed consensus, as current knowledge is always open to well-founded challenge and disagreement. We endorse the need for further independent scientific inquiry and informed public discussion on GM product safety and urge GM proponents to do the same.

After you read the two articles, decide if you believe that we need GM foods to help feed the world. Or better yet, do you want to eat these foods that some call "Frankenfoods"? William Saletan defends biotechnology used in GM crops and believes they bring many advantages to the world's food supply. Claire Robinson, an anti-GM advocate who has been following the scientific debate about GM crops for many years, argues that there are potential health risks associated with GM foods. So, do you think GM foods are potentially dangerous or that we need them to help feed the world?

YES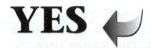

William Saletan

Unhealthy Fixation: The War against Genetically Modified Organisms Is Full of Fearmongering, Errors, and Fraud. Labeling Them Will Not Make You Safer

They Want You to Be Overwhelmed

Is genetically engineered food dangerous? Many people seem to think it is. In the past five years, companies have submitted more than 27,000 products to the Non-GMO Project, which certifies goods that are free of genetically modified organisms. Last year, sales of such products nearly tripled. Whole Foods will soon require labels on all GMOs in its stores. Abbott, the company that makes Similac baby formula, has created a non-GMO version to give parents "peace of mind." Trader Joe's has sworn off GMOs. So has Chipotle.

Some environmentalists and public interest groups want to go further. Hundreds of organizations, including Consumers Union, Friends of the Earth, Physicians for Social Responsibility, the Center for Food Safety, and the Union of Concerned Scientists, are demanding "mandatory labeling of genetically engineered foods." Since 2013, Vermont, Maine, and Connecticut have passed laws to require GMO labels. Massachusetts could be next.

The central premise of these laws—and the main source of consumer anxiety, which has sparked corporate interest in GMO-free food—is concern about health. Last year, in a survey by the Pew Research Center, 57 percent of Americans said it's generally "unsafe to eat genetically modified foods." Vermont says the primary purpose of its labeling law is to help people "avoid potential health risks of food produced from genetic engineering." Chipotle notes that 300 scientists have "signed a statement rejecting the claim that there is a scientific consensus on the safety of GMOs for human consumption." Until more studies are conducted, Chipotle says, "We believe it is prudent to take a cautious approach toward GMOs."

The World Health Organization, the American Medical Association, the National Academy of Sciences, and the American Association for the Advancement of Science have all declared that there's no good evidence GMOs are unsafe. Hundreds of studies back up that conclusion. But many of us don't trust these assurances. We're drawn to skeptics who say that there's more to the story, that some studies have found risks associated with GMOs, and that Monsanto is covering it up.

I've spent much of the past year digging into the evidence. Here's what I've learned. First, it's true that the issue is complicated. But the deeper you dig, the more fraud you find in the case against GMOs. It's full of errors, fallacies, misconceptions, misrepresentations, and lies. The people who tell you that Monsanto is hiding the truth are themselves hiding evidence that their own allegations about GMOs are false. They're counting on you to feel overwhelmed by the science and to accept, as a gut presumption, their message of distrust.

Second, the central argument of the anti-GMO movement—that prudence and caution are reasons to avoid genetically engineered, or GE, food—is a sham. Activists who tell you to play it safe around GMOs take no such care in evaluating the alternatives. They denounce proteins in GE crops as toxic, even as they defend drugs, pesticides, and non-GMO crops that are loaded with the same proteins. They portray genetic engineering as chaotic and unpredictable, even when studies indicate that other crop improvement methods, including those favored by the same activists, are more disruptive to plant genomes.

. . .

Third, there are valid concerns about some aspects of GE agriculture, such as herbicides, monocultures, and patents. But none of these concerns is fundamentally about genetic engineering. Genetic engineering isn't a thing. It's a process that can be used in different ways to create different things. To think clearly about GMOs, you have to distinguish among the applications and focus on the substance of each case. If you're concerned about pesticides and transparency, you need to know about the toxins to which your food has been exposed. A GMO label won't tell you that. And it can lull you into buying a non-GMO product even when the GE alternative is safer.

If you're like me, you don't really want to wade into this issue. It's too big, technical, and confusing. But come with me, just this once. I want to take you backstage, behind those blanket assurances about the safety of genetic engineering. I want to take you down into the details of four GMO fights, because that's where you'll find truth. You'll come to the last curtain, the one that hides the reality of the anti-GMO movement. And you'll see what's behind it.

The Papaya Triumph

Twenty years ago Hawaiian papaya farmers were in trouble. Ringspot virus, transmitted by insects, was destroying the crop. Farmers tried everything to stop the virus: selective breeding, crop rotation, quarantine. Nothing worked. But one scientist had a different idea. What if he could transfer a gene from a harmless part of the virus, known as the coat protein, to the papaya's DNA? Would the GE papaya be immune to the virus?

The scientist, Dennis Gonsalves of Cornell University, got the idea, in part, from Monsanto. But Monsanto wasn't interested in papaya. Although papaya is an important staple in the developing world, it isn't a big moneymaker like soybeans or cotton. So Monsanto and two other companies licensed the technology to an association of Hawaiian farmers. The licenses were free but restricted to Hawaii. The association provided the seeds to farmers for free, and later at cost.

Today the GE papaya is a triumph. It saved the industry. But it's also a cautionary tale. The papaya, having defeated the virus, barely survived a campaign to purge GE crops from Hawaii. The story of that campaign teaches a hard lesson: No matter how long a GMO is eaten without harming anyone, and no matter how many studies are done to demonstrate its safety, there will always be skeptics who warn of unknown risks.

In 1996 and 1997, three federal agencies approved the GE papaya. The U.S. Department of Agriculture reported "no deleterious effects on plants, nontarget organisms, or the environment" in field trials. The Environmental Protection Agency pointed out that people had been eating the virus for years in infected papaya. "Entire infectious

particles of Papaya Ringspot Virus, including the coat protein component, are found in the fruit, leaves and stems of most plants," the EPA observed. The agency cited the long history of mammalian consumption of the entire plant virus particle in foods, without causing any deleterious human health effects. Virus-infected plants currently are and have always been a part of both the human and domestic animal food supply and there have been no findings which indicate that plant viruses are toxic to humans and other vertebrates. Further, plant viruses are unable to replicate in mammals or other vertebrates, thereby eliminating the possibility of human infection.

These arguments didn't satisfy everyone. In 1999, a year after the new papaya seeds were released to farmers, critics said the viral gene might interact with DNA from other viruses to create more dangerous pathogens. In 2000, vandals destroyed papaya trees and other biotech plants at a University of Hawaii research facility, calling the plants "genetic pollution." In 2001 the U.S. Public Interest Research Group identified Hawaii as the state most commonly used for outdoor GE crop tests, and it called for a nationwide moratorium on such tests. "The science of genetic engineering is radical and new," said U.S. PIRG, and GE crops had "not been properly tested for human health or environmental impact."

. . .

A Dutch study published in December 2002 seemed to vindicate this anxiety. According to the paper, a short stretch of the ringspot virus coat protein, now incorporated in the GE papaya, matched a sequence in an allergenic protein made by worms. The resemblance was only partial, and, as the authors noted, it didn't show that the protein triggered allergies, much less that the papaya did so. But anti-GMO activists didn't wait. The Institute of Science in Society published a "Biosafety Alert" titled "Allergenic GM Papaya Scandal." Greenpeace flagged the Dutch study and warned that "the interaction of GE papaya with other viruses . . . can produce new strains of viruses." The organization accused the papaya's developers of "playing with nature."

Some of these early alarms were disconcerting. But scientifically, they made no sense. Start with the distinction between "nature" and "genetic pollution." Nature had invented the ringspot virus. Millions of people had eaten it without any reports of harm. And breeders had been tinkering with nature for millennia.

Anti-GMO activists decried genetic engineering as imprecise and random. They ignored the far greater randomness of mutation in nature and the far greater imprecision of traditional breeding. Furthermore, after five years of commercial sale and consumption, there was no sign that GE papayas had hurt anyone. But the alarmists continued to fret about unforeseen interactions and doomsday mutations, ignoring research that didn't bear out these fantasies.

Take the "Allergenic GM Papaya Scandal." The protein made by the papaya's new gene consisted of about 280 amino acids. Out of that 280, the number of consecutive amino acids it shared with a putative allergen was six. By this standard, a study found that 41 of 50 randomly selected proteins in ordinary corn would also have to be declared allergenic. But GMO opponents ignored this study. They also ignored a second paper, which concluded that the putative worm allergen used in the papaya comparison was not, in fact, intrinsically allergenic.

Years passed, people ate papayas, and nothing bad happened. But the activists wouldn't relent. In 2004, Greenpeace vandals tore up a GE papaya orchard in Thailand, calling the plant a "time bomb" and claiming that it had devastated farmers in Hawaii. In 2006, Greenpeace issued another report condemning the fruit. In reality, the source of farmers' troubles was Greenpeace itself. The organization was working to block regulatory approval and sales of the GE papaya—and then blaming the papaya for farmers' financial woes.

From 2006 to 2010, USDA scientists, prodded by Japanese regulators, subjected the papaya to several additional studies. They verified that its new protein had no genetic sequence in common with any known allergen, using the common standard of eight consecutive amino acids rather than six. They demonstrated that the protein, unlike allergens, broke down in seconds in gastric fluid. They found that conventional virus-infected papayas, which people had been eating all along, had eight times as much viral protein as the GE papaya. In May 2009, after a decade of scrutiny, Japan's Food Safety Commission approved the GE papaya. Two years later, after resolving environmental questions, Japan opened its market to the fruit.

Chinese researchers performed additional tests. For four weeks they fed GE papayas to a group of rats. Meanwhile, they fed conventional papayas to another group of rats. The study found no resulting differences between the rats. It confirmed that coat protein fragments dissolved quickly in gastric fluid and left no detectable traces in organs.

By this point the GE papaya had been investigated and eaten for 15 years. GMO skeptics had two choices. They could acknowledge that their nightmares hadn't come true. Or they could reject the evidence and cling to their faith in a GMO apocalypse.

. . .

That dilemma split the anti-GMO camp in 2013, when the Hawaii County Council, which governed Hawaii's largest island, considered legislation to ban GE crops. The council's hearings, preserved on video by Occupy Hawaii (which favored the proposed ban), document a yearlong struggle between ideology and science. As council members heard testimony and studied the issue, they learned that the GE papaya didn't fit GMO stereotypes. It had been created by public-sector scientists, not by a corporation. It had saved a beloved crop. It had passed extensive scrutiny in Japan and the U.S. It didn't cross-pollinate nearby fields. It also reduced pesticide use, because farmers no longer had to exterminate the aphids that spread the virus.

One council member, Margaret Wille, yielded to the evidence. Wille was Hawaii's leading anti-GMO politician. She had introduced the proposed GMO ban. But after listening to the arguments, she exempted the GE papaya from her bill, noting that it was embedded in local agriculture and had been vetted in safety and cross-pollination tests. In effect, she acknowledged two things. First, the legitimate worries of biotech critics, such as pesticide use and corporate control of agriculture, didn't apply to all GE crops. And second, with the passage of time, novelties became conventional.

Other antagonists held their ground. Chief among them was Jeffrey Smith, the world's most prolific anti-GMO activist. In September 2013, Smith was given 45 minutes to testify before the council as an expert witness, though he had no formal scientific training. (When he was asked whether he should be addressed as Dr. Smith, he sidestepped the question by answering, "No, Jeffrey's fine.") Smith told the council that RNA from the GE papaya might disrupt genes in people and that proteins from the papaya might interfere with human immunity, leading to HIV and hepatitis. He also said the protein might cause cancer.

To support his testimony, Smith cited a March 2013 paper about regulation of GE crops. He said the paper "showed that the evaluation of this technology is sorely inadequate to protect against environmental problems and human health problems. And the papaya was one example cited in that study." But the paper made no claim about papayas. It simply listed them in a table of GE crops, alongside a theoretical critique of the technology.

Smith told the council that "there hasn't been any animal feeding studies on the papaya." Hector Valenzuela, a University of Hawaii crop specialist who also testified as an expert, said the same thing: that scientists hadn't "conducted a single study" to assess the safety of GE papaya. Neither man mentioned the Chinese papaya feeding study in rats—published two months before the theoretical paper Smith had cited—which had found none of the harms Smith alleged.

To explain why scientific organizations and regulatory agencies had declared GE foods safe, the anti-GMO witnesses offered conspiracy theories. They said the Food and Drug Administration had been captured by Monsanto. So had the American Association for the Advancement of Science. When the *New York Times'* Pulitzer Prize-winning science reporter Amy Harmon detailed the safety evidence behind the GE papaya, incredulous council members dismissed her article as a "skewed" account by "the political powers that be."

As for Japan's approval of the papaya, Valenzuela advised the council to look at U.S. government cables released by WikiLeaks. He said the cables showed "the lengths that the State Department goes to twist arms behind the scenes." This was a clear insinuation that U.S. officials had coerced Japan's decision. Smith mentioned the cables, too. But the cables showed no conspiracy. Nearly 6,000 of the leaked cables had been sent from U.S. embassies and consulates in Japan. They covered the years 2005 to 2010, during which Japanese regulators had debated and approved the GE papaya. Food & Water Watch, an environmental group, had searched the cables for references to pressure or lobbying by U.S. officials on behalf of GMOs. The group's report, issued in May 2013, cited no cables that indicated any such activity in Japan.

No allegation was too far-fetched for the anti-GMO witnesses, including several who called themselves experts. They said GMOs were especially dangerous to dark-skinned people. They suggested that vaccines were harmful, too. They said GE flowers should be banned because children might eat them.

What they wouldn't say, regardless of the evidence, was that the GE papaya was safe. Brenda Ford, a council member and sponsor of another anti-GMO bill, told her colleagues that they didn't have to answer that question, even when they were directly asked. Ford described genetic engineering as "random hits" on chromosomes. She said the science was still "in its infancy." Smith, in his testimony, suggested that gene transfer in agriculture should be studied for 50 to 150 years before allowing its use outdoors.

In the end, the papaya survived. Ford's bill died. Wille's bill was signed into law but was tied up in court. The new law makes an exception for papayas. But GMO labels don't. They don't tell you that the fruit you're looking at in your grocery store was engineered to need fewer pesticides, not more. They don't tell you about all the research that went into checking its safety. They don't tell you that

people have been eating it with no ill effects for more than 15 years. They don't tell you that when you buy it, your money goes to Hawaiian farmers, not to Monsanto.

Some people, to this day, believe GE papayas are dangerous. They want more studies. They'll always want more studies. They call themselves skeptics. But when you cling to an unsubstantiated belief, even after two decades of research and experience, that's not skepticism. It's dogma.

Organics Are Not Safer

In 1901 a Japanese biologist discovered that a strain of bacteria was killing his country's silkworms. Scientists gave the bacteria a name: *Bacillus thuringiensis*. It turned out to be handy for protecting crops from insects. Farmers and environmentalists loved it. It was natural, effective, and harmless to vertebrates.

In the mid-1980s, Belgian researchers found a better way to produce the insecticide. They put a gene from the bacteria into tobacco plants. When bugs tried to eat the plants, they died. Now farmers wouldn't need the bacteria. Plants that had the new gene, known as Bt, could produce the insecticidal protein on their own.

Environmentalists flipped. What upset them wasn't the insecticide but the genetic engineering. Thus began the strange backlash against Bt crops. A protein that everyone had previously agreed was innocuous suddenly became a menace. To many critics of biotechnology, the long history of safe Bt use was irrelevant. What mattered was that Bt was now a GMO. And GMOs were evil.

In 1995 the EPA approved Bt potatoes, corn, and cotton. The agency noted that the toxin produced by these crops was "identical to that produced naturally in the bacterium" and "affects insects when ingested, but not mammals." But opponents weren't mollified. In 1999 a coalition led by Greenpeace, the Center for Food Safety, the Pesticide Action Network, and the International Federation of Organic Agriculture Movements sued the EPA to revoke its approvals. The suit said Bt crops might create insecticide-resistant insects and cause "direct harm to non-target organisms."

The coalition claimed to speak for environmental caution. But its caution was curiously selective. Thirty of the 34 farmers who were identified in the lawsuit as victims and plaintiffs affirmed that they sprayed Bt on their own crops. Fourteen of the 16 farming organizations listed as plaintiffs said they had members who used Bt spray. One plaintiff, according to the lawsuit, was a "supplier of organic fertilizers and pest controls" whose business "consists of selling foliar Bt products to conventional apple growers." Another was "one of the largest suppliers of beneficial insects and natural organisms designed to control agricultural pests," including "several Bt products."

Greenpeace and its partners weren't fighting the Bt industry. They were protecting it. They were trying to convince the public that the Bt protein was dangerous when produced by plants but perfectly safe when produced by bacteria and sprayed by farmers.

The anti-GMO lobby says Bt crops are worse than Bt sprays, in part because Bt crops have too much of the bacterial toxin. In 2007, for instance, Greenpeace promoted a court petition to stop field trials of Bt eggplant in India. The petition told the country's highest court, "The Bt toxin in GM crops is 1,000 times more concentrated than in Bt sprays." But Greenpeace's internal research belied that statement. A 2002 Greenpeace report, based on Chinese lab tests, found that the toxin level in Bt crops was severely "limited." In 2006, when Greenpeace investigators examined Bt corn in Germany and Spain, they got a surprise: "The plants sampled showed in general very low Bt concentrations."

An honest environmental organization, having discovered these low concentrations, might have reconsidered its opposition to Bt crops. But Greenpeace simply changed its rationale. Having argued in its 1999 lawsuit that Bt crops produced too much toxin, Greenpeace now reversed itself. In its report on the German and Spanish corn, the organization complained that Bt crops produced too little toxin to be effective. It argued, in essence, that the Bt in transgenic crops was unsafe for humans but insufficient to kill bugs.

Anti-GMO activists also claim that the insecticidal protein is "activated" in Bt crops but not in Bt sprays, and that this makes Bt crops more dangerous to people. That's misleading. "Activation" just means that the protein is truncated, which helps it bind to the guts of insects. And each Bt plant is different. A global database of GE crops, maintained by the Center for Environmental Risk Assessment, shows that some Bt proteins are fully truncated while others are partially truncated. Even the fully truncated proteins are just "semi-activated," according to a technical assessment that was sent to Greenpeace by its own consultants 15 years ago. Unless you're a bug, Bt isn't active.

In its 1999 lawsuit, Greenpeace said Bt crops were dangerous because their toxins were "not readily degraded in the environment." The organization and its allies have repeated this allegation many times since. But when it's convenient, Greenpeace says the opposite. Its 2006 petition to block Bt crops in New Zealand speculated that the concentration of toxin in Bt cotton might be too low

"because the Bt protein is degraded, linked to heat stress." The petition added that the plant's defense mechanisms "may also reduce the insecticidal activity of Bt."

In fact, the 2006 petition suggested that the low concentration of Bt in Indian cotton was allowing insects to flourish, leading to crop losses, and causing farmers to fall into debt and kill themselves. The suicide allegation was just another anti-GMO fiction. But it allowed Greenpeace to claim that the Bt in transgenic crops was killing people in two ways: by being more persistent and potent than the Bt in sprays, and by being less persistent and potent than the Bt in sprays.

The strangest part of the case against Bt crops is the putative evidence of harm. Numerous studies have found that Bt is one of the world's safest pesticides. Still, if you run enough experiments on any pesticide, a few will produce correlations that look worrisome. But that's just the first step in challenging a scientific consensus. Experts then debate whether the correlations are causal and whether the effects are important. They ask for better, controlled experiments to validate the pattern. That's where the case against Bt crops and other GMOs has repeatedly failed.

But that isn't what's strange. What's strange is that so much of the ostensible evidence against Bt crops is, at best, evidence against Bt sprays.

. . .

In its 2006 petition to regulators in New Zealand, Greenpeace argued that Bt crops, by applying evolutionary pressure, would generate Bt-resistant insects, thereby depriving organic farmers of their rightful "use of Bt as a pesticide." The petition also warned that the "Bt toxin can persist in soils for over 200 days" and that this "could cause problems for non-target organisms and the health of the soil ecosystem." But two of the three experiments cited as evidence for the soil warning weren't done with Bt crops. They were done with DiPel, a commercial Bt spray compound. Greenpeace was asking New Zealand to protect Bt spray from Bt crops based on studies that, if anything, indicted Bt spray.

The 2007 petition against Bt eggplant in India repeated this fallacy. "The natural bacterium Bt is very important in advanced organic agriculture," said the petition. For this reason, it argued, the evolution of Bt-resistant insects due to Bt crops "would be a serious threat to many types of agriculture on which a country such as India inevitably & rightly relies." But an addendum to the petition cited, as evidence of Bt's perils, studies that were done with Javelin, Foray, and VectoBac—three Bt spray compounds.

This paradox pervades the anti-GMO movement: alarmism about any possibility of harm from Bt crops, coupled with relentless flacking for the Bt spray industry. "Farmers have always used Bt sparingly and usually as a last resort," says the Organic Consumers Association. But that doesn't square with the product literature for commercial Bt sprays. One brochure recommends "motorized boom sprayers" and says "aerial applications are also commonplace in many crops." Another explains that "many avocado orchards are sprayed by helicopter." Saturation is a point of emphasis: "Sprays should thoroughly cover all plant surfaces, even the undersides of leaves."

Greenpeace says you needn't worry, because "Bt proteins from natural Bt sprays degrade" within two weeks. But this is a false assurance, because farmers compensate for the degradation by reapplying the spray. A typical brochure recommends reapplication "every 5–7 days." That's plenty of time to get the toxin to your mouth, since the product literature tells growers that "ripe fruit can be picked and eaten the same day that it is sprayed." In YouTube videos, organic farmers deliver the same instructions: You should spray your vegetables with Bt every four days, coating each surface, and you can eat the food right after you spray it.

Bt sprays, unlike Bt crops, include live bacteria, which can multiply in food. Several years ago researchers examined vegetables for sale in Denmark. They found 23 strains of Bt identical to the kind used in commercial sprays. In China a similar study of milk, ice cream, and green tea beverages found 19 Bt strains, five of them identical to the kind used in sprays. In Canada nasal swabs of people living inside and outside zones where Bt was being applied found the bacteria in 17 percent of samples taken before crops were sprayed, as well as 36 percent to 47 percent of samples taken afterward.

Nobody monitors how much Bt is applied worldwide. Last fall the *Wall Street Journal* estimated that annual sales of biopesticides were roughly $2 billion. Bt has been said to account for 57 percent to 90 percent of that market. In 2001, Bt was reportedly applied in the U.S. to more than 40 percent of tomatoes and 60 percent of brassica crops, which include broccoli, cauliflower, and cabbage. Since then, biopesticide sales have risen substantially. In Europe the annual growth rate since 2000 has been nearly 17 percent. Every market analysis predicts that biopesticides will grow at a much faster rate than the overall insecticide market, in part because governments are promoting them. The Journal projects that by 2020, 10 percent of global pesticide sales will be Bt and other biological formulas.

One result of this paradox—GMOs under attack, while biopesticides flourish—is that you can think you're eating less Bt, when in fact you're eating more. Suppose you live in Germany. According to a 2014 congressional research report, Germany has some of the world's strictest GMO policies. It requires labels, discourages GMO cultivation, and has prohibited even some crops approved by the European Union. But U.N. data show that during the most recent 10-year reporting period, for every 1,000 hectares of arable German land, an annual average of 125 metric tons of biological and botanical pesticides (the category that includes Bt) were sold for agricultural use in crops and seeds. That works out to more than 100 pounds per acre per year. By comparison, no Bt corn variety produces more than 4 pounds of toxin per acre.

And guess who's selling all that Bt: the same companies Greenpeace condemns for peddling chemical pesticides and GMOs. Since 2012 the top four companies on Greenpeace's list of global pesticide villains—Monsanto, Syngenta, Bayer, and BASF—have spent about $2 billion to move into the biopesticide market. Another agrochemical giant, DuPont, has invested $6 billion. If you're boycotting GMOs or buying organic to escape Bt and fight corporate agriculture, think again. Monsanto is one step ahead of you.

Anti-GMO zealots refuse to face the truth about Bt. Two years ago the Organic Consumers Association and its allied website GreenMedInfo published the headline "New Study Links GMO Food to Leukemia." Today that headline remains uncorrected, even though the study was done with Bt spore crystals, which are components of Bt spray, not Bt crops. (The study is a mess. Most of what was fed to the test animals wasn't Bt toxin, and the write-up, for undisclosed reasons, was withdrawn from an established journal and published instead in a journal that had never before existed.) Meanwhile, last year, Greenpeace published a catalog of "exemplary" agriculture, in which it celebrated a Spanish farm where "the use of Bacillus thuringiensis is being expanded to a greater cultivated surface area." Both organizations encourage you to buy organic, neglecting to mention the dozens of Bt insecticides approved for use in organic agriculture.

GMO labels won't clear this up. They won't tell you whether there's Bt in your food. They'll only give you the illusion that you've escaped it. That's one lesson of the Non-GMO Project, whose voluntary labels purport to give you an "informed choice" about what's in your food. Earlier this year, Slate interns Natania Levy and Greer Prettyman contacted the manufacturers of 15 corn products bearing the Non-GMO Project label. They asked each company whether its product included any ingredients sprayed with biopesticides. Five companies didn't reply. Two told us, falsely, that their organic certification meant they didn't use pesticides or anything that could be harmful. One sent us weasel words and repeated them when we pressed for a clearer answer. Another told us it adhered to legal limits. Three confessed that they didn't know. None of the manufacturers could give us a clear assurance that its product hadn't been exposed to Bt.

That's the fundamental flaw in the anti-GMO movement. It only pretends to inform you. When you push past its dogmas and examine the evidence, you realize that the movement's fixation on genetic engineering has been an enormous mistake. The principles it claims to stand for—environmental protection, public health, community agriculture—are better served by considering the facts of each case than by treating GMOs, categorically, as a proxy for all that's wrong with the world. That's the truth, in all its messy complexity. Too bad it won't fit on a label.

A Humanitarian Project Zealots Hate

Right now, across the world, a quarter of a billion preschool-age children are suffering from vitamin A deficiency. Every year, 250,000 to 500,000 of these kids go blind. Within a year, half of the blinded children will die. Much of the affliction is in Southeast Asia, where people rely on rice for their nutrition. Rice doesn't have enough beta carotene—the compound that, when digested, produces vitamin A.

Twenty-five years ago, a team of scientists, led by Ingo Potrykus of the Swiss Federal Institute of Technology, set out to solve this problem. Their plan was to engineer a new kind of rice that would make beta carotene.

The idea sounded crazy. But to Potrykus it made more sense than what some governments were already doing: giving each person two high-dose vitamin A pills a year. Wouldn't it be smarter to embed beta carotene in the region's staple crop? That way, people could grow the nutrient and eat it every day, instead of relying on occasional handouts. This was a sustainable solution. It would use biotechnology to prevent suffering, disability, and death.

In 1999, Potrykus and his colleagues achieved their first breakthrough. By transferring genes from daffodils and bacteria, they created the world's first beta carotene rice. The yellow grains became known as "Golden Rice." President Clinton celebrated the achievement and urged GMO skeptics to do the same. He acknowledged that genetic engineering "tends to be treated as an issue of the interest of the agribusiness companies, and earning big profits, against food safety." But in the case of vitamin A deficiency, the greater risk to health lay in doing nothing. "If we could get more of this Golden Rice . . . out to the

develop[ing] world," said Clinton, "it could save 40,000 lives a day."

Anti-GMO groups were confounded. This humanitarian project undermined their usual objections to genetic engineering. In 2001, Benedikt Haerlin, Greenpeace's anti-GMO coordinator, appeared with Potrykus at a press conference in France. Haerlin conceded that Golden Rice served "a good purpose" and posed "a moral challenge to our position." Greenpeace couldn't dismiss the rice as poison. So it opposed the project on technical grounds: Golden Rice didn't produce enough beta carotene.

The better approach, according to biotechnology critics, was to help people cultivate home gardens full of beans, pumpkins, and other crops rich in vitamin A. Where that wasn't feasible or sufficient, Greenpeace recommended supplementation (distributing vitamin A pills) or food fortification, by mixing vitamin A into centrally processed ingredients such as sugar, flour, and margarine.

Greenpeace was right about Golden Rice. At the time, the rice didn't provide enough beta carotene to cure vitamin A deficiency. But neither did the alternatives. Gordon Conway, the president of the Rockefeller Foundation, which was funding the project, explained some of the difficulties in a 2001 letter to Greenpeace:

> Complete balanced diets are the best solution, but the poorer families are, the less likely it is that their children will receive a balanced diet and the more likely they will be dependent on cheap food staples such as rice. This is particularly true in the dry seasons when fruits and vegetables are in short supply and expensive.

Conway echoed the skepticism of UNICEF nutritionists, who doubted that plants native to the afflicted countries could deliver enough digestible beta carotene. To Potrykus, the notion of home gardens for everyone—Let them eat carrot cake—reeked of Western ignorance. "There are hundreds of millions of landless poor," Potrykus pointed out. "They don't have a house to lean the fruit tree against."

Potrykus and Conway wanted to try everything to alleviate vitamin A deficiency: diversification, fortification, supplementation, and Golden Rice. But the anti-GMO groups refused. They called Golden Rice a "Trojan horse" for genetic engineering. They doubled down on their double standards. They claimed that people in the afflicted countries wouldn't eat yellow rice, yet somehow could be taught to grow unfamiliar vegetables. They portrayed Golden Rice as a financial scheme, but then—after

Potrykus made clear that it would be given to poor farmers for free—objected that free distribution would lead to genetic contamination of local crops. Some anti-GMO groups said the rice should be abandoned because it was tied up in 70 patents. Others said the claim of 70 patents was a fiction devised by the project's leaders to justify their collaboration with AstraZeneca, a global corporation.

While critics tried to block the project, Potrykus and his colleagues worked to improve the rice. By 2003 they had developed plants with eight times as much beta carotene as the original version. In 2005 they unveiled a line that had 20 times as much beta carotene as the original. GMO critics could no longer dismiss Golden Rice as inadequate. So they reversed course. Now that the rice produced plenty of beta carotene, anti-GMO activists claimed that beta carotene and vitamin A were dangerous.

In 2001, Friends of the Earth had scoffed that Golden Rice would "do little to ameliorate VAD [vitamin A deficiency] because it produces so little beta-carotene." By November 2004 the group had changed its tune. Crops that yielded beta carotene could "cause direct toxicity or abnormal embryonic development," it asserted. Another anti-GMO lobby, the Institute of Science in Society, documented its own shift in a 2006 report:

> ISIS critically reviewed golden rice in 2000. Among the observations was that the rice produced too little beta-carotene to relieve the existing dietary deficiency. Since then, golden rice strains have been improved, but still fall short of relieving dietary deficiency. On the other hand, increasing the level of beta-carotene may cause vitamin A overdose to those [whose] diets provide adequate amounts of the vitamin. In fact, both vitamin A deficiency and supplementation may cause birth defects.

To support the new alarmism, David Schubert, an anti-GMO activist and neurobiologist at the Salk Institute, drafted a paper on the ostensible perils of boosting vitamin A. In 2008 he got it published in the *Journal of Medicinal Food*. In the article he noted that beta carotene and dozens of related compounds, known as carotenoids, could produce other compounds, called retinoids, which included vitamin A. He declared that all retinoids "are likely to be teratogenic"—prone to causing birth defects—and, therefore, "extensive safety testing should be required before the introduction of golden rice."

. . .

Schubert systematically distorted the evidence. To suggest that Golden Rice might be toxic, he cited a study that had been reported in the New England Journal of Medicine in 1994. Schubert said the study found that "smokers who supplemented their diet with beta-carotene had an increased risk of lung cancer." He neglected to mention that the daily beta carotene dose administered in the study was the equivalent of roughly 10 to 20 bowls of Golden Rice. He also failed to quote the rest of the paper, which emphasized that in general, beta carotene was actually associated with a lower risk of lung cancer. Furthermore, he claimed that a 2004 report by the National Research Council said genetic engineering had "a higher probability of producing unanticipated changes than some genetic modification methods." In reality, the NRC report said genetic engineering has a higher probability of producing unanticipated changes than some genetic modification methods, such as narrow crosses, and a lower probability than others, such as radiation mutagenesis. Therefore, the nature of the compositional change merits greater consideration than the method used to achieve the change.

By omitting the second half of the sentence—"and a lower probability than others"—Schubert made the NRC report appear to raise alarms about GMOs, when in fact the report had explained why alarmism about GMOs was wrongheaded.

Schubert gave opponents of Golden Rice what they needed: the illusion of scientific support. Every anti- GMO lobby cited his paper. The movement's new position, as expressed by Ban GM Food, was that "Golden Rice is engineered to overproduce beta carotene, and studies show that some retinoids derived from beta carotene are toxic and cause birth defects."

But the new position, like the old one, relied on double standards. To begin with, every green plant produces carotenoids. For years, anti-GMO groups had argued that instead of eating Golden Rice, people should grow other plants rich in beta carotene. They had also encouraged the use of selective breeding to increase carotenoid levels. If carotenoids were toxic, wouldn't these plants deliver the same poison?

GMO critics didn't seem to care how much beta carotene people ate, as long as the food wasn't genetically engineered. They demanded extra safety tests on Golden Rice, on the grounds that "large doses of beta-carotene can have negative health effects." But they shrugged off such vigilance in the case of home gardens, saying it was "not necessary to count the amount" of each vitamin consumed. They also advocated the mass administration of vitamin A through high-dose capsules and chemical manipulation of the food supply. By their own alarmist standards—which, fortunately, were unwarranted—this would have been reckless. The human body derives from beta carotene sources, such as Golden Rice, only as much vitamin A as it needs.

In the context of GMOs, Greenpeace claimed to stand for freedom. Its 2009 statement "Hands off our rice!" said "keeping rice GE-free" was an issue of "consumer choice" and "human rights." The statement complained that GE rice was "controlled by multinational corporations and governments" and "severely limits the choice of food we can eat." But as long as GMOs weren't involved, Greenpeace was all for corporate and government control. It lauded the distribution of vitamin A and beta carotene capsules in "mass immunization campaigns." It praised health officials and food-processing companies for putting vitamin A and beta carotene in sugar, margarine, and biscuits. It suggested that governments could "make fortification compulsory."

In the Philippines, where Greenpeace was fighting to block field trials of Golden Rice, its hypocrisy was egregious. "It is irresponsible to impose GE 'Golden' rice on people if it goes against their religious beliefs, cultural heritage and sense of identity, or simply because they do not want it," Greenpeace declared. But just below that pronouncement, Greenpeace recommended "vitamin A supplementation and vitamin fortification of foods as successfully implemented in the Philippines." Under Philippine law, beta carotene and vitamin A had to be added to sugar, flour, and cooking oil prior to distribution. The government administered capsules to preschoolers twice a year, and to some pregnant women for 28 consecutive days. If Greenpeace seriously believed that retinoids caused birth defects and should be a matter of personal choice, it would never have endorsed these programs.

Despite this, the anti-GMO lobby went ballistic when scientists fed Golden Rice to 24 children during clinical trials in China. The trials, conducted in 2008, were designed to measure how much vitamin A the rice could generate in people who suffered from vitamin A deficiency. One group of kids was given Golden Rice, a second group was given beta carotene capsules, and a third was given spinach. The researchers found that a single serving of Golden Rice, cooked from 50 grams of grains, could supply 60 percent of a child's recommended daily intake of vitamin A. In a separate study, they found that an adult-sized serving could do the same for adults. Golden Rice was as good as capsules, and better than spinach, at delivering vitamin A.

When Greenpeace found out about the trials, it enlisted the Chinese government to stop them. It accused the researchers of using the kids as "guinea pigs." In a letter to Tufts University, which was responsible for the trials, Schubert and 20 other anti-GMO scientists protested:

Our greatest concern is that this rice, which is engineered to overproduce beta carotene, has never been tested in animals, and there is an extensive medical literature showing that retinoids that can be derived from beta carotene are both toxic and cause birth defects.

In these circumstances the use of human subjects (including children who are already suffering illness as a result of Vitamin A deficiency) for GM feeding experiments is completely unacceptable.

For all the scare talk about beta carotene, Schubert and his colleagues never mentioned the kids who were given beta carotene capsules in the studies. Nor did Greenpeace. Their sole concern was the rice.

Supporters of Golden Rice were baffled. In a letter to the *Daily Mail*, six scientists wrote, "The experiments were no more dangerous than feeding the children a small carrot since the levels of beta- carotene and related compounds in Golden Rice are similar." But anti-GMO groups were determined to discredit the studies. They discovered that although the consent forms given to the children's parents said Golden Rice "makes beta carotene," the forms didn't specify that this had been achieved through gene transfer.

Greenpeace was outraged. Its press release titled "Greenpeace alarmed at US-backed GMO experiments on children" quoted a Greenpeace official in Asia: "The next 'golden rice' guinea pigs might be Filipino children. Should we allow ourselves to be subjects in a human experiment?" In another press release, Greenpeace questioned whether the Chinese parents were "properly informed of the risks." Yet in the same statements, Greenpeace praised the Philippines for administering vitamin A to pregnant women and for putting beta carotene in the food supply.

Eventually, Tufts commissioned three reviews of the clinical trials. Two were internal; the third was external. The findings, released in 2013, confirmed that the reviews had "identified concerns" about "inadequate explanation of the genetically-modified nature of Golden Rice." But the more important verdict was that "the study data were validated and no health or safety concerns were identified." The university explained:

These multiple reviews found no concerns related to the integrity of the study data, the accuracy of the research results or the safety of the research subjects. In fact, the study indicated that a single serving of the test product, Golden Rice, could provide greater than 50 percent of the recommended daily intake of vitamin A in these children, which could significantly improve health outcomes if adopted as a dietary regimen.

This verdict didn't suit opponents of Golden Rice. So they ignored it. For 16 years they've ignored every fact or finding that doesn't fit their story. Their enmity is unappeasable; their alarmism is unfalsifiable. Take the question of allergies. In 2006, scientists found no allergens among the proteins in Golden Rice. The critics refused to accept this finding. They demanded additional tests. They said climate change could undermine the rice's "genetic stability." They claimed that unforeseen environmental interactions could cause unintended changes in the rice after several generations, and therefore, regulators should indefinitely delay its approval.

The critics openly advocate unattainable standards. ISIS says the "instability of transgenic lines" makes "proper safety assessment well-nigh impossible." Greenpeace says of Golden Rice:

> It would not be a surprise if additional unexpected changes in the plant occurred, posing new risks to the environment or human health. . . . However, it is virtually impossible to look for unexpected effects—by definition, one cannot know what these effects might be, or where to look for them!

And these standards apply only to GMOs. They don't apply to alternatives favored by the anti-GMO movement. Three years ago Greenpeace recommended marker-assisted selection—essentially, breeding guided by genetic analysis—as a better way to increase levels of beta carotene and other nutrients. One argument quoted in the Greenpeace report was that genetic engineering caused "unpredictable integration sites, copy numbers and often spontaneous rearrangements and losses"—in short, that it screwed up the DNA of the altered organism. Shortly afterward, a study found that Greenpeace had it backward: In rice, marker-assisted selection caused more genetic and functional disruption than genetic engineering did. Nevertheless, Greenpeace continues to claim that genetic engineering, unlike marker-assisted selection, creates "novel traits with novel hazards."

. . .

There's no end to the arguments and demands of anti-GMO watchdogs. They want more studies—"systematic trials with different cooking processes"—to see how much vitamin A the rice delivers. They want studies to assess how much beta carotene the rice loses when stored at various temperatures. If the rice delivers enough vitamin A, they say that's a problem, too, because people won't feel the need to eat other plants and will consequently develop other kinds of malnutrition. They claim that criminals will counterfeit the rice, using yellow spices or naturally yellow grains, so people will think they're getting vitamin A when they aren't.

Sixteen years after it was invented, Golden Rice still isn't commercially available. Two years ago anti-GMO activists destroyed a field trial of the rice in the Philippines. Last year they filed a petition to block all field tests and feeding studies. Greenpeace boasted, "After more than 10 years of research 'Golden' Rice is nowhere near its promise to address Vitamin A deficiency." And a million more kids are dead.

A Legitimate Concern

Up to this point, we've been focusing on health concerns about GMOs. The stories of papaya, Bt, and Golden Rice demonstrate, in several ways, that these concerns are unfounded. One thing we've learned is that fear of GMOs is unfalsifiable. Hundreds of studies have been done, and tons of GE food have been eaten. No amount of evidence will convince the doomsayers that GMOs are safe. You can't live your life clinging to such unappeasable fear. Let it go.

Another thing we've learned is that it makes no sense to avoid GMOs based on standards that nobody applies to non-GMO food. Yes, it's conceivable that you could overdose on vitamin A or ingest a viral or insecticidal protein from eating fruits, grains, or vegetables. But GMOs don't make any of these scenarios more likely or more dangerous. In fact, if you look at illness or direct fatalities—or at correlations between food sales and disease trends, which anti-GMO activists like to do—you can make a better case against organic food than against GMOs.

A third lesson is that GMO segregation, in the form of labels or GMO-free restaurants, is misguided. GMO labels don't clarify what's in your food. They don't address the underlying ingredients—pesticides, toxins, proteins—that supposedly make GMOs harmful. They stigmatize food that's perfectly safe, and they deflect scrutiny from non-GMO products that have the same disparaged ingredients.

The people who push GMO labels and GMO-free shopping aren't informing you or protecting you. They're using you. They tell food manufacturers, grocery stores, and restaurants to segregate GMOs, and ultimately not to sell them, because people like you won't buy them. They tell politicians and regulators to label and restrict GMOs because people like you don't trust the technology. They use your anxiety to justify GMO labels, and then they use GMO labels to justify your anxiety. Keeping you scared is the key to their political and business strategy. And companies like Chipotle, with their non-GMO marketing campaigns, are playing along.

But safety isn't the only concern that's been raised about GMOs. There are other criticisms, and one of them is worth your attention. It addresses the world's most common agricultural application of genetic engineering: herbicide tolerance.

Three-quarters of the corn and cotton grown in this country is engineered to resist insects. These crops have the bacterial Bt gene, which makes them lethal to bugs that eat them. Slightly more than that, about 80 percent to 85 percent of corn and cotton, is engineered to withstand weed-killing chemicals, especially glyphosate, which is sold as Roundup. (The two traits are usually packaged together.) The percentages are similar for soy. Worldwide, insect-resistant crops are grown on about 50 percent of the land allotted to GMOs, while herbicide-tolerant crops are grown on more than 80 percent.

Both applications are considered pesticidal, because weeds, like bugs, are pests. And this is crucial to understanding the debate over whether GMOs, as a whole, have raised or lowered the level of pesticide use. One study, published in 2012 by Charles Benbrook, the most sensible critic of GMOs, calculates that GMOs increased pesticide use in the United States by 7 percent. An international analysis of multiple studies, published last year, calculates that GMOs decreased pesticide use by 37 percent. But the two assessments agree on a fundamental distinction: While bug-resistant GMOs have led to lower use of insecticides, herbicide-tolerant GMOs have led to higher use of weedkillers.

Two factors seem to account for the herbicide increase. One is direct: If your crops are engineered to withstand Roundup, you can spray it profusely without killing them. The other factor is indirect: When every farmer sprays Roundup, weeds adapt to a Roundup-saturated world. They evolve to survive. To kill these herbicide-resistant strains, farmers spray more weedkillers. It's an arms race.

Despite an ongoing debate about the effects of glyphosate, experts agree that it's relatively benign. Benbrook has called it one of the safest herbicides on the market. He concludes: "In light of its generally favorable environmental and toxicological properties, especially compared to some of the herbicides displaced by glyphosate, the dramatic increase in glyphosate use has likely not markedly increased human health risks."

But the arms race could change that. As weeds evolve to withstand Roundup, farmers are deploying other, more worrisome herbicides. And companies are engineering crops to withstand these herbicides so that farmers can spray them freely.

Chipotle complains that GMOs "produce pesticides" and "create herbicide resistant super-weeds." The company says Benbrook's study showed that "pesticide and herbicide use increased by more than 400 million pounds as a result of GMO cultivation." (Chipotle, unlike Benbrook and other experts, uses the term pesticide to mean insecticide.) But this is misleading in two ways. First, by pooling the data, Chipotle has hidden half of what Benbrook found: that Bt crops reduced insecticide use and thereby, in terms of their contribution to the bottom line, reduced the combined use of pest-killing chemicals. And second, the problem that's driving the herbicide arms race isn't genetic engineering. It's monoculture.

Everyone who has studied the problem carefully—Benbrook, the USDA, the National Research Council—comes to the same conclusion: By relying too much on one method of weed control, we've helped weeds evolve to defeat it. To confound evolution, you have to make evolutionary pressures less predictable. That means switching herbicides so weeds that develop resistance to one herbicide will be killed by another. It also means alternating crops, so weeds have to compete with different plants and grow under different tilling, watering, and harvest conditions. Industry and regulators, belatedly, are beginning to address this problem. As part of its product approval and renewal process, the EPA, backed by the USDA, is requiring producers of herbicides and herbicide-tolerant crops to monitor and report use of their chemicals, work with farmers to control excessive use, and promote non-herbicidal weed control methods.

GMOs are part of the problem. Herbicide-tolerant crops let farmers spray weedkillers more often and more thoroughly without harming their crops. It's no accident that Monsanto, which sells Roundup-ready seeds, also sells Roundup. But GMOs didn't invent monoculture, and banning them won't make it go away. Farmers have been cultivating homogeneity for millennia. Roundup has been used for more than 40 years.

Chipotle illustrates the folly of renouncing GMOs in the name of herbicide control. According to its new policy, "All corn-based ingredients in Chipotle's food that formerly may have been genetically modified have been removed or replaced with non-GMO versions, while all soy-derived ingredients that may have been genetically modified were replaced with alternatives, such as rice bran oil and sunflower oil."

But shifting to sunflower oil is demonstrably counterproductive. As NPR's Dan Charles points out, "many sunflower varieties, while not genetically modified, also are herbicide-tolerant. They were bred to tolerate a class of herbicides called ALS inhibitors. And since farmers start[ed] relying on those herbicides, many weeds have evolved resistance to them. In fact, many more weeds have become resistant to ALS inhibitors than to glyphosate."

That's just one example of how tricky it is to assess the effects of swearing off GMOs. Roundup isn't the only herbicide, genetic engineering isn't the only technology that creates herbicide tolerance, and your health (which is no more likely to be affected by a given herbicide in GE food than in non-GE food) is just one of many factors to consider. To judge the environmental wisdom of switching from a GMO to a non-GMO product, you'd have to know which pesticides each product involves and how those pesticides affect species that live where the crops are grown. None of that is on the label.

You'd also have to consider the environmental benefits of agricultural efficiency. By making cropland more productive, with less output lost to weeds and insects, GMOs reduce the amount of land that has to be farmed and the amount of water that's wasted. Herbicide-tolerant crops even mitigate climate change by reducing the need to till fields, which erodes soil and releases greenhouse gases.

The more you learn about herbicide resistance, the more you come to understand how complicated the truth about GMOs is. First you discover that they aren't evil. Then you learn that they aren't perfectly innocent. Then you realize that nothing is perfectly innocent. Pesticide vs. pesticide, technology vs. technology, risk vs. risk—it's all relative. The best you can do is measure each practice against the alternatives. The least you can do is look past a three-letter label.

Better GMOs

Twenty years after the debut of genetically engineered food, it's a travesty that the technology's commercial applications are still so focused on old-fashioned weedkillers. Greenpeace and Chipotle think the logical response to this travesty is to purge GMOs. They're exactly wrong. The relentless efforts of Luddites to block testing, regulatory approval, and commercial development of GMOs are major reasons why more advanced GE products, such as Golden Rice, are still unavailable. The best way to break the herbicide industry's grip on genetic engineering is to support the technology and push it forward, by telling policymakers, food manufacturers, and seed companies that you want better GMOs.

The USDA's catalog of recently engineered plants shows plenty of worthwhile options. The list includes drought-tolerant corn, virus-resistant plums, non-browning apples, potatoes with fewer natural toxins, and soybeans that produce less saturated fat. A recent global inventory by the U.N. Food and Agriculture Organization discusses other projects in the pipeline: virus-resistant beans, heat-tolerant sugarcane, salt-tolerant wheat, disease-resistant cassava, high-iron rice, and cotton that requires less nitrogen fertilizer. Skim the news, and you'll find scientists at work on more ambitious ideas: high-calcium carrots, anti-oxidant tomatoes, nonallergenic nuts, bacteria-resistant oranges, water-conserving wheat, corn and cassava loaded with extra nutrients, and a flaxlike plant that produces the healthy oil formerly available only in fish.

That's what genetic engineering can do for health and for our planet. The reason it hasn't is that we've been stuck in a stupid, wasteful fight over GMOs. On one side is an army of quacks and pseudo-environmentalists waging a leftist war on science. On the other side are corporate cowards who would rather stick to profitable weed-killing than invest in products that might offend a suspicious public.

The only way to end this fight is to educate ourselves and make it clear to everyone—European governments, trend-setting grocers, fad-hopping restaurant chains, research universities, and biotechnology investors—that we're ready, as voters and consumers, to embrace nutritious, environmentally friendly food, no matter where it got its genes. We want our GMOs. Now, show us what you can do.

WILLIAM SALETAN is a national correspondent for Slate.com and writes its "Human Nature" column. He is also the author of *Bearing Right*.

Claire Robinson   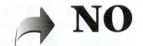 **NO**

Lessons in Critical Thinking
and William Saletan—Part 1

In a recent incisive article on the GMO debate, Timothy Wise of Tufts University laments the "current vehemence" of the battle. He singles out *Slate* magazine's William Saletan as one of the more extreme examples of those ready to tar "anyone who dares call for precaution with the stain of being another science-denying zealot." Wise accuses pundits like Saletan of "polarizing" the debate so much that they actually contribute to the suppression of scientific inquiry.

This couldn't contrast more with how Saletan himself sees things. He responded to my three-part critique of his recent GMO promotional in *Slate* with a lecture on "how to think critically." The implication is that this is something he is rather good at, whereas I and other GMO opponents are not.

So let's take a look at the supposed gold standard of critical thinking, as exemplified by Saletan. And because we all have a life beyond the wit and wisdom of gullible journalists, I'll restrict myself to a few major lessons in critical thinking in which Saletan gets a big "F" for "fail."

1. If you're charged with sins of omission, don't omit to answer the charge

The first part of my critique focused on how Saletan dealt with the topic of GM golden rice. I pointed out that he blamed the critics of golden rice for the blindness and death of a million or so malnourished children. That's a damning accusation and it is this aspect of Saletan's article that has led to GMO critics, like the journalist Michael Pollan and the Union of Concerned Scientists, being directly accused by Jon Entine of having "blood on your hands. Literally."

But the blood Entine is pointing at is fake blood, thrown by Saletan. As I pointed out, Saletan's article totally fails to make clear that the real reasons golden rice is still unavailable are:

1. It has failed its field trials
2. It hasn't been safety tested

3. It hasn't even been shown to help the malnourished.

And even the body overseeing the rolling out of golden rice, the staunchly pro-GMO IRRI, has never once to my knowledge tried to argue that the critics of golden rice are responsible for these failings.

So how does Saletan answer the charge that he omitted to tell his readers the real reasons for golden rice not being in use? He deals with it by omitting any mention of it at all in his response. Instead, he accuses me of having been corrupted by a "political agenda" that has somehow skewed my thinking on golden rice.

So let me spell out the gravity of the charge that Saletan is ducking. He stands accused of omitting key information from his account of golden rice in order, in effect, to manufacture a crime against humanity. This sort of fakery is almost as repellent as that of the revisionists who distort history in order to massage away real crimes against humanity.

What Saletan is doing is nothing new. It is something that has been done over and over again to environmentalists, starting with Rachel Carson who has been repeatedly accused of causing the deaths of millions through having encouraged a global—but entirely fictitious—DDT ban. And ironically, those mounting these kind of vicious attacks on environmental critics have a very real political agenda: to demonize those who stand in the way of powerful vested interests.

2. Don't rely on authority

Saletan is correct in saying that I don't believe in appeals to authority as evidence for GMO safety. I do believe in examining rigorously obtained data and checking primary sources—two things that Saletan has repeatedly failed to do.

Saletan says he also doesn't believe in relying on authority and claims to look at "the evidence, not the assurances," since this is "what debunks the arguments against these GMOs."

Yet it is just this "evidence" on three of his topics—GM golden rice, GM food safety, and GM papaya, that I systematically debunked in my articles by following his claims to their source. His claims on organic food have also been debunked by a knowledgeable organic grower.

Far from relying on evidence, Saletan has taken industry talking points at face value. He has also, despite his protestations, relied on vague appeals to authorities that have issued statements saying GM foods are as safe as non- GM foods. These in turn lack reliable data on which such conclusions could reasonably be based. Given that human studies on the effects of eating GMOs are non-existent, long-term animal feeding studies with GMOs are rare, and some animal feeding studies have found GMOs to be unexpectedly toxic or allergenic, claims of GMO safety are at best baseless and at worst lies.

3. Don't misrepresent authority

Saletan claims I try to "drown out" evidence with my own appeals to authority, "citing bogus 'science-related organizations' such as the American Academy of Environmental Medicine" (AAEM), which Saletan smears as "a quack group dressed up as an association of scholarly referees." As evidence for this smear, Saletan refers to a blog article written by Stephen Barrett, a man who was judged by a California court as "biased" and as having "little, if any, credibility" on the topics he claimed to be an expert in.

In reality, for the benefit of Saletan and others who believe in authority, I pointed to 124 science- or health-related organisations that had expressed doubts about the safety of GMOs and/or asked for mandatory labeling. Of these 124, the AAEM is one. Others include the British Medical Association, the American Public Health Association, the Australia Public Health Association, and the German Medical Association. Perhaps Saletan would like to tell us, based on evidence, how many "quacks" these organisations have among their membership.

4. Don't defend the indefensible

Saletan attacks me for criticizing his defence of glyphosate as "relatively benign." He backs up this defence by saying there are even more toxic herbicides out there. But that's equivalent to claiming that arsenic is "relatively benign" because it's less toxic than mercury. Less toxic, yes. Benign, even qualified with Saletan's "relatively," no.

A probable human carcinogen—as glyphosate has been judged to be by the World Health Organisation's cancer agency IARC—is just that. It "probably" can cause cancer. An unbiased assessment would replace Saletan's ludicrous claim, "experts agree that [glyphosate is] relatively benign," with "qualified experts agree that glyphosate is a probable carcinogen." In fact, we now know that the IARC experts came close to classifying glyphosate as a "known carcinogen," so strong was the evidence against it.

Saletan tries to make light of that evidence by quoting one expert as saying of IARC's classification: "the evidence cited here appears a bit thin." But what he doesn't tell his readers is that at the point that comment was made, IARC had only published a summary judgment and hadn't yet published its 92–page monograph of evidence—something that it has now done.

5. Keep up with new information

It's telling that in defending glyphosate, Saletan has to exploit statements made in the past by pesticides expert Chuck Benbrook. In his original article, Saletan first talks up Benbrook as "the most sensible critic of GMOs" and then says he has vouched for the relative safety of glyphosate. He quotes Benbrook as saying that "the dramatic increase in glyphosate use has likely not markedly increased human health risks." But what he doesn't point out to his readers is that this comment was made several years ago, before some of the most damning evidence on glyphosate was published and long before the IARC reached its verdict on the link to cancer.

If Saletan had actually bothered to check with Benbrook what his current view on glyphosate safety was, he would have discovered it was a world away from what Saletan was claiming. Just this week the *New England Journal of Medicine* published an article co-authored by Benbrook in which he says that the IARC classification has helped "dramatically" change "the GMO landscape". He argues that the strong glyphosate link to cancer in combination with the massive increase in use of glyphosate that GM crops are encouraging could mean "GM foods and the herbicides applied to them may pose hazards to human health that were not examined in previous assessments."

Reuters quotes Benbrook as saying, "There is growing evidence that glyphosate is genotoxic and has adverse effects on cells in a number of different ways. It's time to pull back . . . on uses of glyphosate that we know are leading to significant human exposures while the science gets sorted out."

The main expert that Saletan deployed in his defence of glyphosate sees previous regulatory assessments as having relied on flawed and outdated research.

Nothing could better describe what Saletan has served up to his readers.

6. Read the studies

Saletan names me among those who are "clinging to the same old discredited attacks on GMO safety." His source for the alleged discreditation is an article by the journalist Amy Harmon. Harmon in turn cites the GENERA list of studies on the pro-GMO group Biofortified's website, one of several Big Lists of Studies cited by GMO proponents as evidence of GMO safety. Unfortunately though, the GENERA list is nothing of the sort. It includes studies that found the GMO unexpectedly toxic. And an investigation by Food & Water Watch found that the most common funder of studies in the GENERA database [was either (the uncertainty being due to lack of clarity in the GENERA coding system) Monsanto or the U.S. government. The latter is not impartial on GM crops, having a declared mission to promote the growth of the biotechnology industry.]

Of course, Saletan would argue that I can't criticize the biasing effect of Monsanto funding because (as he noted) I sit on an NGO board that has someone from the Organic Consumers Association on it and therefore, it seems, I have a business agenda. Go figure.

And while Harmon and Saletan have fiercely defended the safety of GM papaya in Hawaii and ridiculed those who doubt it, both authors have failed to look at what is apparently the only animal feeding study with this GMO. As I pointed out before, this study showed problems with the GMO, which Saletan is apparently reluctant to confront. What does Saletan make of the immune responses, such as raised white blood cell and lymphocyte counts, and biochemical changes in rats that ate the GM papaya for the short period of 28 days—in a study perversely conducted years after the GM papaya had been introduced on the market? Doctors advise that raised white blood cell and lymphocyte counts can indicate infection, inflammation, tissue damage, or cancer. Does Saletan believe he knows

differently? Let him produce his evidence. If it stands up, maybe we'll rewrite the medical textbooks.

In contrast with Saletan's uninformed views on GMO safety, a recent peer-reviewed article, "An illusory consensus behind GMO health assessment," by Prof Sheldon Krimsky of Tufts University, examined animal feeding studies with GMOs and reviews of such studies. He found 26 studies that found adverse effects or health uncertainties from GMOs (there are many more, but Krimsky doesn't claim his list is exhaustive) and eight reviews that were "mixed in their assessment of the health effects of GMOs." Krimsky concluded, "When there is a controversy about the risk of a consumer product, instead of denying the existence of certain studies, the negative results should be replicated to see if they hold up to rigorous testing."

For those who counter that these are only 26 studies and/or like to wave vaguely towards Big Lists of Studies supposedly showing GMO safety, I can point them to a list of over 1800 studies, surveys, and analyses that suggest actual and potential adverse impacts of GM crops and foods and their related pesticides.

We look forward to reading Saletan's response to a representative sample of these studies. It will be a useful lesson for him in critical thinking—a skill that seems to have deserted him when it comes to GMOs.

Claire Robinson is an editor at GMWatch, a U.K.-based news and public information service on issues relating to genetic modification. She was formerly the research director at the sustainability nonprofit Earth Open Source and is a co-author of the book *GMO Myths and Truths*.

EXPLORING THE ISSUE

Does the World Need Genetically Modified Foods?

Critical Thinking and Reflection

1. Explain why foods in the U.S. are genetically modified and which foods are produced with GM seeds.
2. Explain what the Bt gene is and why it was developed.
3. List and discuss the two strongest reasons that Saletan has in favor of GM crops.
4. List and discuss the two strongest reasons that Robinson has against GM crops.
5. Currently the FDA does not require food manufacturers to print on the food label if a food contains GM products. (The UK does require labeling.) Write a 1-page letter to your senator requesting that GM become a part of the requirements on food labels OR a letter expressing your support of GM seeds.

Is There Common Ground?

Saletan and Robinson are at far ends on the issue of GMOs. Saletan's article is based on the one year he spent researching the literature about GMOs. Even as a Swarthmore College graduate, he admits that the "issue is complicated" but feels there is much "fraud in the case against GMO." He also believes there is fraud in the accusation that "Monsanto is hiding the truth." Saletan believes that groups, such as GMWatch and Claire Robinson, are "counting on you to feel overwhelmed by the science and to accept, as a gut presumption, their message of distrust."

In contrast, Claire Robinson is co-editor of *GMWatch*, a site founded in 1998, shortly after GM crops were introduced in our food supply. Additionally, Robinson is co-author of the book *GMO Myths and Truths*. Which of the two authors do you think has had more experience and

exposure to GMO research? Which of the two supports his or her case?

Additional Resources

Delaney B. Safety assessment of foods from genetically modified crops in countries with developing economies. *Food Chem Toxicol.* 2015;86:132–43.

Lucht JM. Public acceptance of plant biotechnology and GM crops. *Viruses.* 2015;7(8):4254–81.

Marinho CD, Martins FJ, Amaral Júnior AT, et al. Genetically modified crops: Brazilian law and overview. G*enet Mol Res.* 2014;13(3):5221–40.

Wunderlich S, Gatto KA. Consumer perception of genetically modified organisms and sources of information. *Adv Nutr.* 2015;6(6):842–51.

Internet References . . .

Environmental Protection Agency (EPA)

www3.epa.gov

European Network of Scientists for Social and Environmental Responsibility (ENSSER)

www.ensser.org

GMO Myths and Truths

gmomythsandtruths.earthopensource.org

GMWatch

gmwatch.org

Slate

www.slate.com

Selected, Edited, and with Issue Framing Material by:
Janet M. Colson, *Middle Tennessee State University*

ISSUE

Are Probiotics and Prebiotics Beneficial in Promoting Health?

YES: **Anneli Rufus**, from "Poop Is the Most Important Indicator of Your Health," *AlterNet* (2010)

NO: **Matt Wood**, from "Do Probiotics Work?" *Science Life* (2014)

Learning Outcomes

After reading this issue, you will be able to:

- Explain what prebiotics and probiotics are and list sources of each.
- Describe how prebiotics and probiotics function within the body.
- Identify the therapy that allows doctors to recolonize patients' bowels with beneficial bacteria.
- Discuss how to determine if a food contains adequate amounts of beneficial bacteria.
- Describe health conditions for which prebiotics have proven to be beneficial and conditions for which they are not beneficial.
- Identify the strains of probiotics (bacteria) that have been validated through clinical trials and published in peer-reviewed journals to show efficacy for treating certain health conditions.

ISSUE SUMMARY

YES: Journalist Anneli Rufus describes how chemicals added to today's food supply destroy the good bacteria (probiotics) and various ways to restore the bacteria to the body. She also encourages us to start looking for prebiotic-fortified foods, because it is hard to get an adequate amount from foods.

NO: Matt Wood discusses what the scientific studies show about the two biotics but points out some negative effects of prebiotics and the short list of probiotics shown to actually be beneficial to health.

Even though the terms are relatively new, the concept of probiotics and prebiotics has been around for centuries. German researchers Jürgen Schrezenmeir and Michael de Vrese provide a brief history of the two biotics in the February 2001 supplement to the *Journal of Clinical Nutrition*. Their article "Probiotics, Prebiotics, and Synbiotics— Approaching a Definition," traces probiotics back to the *Old Testament* and the description of sour milk:

> There is a long history of health claims concerning living microorganisms in food, particularly lactic acid bacteria. In a Persian version of the *Old Testament* (Genesis 18:8) it states that "Abraham owed his longevity to the consumption of sour milk." In

76 BC the Roman historian Plinius recommended the administration of fermented milk products for treating gastroenteritis. . . . Metchnikoff [1907] claimed that the intake of yogurt containing *lactobacilli* results in a reduction of toxin-producing bacteria in the gut and that this increases the longevity of the host. Tissier [1905] recommended the administration of bifidobacteria to infants suffering from diarrhea, claiming that bifidobacteria supersede the putrefactive bacteria that cause the disease. He showed that bifidobacteria were predominant in the gut flora of breast-fed infants.

Schrezenmeir and de Vrese report that the actual term "probiotic" was first used by "Lilly and Stillwell in

1965 to describe 'substances secreted by one microorganism which stimulates the growth of another' and thus was contrasted with the term antibiotic." The term "prebiotic" was introduced in 1995 by Gibson and Roberfroid who define it as:

> . . . nondigestible food ingredients that beneficially affect the host by selectively stimulating the growth and/or activity of one or a limited number of bacterial species already resident in the colon, and thus attempt to improve host health. Intake of prebiotics can significantly modulate the colonic microbiota by increasing the number of specific bacteria and thus changing the composition of the microbiota. Nondigestible oligosaccharides in general, and fructooligosaccharides in particular, are prebiotics. They have been shown to stimulate the growth of endogenous bifidobacteria, which, after a short feeding period, become predominant in human feces. Moreover, these prebiotics modulate lipid metabolism, most likely via fermentation products.

And, to complicate things, they define "synbiotic" as a product that contains probiotics and prebiotics, because the two work *synergistically*. Although the terms are spelled about the same, the term "symbiotic" refers to two or more organisms (especially of different species) living together but not necessarily in a relation beneficial to each.

Before the media and food industry began to capitalize on the term "probiotic," we called the bacteria that live in our GI tract "friendly bacteria" or "gut microflora." The bacteria are beneficial because they may synthesize certain vitamins, reduce GI problems, and/or control the level of pathogenic bacteria. A tremendous amount of research is being conducted on other aspects of these bacteria related to health. Some even think they may have a role in treating obesity. The main sources of probiotics are fermented products like yogurt, buttermilk, sweet acidophilus milk, sauerkraut, kefir, and tempeh.

The only thing new about prebiotics is the name. They are naturally occurring and have been in our diets from the beginning of time. Many people think that the "non-digestible food ingredient" is anything that contains fiber. But not all fibers have prebiotic activity. To be considered a prebiotic, the substance must resist digestion and travel to the colon where the bacteria reside, and it must be a food that the bacteria will eat. The two main substances that are classified as prebiotics are inulin and oligofructose. The table below is adapted from a 1999 article by Moshfegh et al. published in the *Journal of Nutrition*. (A more extensive list is in the article.) It is easy to see that traditional American foods are low in these two prebiotics. Keep in mind that 100 grams is almost a half-cup. And eating a half-cup of dried garlic or onions would be pretty potent.

The average American consumes about 5 grams of prebiotics per day, whereas people in other parts of the world average twice as much. The Committee for the Dietary Guidelines for 2010 believes that "the gut microbiota do play a role in health, although the research in this area is still developing." Therefore, a recommended intake for the two has not been established. Food manufactures have been adding it to foods for a few years, mainly in the form of chicory root.

Do we need to increase our probiotic and prebiotic intake? Will the two biotics make us healthier, happier, and thinner? Anneli Rufus says, yes. She describes the many benefits of probiotics and explains some unusual ways to ingest them. Matt Wood is a bit skeptical about the current body of knowledge related to the biotics. He says that our current understanding about them is not advanced to the stage for widespread use in treating disease.

Inulin and Oligofructose Content of Common Foods		
Food (100 g)	Inulin (g)	Oligofructose (g)
Chicory root	41.6	22.9
Jerusalem artichoke	18.0	13.5
Dandelion greens (raw)	13.5	10.8
Garlic (dried)	28.2	11.3
Garlic (raw)	12.5	5.0
Onion (dried)	18.3	18.3
Onion (raw)	4.3	4.3
Wheat bran	2.5	2.5
Asparagus	2.5	2.5
Banana	0.5	0.5

Source: Adapted from Moshfegh et al., *J Nutr.* 1999.

TIMELINE

76 B.C. Plinus recommends fermented milk to treat GI problems.

1907 Russian scientist Elie Metchnikoff proposes that yogurt increases longevity.

1965 Lilly and Stillwell coin the term "probiotics."

1995 Gibson and Roberfroid introduce the term "prebiotic."

DEFINITIONS

Antibiotic A substance produced by various microorganisms that are used to destroy disease-causing bacteria.

Ferment The process by which bacteria or yeast convert sugar (from milk, fruits, or vegetables) to an acid, typically lactic acid.

Prebiotic A non-digestible food ingredient that bacteria in the colon use as a source of food.

Probiotic A live microorganism, which when administered in adequate amounts, confers a health benefit.

Symbiotic Two or more organisms (especially of different species) living together not necessarily in a relation beneficial to each.

Synbiotic A food that contains a probiotic and prebiotic.

YES ⤶

Anneli Rufus

Poop Is the Most Important Indicator of Your Health

*L*ike it or not, our bowels are the ID cards of our bodies, charting our recent histories with terrifying accuracy. So, how do we ensure a healthy gut?

According to a lawsuit filed this month, Ron and Sarah Bowers bought their son a Subway sandwich in Lombard, Illinois on February 27. After eating it, he had agonizing cramps and diarrhea. According to the suit, what the couple really bought was a shit sandwich.

It had been contaminated with *Shigella sonnei,* a bacteria transmitted via the fecal-oral route and can cause vomiting, dysentery and death. Over 100 people claim to have been sickened at Lombard's Subway, according to attorney Drew Falkenstein, whose firm has filed suit on behalf of Ron and Sarah Bowers and two other customers.

We don't want to think about excrement. We don't want to see it, smell it or touch it. We definitely don't want to eat it with chicken teriyaki, on toast. Yet intestinal goings-on are in our faces everywhere these days, whether the news is about probiotics and prebiotics appearing in new food products or yet another outbreak of norovirus—the painful gastroenteritis that is spread via fecally contaminated food, water and surfaces and has sickened thousands of cruise-ship passengers in eight unprecedentedly massive outbreaks so far this year.

And "poopular culture" is upon us: Witness *Slumdog Millionaire*'s outhouse-plunge scene. Witness Oprah's "Everybody Poops" episode, in which Dr. Mehmet Oz avows that excrement should enter the toilet with not a plop but a swoosh "like a diver from Acapulco." In a scene from the forthcoming film *Life As We Know It*, a young mom portrayed by Katherine Heigl is interrupted by visitors while changing a diaper. "Sweetie," one of the visitors tells her, "you have shit on your face."

In a dirty, crowded world where germs are outsmarting drugs by leaps and bounds and our health care options may or may not be mired in red tape for years, we're being forced to face feces. Which is kind of a good thing. They're the ID cards our bodies issue, charting with terrifying accuracy where we've been and what we've done. *The bowel knows.*

Good Bugs vs. Bad Bugs

"A gram of feces can contain 10 million viruses, one million bacteria, 1,000 parasite cysts and 100 worm eggs," asserts Rose George, author of *The Big Necessity: The Unmentionable World of Human Waste and Why It Matters* (Metropolitan, 2008). She despairs over the fact that 2.6 billion people "have no access to any latrine, toilet bucket or box. . . . They do it in plastic bags and fling them through the air in narrow slum alleyways." Four out of every 10 human beings, George laments, "live in situations where they are surrounded by human excrement."

In the developed world, our relationship with our bowels mostly entails controlling the flora that live in them. *Lactobacillus. Peptococcus. Streptococcus.* A hundred trillion microbes belonging to as many as 1,000 different species coexist at any given time in a single gut, which measures over three yards. What are they doing down there? Battling it out, rendering us well or ill.

Over 70 percent of the human body's immune cells are found in the gut's mucosal lining. A healthy gut means more immunity, and a healthy gut is a gut in which good bacteria outnumber bad. And they're all hitchhikers that rushed in from outside, mounting an invasion that began the instant our placentas broke. "We're all bacteria-free until then," says Emory University School of Medicine associate professor Andrew Gewirtz, the senior author of a study released this month on the effects of imbalanced gut flora. Once the placenta breaks, Gewirtz says, "the colonization begins."

Garnering such headlines in the mainstream media as "You can blame bacteria in your stomach for those unwanted pounds" and "Germs are making you fat," his study found that mice whose guts contained too many of the class of bacteria known as *Firmicutes* ate much more than other mice, experienced metabolic changes and became obese.

This finding undermines the assumption that obesity is driven by laziness and easy access to cheap fattening foods.

"You can't ask the mice" why they ate more, "but how much they ate was clearly not affected by price or marketing schemes," Gewirtz says. Instead, bad bugs can promote excessive appetite and fat storage. They can also make us sick in a million other ways.

The Business of the Gut

"Good bugs form an invisible barrier preventing pathogenic bugs to take root and multiply," says Ann Louise Gittleman, a doctor of holistic nutrition who has appeared on "Dr. Phil" and authored over 30 books including *Fat Flush for Life* (Da Capo, 2009).

She urges us to wage "the new germ warfare" that optimizes "the balance of power in what amounts to a huge fungi kingdom. We have to, because in our bodies we have more bacteria than we have cells."

Because of their crucial role in immune function, the bad ones "can turn into a source of bad health that can affect us from head to toe," creating not just irritable bowel syndrome, colitis and Crohn's disease but conditions such as nasal congestion, itchy skin, bleeding gums, acne and depression that we might not think had anything to do with our bowels, Gittleman says. Online, she sells stool-sample testing kits that come with vials and a discreet white box printed with the address of the lab that does the analysis.

"The intestine is an unappreciated organ. It's a beautiful membrane," asserts vegan physician Michael Klaper, who appeared in the PBS documentaries *Diet for a New America* and *Food for Thought* and has served as an adviser to NASA. "Think of all the intestine does while supporting a population of alien organisms. Miraculous things happen on our gut linings."

At True North Health Education and Fasting Center in Santa Rosa, California, Klaper and his fellow doctors supervise patients undergoing water-only fasts that can last up to 40 days. "Like other organs, the gut could use a rest. We're talking about 22 feet of small intestine. Its lining is a very active membrane and it needs a holiday sometimes, too.

"The body is perfectly capable of going for weeks without food as you burn off your fat stores. Of course, it's no picnic. In the first few days, people are very energetic, as all the energy that would have been used to digest food is put to other purposes. At the end of the second week, they get very quiet, meditative. They're in a different space," said Klaper.

When it's over, "they're very light and clean, and we very gently re-feed them on highly diluted fruit juices and steamed vegetables." However long the fast lasted, refeeding takes half that long. "There's an art to it, of course," Klaper says.

How did we get so messed-up?

"In the old days, our ancestors drank water out of streams and wells. They ate fruit and vegetables harvested in gardens. They lived in close connection with the natural world, and part of the natural world would set up housekeeping in their intestines," he said.

Traditional diets lacking chemical additives kept their gut bugs in balance, "but modern life is an assault on our normal bacterial flora. We put five or six majorly disruptive substances down there every day."

The first of these is chlorine, found in tap water. "Okay, so we don't get cholera or typhoid. That's great. But every time you drink this water, you're drinking a chlorine-dilute solution," he said. That kills good bugs along with bad. Ditto phosphoric acid, a key soft-drink ingredient. "We're a nation of tea and coffee drinkers. What happens in your gut when you're constantly sloshing down a known bactericide?"

Sugar is yet another villain, as are antibiotics, which wipe out nearly every bug in sight—which saves lives but leaves guts thinking *What the hell?*

And they do think, insists Chicago colon therapist Alyce Sorokie, the author of *Gut Wisdom: Understanding and Improving Your Digestive Health* (Career, 2004). "The gut is always speaking to us. It has more emotional receptor sites than anywhere else in the body. The gut is filled with neurons and neuropeptides, the same things that are in our brains, so it can take in information. It can learn. It can respond to events even more rapidly that our brain does," says Sorokie.

"You feel something in the gut, and the vagus nerve brings that 'gut feeling' up the spinal cord to the brain, and the brain makes up a story about it. The brain can always rationalize, but when we feel something in the gut, it's unedited. It's very primal. That's the gut's voice, and the more we don't listen, the louder it gets."

And that is why Sorokie says her clients get emotional during colonics, as filtered water flowing through a hose inserted into the anus bathes the colon, bringing out with it accumulated fecal matter that can be viewed through a clear portion of the mechanism, foot by wiggly, rubbery, slippery, corn-kernel-studded foot.

Releasing stored material from digestive tracts releases stored material from hearts and minds as well, Sorokie says.

"It lets everything come out. These clients say they wish they could bring the hose along with them to their psychotherapy appointments. Nobody wants to think,

'I harbor toxic thoughts and toxic waste within me,' but then there's a liberation: Here it is and there it goes. This was part of me, and now it's not," she said.

Short of anal hoses and doctor-supervised starvation, we can give our bowels a break by eating prebiotics. Found in dandelion greens, Jerusalem artichokes, chicory, milk and a few other natural sources, these are soluble fibers that we can't digest, but our beneficial flora *can*. In other words, prebiotics (which aren't alive) fuel probiotics (which are), making them more active and fighting-fit. So, eating prebiotics is like sprinkling fish-food into a tank full of hungry fish.

"Most people are already comfortable with the idea of fiber in their diets," says microbiologist Mary Ellen Sanders, who belongs to the International Scientific Association of Probiotics and Prebiotics.

"Now you can start to think of eating fiber not just for the traditional fiber effects, but to feed beneficial members of your bacterial community," she explained.

These communities, which are unique to each of us, remained almost a total mystery until recently. Only in the last few years has DNA research brought the identities and functions of much of this flora to light. Up to 80 percent of the various types of human bacterial microbes have still never been grown outside the body under laboratory conditions, Sanders says. "It will be very interesting to see how all this develops in the next five years."

In the meantime, she says eating probiotics and prebiotics "lets us feed the right microbes in the right way." As it would be difficult to eat enough chicory and dandelion greens to get the recommended five to eight daily grams of prebiotics, we can start looking for prebiotic-fortified food products and supplements, often identified by the presence of oligofructose and/or inulin on their labels.

We'll be seeing those words more and more, as products containing prebiotics are among the food industry's fastest-growing sectors. New ones keep popping up, such as the Jamba Juice frozen sorbet and yogurt bars that hit stores this month. The bars' marketing material promises that Coconut-Pineapple Passion Smashin' and its fellow treats-on-sticks "contain prebiotic fiber, allowing customers to satisfy their sweet tooth without feeling guilty."

One hundred trillion microbes are too many to kill, so we're never out of bugs. But when they go way out of balance, a new kind of therapy lets doctors recolonize patients' bowels with what Emory University's Andrew Gewirtz calls "cocktails of good bacteria."

As seen on "Grey's Anatomy" and in real life, the treatment is an extreme measure for people suffering from *Clostridium difficile*, a bad bacteria whose overpopulation causes debilitating intestinal infections when antibiotics wipe out the good bacteria that would normally quell it. (*Clostridium difficile* rates are skyrocketing in American hospitals these days.) Known as fecal bacteriotherapy, fecal transfusion or fecal transplant, the treatment entails inserting a healthy person's feces into the sick person.

Rich in good bacteria, these feces enter the patient's intestine from either end: via enemas or orally, through a tube. "These patients are at the ends of their ropes," says Gewirtz. "They're willing to try something that isn't very pleasant."

So: Bad gut bacteria stay bad when Subway workers don't wash their hands after doing you-know-what. Good gut bacteria stay good even after they exit one body in feces and are more or less fed to another. And in this brave new world, eating shit might save lives.

ANNELI RUFUS is an award-winning author who is the literary editor for the *East Bay Express*. She graduated from Berkley with a degree in English. Rufus is the author of *The Scavengers' Manifesto* (2009), *The Farewell Chronicles: How We Really Respond to Death* (2005), and *Party of One: The Loners' Manifesto* (2002).

Matt Wood

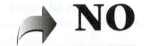 **NO**

Do Probiotics Work?

Walk past the dairy case or health food section of any grocery store and you'll see a variety of yogurts, milk, shakes and even granola bars that say they contain probiotics. These "good" bacteria are added to foods to promote a healthy environment of microorganisms in the digestive tract, supposedly to aid in digestion and promote good gastrointestinal health. Are these claims based in real science, or are they just another food fad to squeeze money out of consumers?

We spoke to Stefano Guandalini, MD, Section Chief of Pediatric Gastroenterology, Hepatology, and Nutrition and Medical Director of the Celiac Disease Center at the University of Chicago, about probiotics and prebiotics, the precursor that provides fuel for the supposedly beneficial bacteria. He and his colleagues published a review paper recently looking at various studies and clinical trials that used pre- and probiotics to treat symptoms of inflammatory bowel disease (IBD) and irritable bowel syndrome (IBS) in children. The following is an edited version of that conversation.

Many people are familiar with the term probiotics, but what are prebiotics?

Prebiotics are basically the metabolic fuel for probiotics. It's a term that encompasses a number of mostly carbohydrates that are present in vegetables and grains, for instance in wheat, artichokes, legumes, etc. They are only partially digested by the human intestinal tract, so they reach the colon where they are fermented by bacteria. We have trillions of bacteria happily living in our colon, and they ferment these substrates. They're happy with them, and so they thrive. The idea of taking prebiotics is that you can encourage the growth of good bacteria in the gut by providing them the food they like.

Can you do that by changing your diet? Or is there a pill you can take?

You can do in both ways. If your diet is rich in things like onions, garlic, wheat, legumes and artichokes, then you

ingest a lot of prebiotics already. But there are also chemically identifiable supplements that also serve the same purpose.

Are prebiotics effective for treating digestive diseases?

In theory these are a good way of promoting a healthy microflora in your gut, and one would expect beneficial effects, but in reality it has been quite disappointing. There's not a lot of practical use for prebiotics as we speak, in terms of clinical effectiveness. The only niche in which we found them to be successful is as an additive to formula for premature babies, because human milk actually contains plenty of prebiotics. Other than that, there hasn't been much practical use. In fact, in our review, we saw that prebiotics have been tried for treating irritable bowel syndrome, but actually with mostly negative results.

With inflammatory bowel disease, it's likely different. Several preparations have been tried with mixed results, but again, nothing sticks out as important or with clinical relevance. So in spite of good conceptual reasons to expect good results, they have not been proven very effective.

How are probiotics different from prebiotics?

Probiotics are microorganisms that, if ingested in adequate amounts, confer a health benefit to the host beyond the nutritional value. In practical terms, it's a class of mostly live bacteria that have been studied for a long time and found useful for treating or preventing a number of clinical conditions.

Our review paper focuses on the efficacy of probiotics for IBS and IBD, including both ulcerative colitis and Crohn's disease. For IBS, we have some good evidence in adults that some probiotics actually seem to be effective in relieving some of the symptoms, mostly the bloating and abdominal pain that accompanies IBS, especially when there is either diarrhea or constipation that goes along with it.

And in the case of ulcerative colitis, there is a growing body of evidence supporting the efficacy of some specific strains as an adjuvant in the course of the therapy. Crohn's disease is different, however. People have tried multiple ways of addressing the problem with different strains of probiotics, different clinical settings, different endpoints, but none of the researchers were able to show any efficacy with probiotics in Crohn's disease patients.

You can go into any grocery store and find yogurt and other foods that have probiotics added to them. Do those products do any good?

Not all probiotics are equal, that's an important thing to stress. People think they can walk into a store and pick any probiotic from the shelf and they're just the same. That is not the case. Different probiotics have different strains and concentrations of bacteria that have different properties. Only a minority of them has been tested properly in clinical trials to find if they were indeed effective.

In reality, yogurt by definition has to have two strains of bacteria—*Lactobacillus bulgaricus* and *Streptococcus thermophilus*—to create the yogurt. However these strains do not pass the gastrointestinal tract intact. They are destroyed by the acidity of the stomach and the enzymes of the pancreas, so nothing reaches the colon and it's not beneficial. However, like you said, some yogurts are now enriched with other live bacteria of different strains. Some of them indeed include strains that survive the passage through the intestinal tract and then can be beneficial, and some make that claim but they don't, and it's hard for the general public to discriminate. Activia, for instance, is one of the good preparations. These yogurts actually do have strains of live *Bifidobacteria* that have been studied and may be beneficial. Yakult, containing well-studied strains of *Lactobacilli*, is another one that does the same.

Is a food product the best way to treat symptoms of IBS or IBD, or do you need a special preparation in a pill?

The best way is to use specific strains that have been validated through clinical trials and published in peer-reviewed journals to show efficacy, and if possible reproduced by different groups using the same preparations. So the list of probiotics that have gone through this process is actually very short:

- There is a product called Align, based on a specific *Bifidobacterium*, which is mostly for adults with IBS.
- For infants and colicky babies there is some proof of effectiveness for a product called Biogaia, which has the bacterium *Lactobacillus reuteri* in it.

- Then we have Culturelle with *Lactobacillus GG*, another one with a long record of scientific, well conducted studies, which has been found effective in treating diarrheal diseases.
- Florastor, which contains a yeast [*Saccharomyces boulardii*] instead of bacteria, is also effective in treating and preventing antibiotic associated diarrhea. Children who get antibiotics often develop diarrhea, and in many cases that can be prevented by the use of Florastor.
- Finally there is a preparation called VSL #3, which is a highly concentrated preparation of 8 different strains of probiotics. This has received a great deal of attention by the scientific world to treat a number of conditions. It seems to be effective for ulcerative colitis, both in adults and children, and it has been found effective in irritable bowel syndrome as well.

Outside of this incredibly short list, however, there is nothing else. There is no other probiotic that has been found to be effective in rigorous, controlled clinical trials. This is not to say they aren't working, it's just to say we don't have any scientific proof yet.

Are probiotics safe?

One thing that all these probiotics have in common is that they are relatively safe. They are very tolerable and basically create no side effects. One caveat is for premature babies and people with profoundly depressed immune systems. Some of these preparations might be contaminated by yeasts, which can be dangerous in those cases. But with these two exceptions, probiotics have been used in large amounts for generations now. So they are safe, but if there is no clear cut indication, I wouldn't necessarily recommend them. That's a question I often get from patients, "Could we use probiotics?" And if it's not to treat a specific condition and they just think it will improve health, I tell them it's not necessary.

Where is the research on prebiotics and probiotics headed?

It's interesting. There was a boom for years and then it died down quite a bit. From a laboratory standpoint, we don't understand a lot about how the probiotics work. So I think the attention of scientists now is more focused on understanding the mechanisms of the interactions between these bacteria and the host, which are different between different individuals. Each one of us has a unique composition of intestinal flora. The same probiotics may have a different effect for you and me, because they interact with trillions of other bacteria, which are different for each person. So all of these nuances are going back to basic science before moving further to the clinical arena.

That seems to be a theme of microbiome research. Everyone agrees on its profound effect on our health, but getting to where you could change something meaningfully to treat a disease is a different thing.

Right, we are not there yet. It's very complicated. As we have said many times, the genome of the microbes is thousands of times more complex and more numerous than the human genome. When we are talking about personalized medicine, we are really talking about the microbiome: how to understand all the subtle interactions with the human host, and how to possibly exploit this for health reasons. It's an incredibly interesting area, and my colleagues here at the University of Chicago, David Rubin, Eugene Chang, Cathryn Nagler, Bana Jabri and others are actively working on this. We aren't there yet, but we will. I have great enthusiasm in this. I think this is the medicine of the future.

MATT WOOD is the editor of the *Science Life* blog and the manager of Digital and Social Media for the University of Chicago Medicine News Office.

EXPLORING THE ISSUE

Are Probiotics and Prebiotics Beneficial in Promoting Health?

Critical Thinking and Reflection

1. Define the following: probiotic, prebiotic, and synbiotic. List three foods that are considered to be a good source of each.
2. Explain why our current food supply is lower in beneficial bacteria (probiotics) and how we can restore the levels.
3. Record all the foods you eat for one day. Determine which foods provide probiotics and which provide prebiotics.
4. Go to the grocery store and find five products whose labels claim they "contain live active cultures." What types of bacteria are in the products and what health claims are on the label, if any? How does one determine if the bacteria will actually survive the journey from the food processing plant to your large intestine?
5. Refer to the definition of synbiotic. Describe three things that meet the criteria of synbiotic and state which component of the food provides probiotic activity and which provides prebiotic components.

Is There Common Ground?

Both Rufus and Wood agree about the definitions and food sources of prebiotics and probiotics and that they exert some benefit to the body. Perhaps Rufus takes a more colorful approach as she describes how vital "poop" is to our overall health. For example, her description of a Subway sandwich contaminated with *Shigella sonnei*, probably transmitted by a careless employee who didn't wash his hands properly. Even though human feces is not typically considered a pleasant topic of conversation—especially around the dinner table—it has gained popularity in the media. Even Oprah had an "Everybody Poops" episode feathering Dr. Oz. Rufus describes the various types of colonies of bacteria, viruses, parasites, and worms found in feces. She points out the beneficial things about "good bacteria."

Wood agrees with much of Rufus' general theme, but takes a more scientific approach. As the media specialist for the University of Chicago School of Medicine, he has expert gastroenterologists and other medical staff who are currently conducting research using various strains of bacteria to determine their effects on specific disease conditions.

Additional Resources

Gibson GR, Roberfroid MB. Dietary modulation of the human colonic microbiota: Introducing the concept of prebiotics. *J Nutr.* 1995;125:1401–12.

Marchesi JR, Adams DH, Fava F, et al. The gut microbiota and host health: A new clinical frontier. *Gut.* 2015. doi:+10.1136/gutjnl-2015-309990.

Moshfegh AJ, Friday JE, Goldman JP, Ahuja JK. Presence of inulin and oligofructose in the diets of Americans. *J Nutr.* 1999;129(7 Suppl):1407S–11S.

Schrezenmeir J, de Vrese M. Probiotics, prebiotics, and synbiotics—approaching a definition. *Am J Clin Nutr.* 2001;73(2) 361s–64s.

Internet References . . .

Institute of Food Technologist

www.ift.org

International Scientific Association for
Probiotics and Prebiotics (ISAPP)

www.isapp.net

Probiotics.org

probiotics.org

Selected, Edited, and with Issue Framing Material by:
Janet M. Colson, *Middle Tennessee State University*

ISSUE

Is Modern Wheat Unhealthy?

YES: Kris Gunnars, from "Modern Wheat—Old Diet Staple Turned into a Modern Health Nightmare," *Authority Nutrition* (2014)

NO: Donald D. Kasarda, from "Can an Increase in Celiac Disease Be Attributed to an Increase in the Gluten Content of Wheat as a Consequence of Wheat Breeding?" *Journal of Agricultural and Food Chemistry* (2013)

Learning Outcomes

After reading this issue, you will be able to:

- Outline the role that grains have had in mankind's diet for thousands of years and changes that have occurred in the way wheat is grown and processed.
- Identify various types of wheat such as spelt, kamut, diploid, polyploid, durum, soft, hard, winter, and spring.
- Describe changes in the protein content of wheat during the twentieth century.
- State the protein content of various types of wheat.

ISSUE SUMMARY

YES: Kris Gunnars claims that there are profound genetic changes in modern wheat and that it is processed differently than wheat grown in earlier times. He describes how the new wheat is the root of a variety of health problems.

NO: Cereal chemist Donald Kasarda reports that today's wheat has the same level of protein and gluten it had hundreds of years ago and believes modern wheat is not the cause of celiac disease or gluten sensitivity.

$\mathbf{A}$n Internet search using the term "gluten" reveals 135 million sites; using the term "gluten-free foods" finds 95 million, whereas "celiac" finds only 5 million and "gluten sensitivity" uncovers a mere 2.6 million. There is even a gluten-free dating site that was named the "Best Up and Coming" dating site for 2014 and a Canadian-based marketing firm dedicated to help food processors increase sales of gluten-free foods. How have we become so obsessed with gluten and do we really need to avoid it?

Gluten is actually two types of protein (gliadin and glutenin) found in wheat, rye, barley, and triticale that gives dough elasticity and makes bread chewy with a firm crust. Traditional American, European, and Australian diets are loaded with gluten because most breads are made with wheat. Gluten is not found in rice or corn; therefore,

typical rice-based Asian or corn-based Mexican foods may naturally be gluten-free.

People who have the autoimmune disorder celiac disease should avoid gluten, and therefore wheat. (The condition is also known as gluten-sensitive enteropathy and celiac sprue.) Eating gluten damages the inner lining of the small intestine of a person who has celiac and may interfere with nutrient absorption. The University of Chicago Celiac Center reports that celiac affects at least 3 million Americans and the prevalence of celiac in the United States is:

- In average healthy people: 1 in 133
- In people with related symptoms: 1 in 56
- In people with first-degree relatives who are celiac: 1 in 22

- In people with second-degree relatives who are celiac: 1 in 39
- Estimated prevalence for African-, Hispanic-, and Asian-Americans: 1 in 236

Diagnosis of celiac consists of a blood test to determine gluten autoantibodies; the most common one measures the tissue transglutaminase antibodies (TG-IgA). If the test is positive, a biopsy of the small intestine is completed to confirm celiac. Although not used as frequently, genetic markers can be assessed to determine if a person carries the celiac gene.

Non-celiac gluten sensitivity (NCGS) is a second condition related to wheat that produces symptoms similar to those seen in celiac disease. However, unlike celiac disease, it is not an autoimmune disorder and is not genetically linked. Common symptoms of NCGS are mental fatigue, lethargy, and general intestinal problems such as gas, bloating, pain, and cramps. It is unclear if this condition is related to gluten or another factor in the diet, or even another substance in wheat. A third related condition is a true wheat allergy. Most allergies result from a protein in food, and wheat is among the top allergenic foods.

Gluten-free food sales have risen dramatically in the past decade, especially in the United States. *Time* magazine writer Martha White wonders about the gluten craze in her 2013 article "Why We're Wasting Billions on Gluten Free Foods?" White points out, "Many of us [who are] paying a premium to avoid the gluten in our food are doing so without any good medical reason." A 2013 *Statista (The Statistics Portal)* survey found that 36 percent of consumers who choose gluten-free report that they have not been diagnosed with celiac but buy gluten-free for other reasons. So White is right, we opt for gluten-free for no apparent reason.

Along with the gluten-free obsession, some people are simply avoiding wheat, possibly after reading two recent books. In his 2011 best-selling book *Wheat Belly*, cardiologist William Davis, MD, explains his idea that eliminating wheat from our diets can prevent fat storage, shrink the spare tire around the belly, and reverse a host of health problems. A couple of years later, neurologist David Perlmutter, MD, published another best-seller, *Grain Brain*. Perlmutter claims that carbohydrates are destroying our brains. He even links whole grains to dementia, anxiety, headaches, and much more.

So we have physicians, who America should trust for reliable health information, blaming health problems on wheat. Are gluten and wheat unhealthy and should we avoid them? Is today's wheat the cause of celiac disease? Those are the questions in this issue.

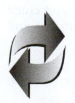

YES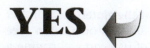

Kris Gunnars

Modern Wheat—Old Diet Staple Turned into a Modern Health Nightmare

Wheat is a highly controversial food these days.

On one hand, we've got people telling us that it is extremely harmful, with one doctor calling it poison.

Then on the other hand, we've got dietitians and the government telling us that whole wheat is an essential part of a "balanced" diet.

Well . . . one inescapable fact is that humans have been consuming wheat, in one form or another, for *thousands* of years.

It is an old food . . . and most diet-related diseases are relatively new.

Therefore, it doesn't make sense to blame old wheat for these new health problems.

However . . . it's important to realize that wheat today is not the same as it was a thousand, one hundred or even 60 years ago.

How Has Wheat Changed?

Wheat today is completely different from the wheat we ate back in the day.

First of all, it is processed differently. New techniques in grain processing in the late 19th century made it possible to create massive amounts of refined wheat for a low cost.

We are now able to separate the nutritious components of the grain (the bran and germ) away from the endosperm, where most of the starchy carbs are contained.

This led to an obvious reduction in nutrient density and gave refined wheat the ability to spike blood sugar very fast.

But we also used to *prepare* our grains differently. They were soaked, sprouted, fermented and bread was baked using slow rise yeast.

Sprouting and fermenting grains leads to many beneficial effects. It increases the amino acid lysine, reduces anti-nutrients (like phytic acid and lectins),

disables enzyme inhibitors and makes nutrients more accessible.

Today, the flour is bleached and the bread is baked with quick rise yeast. The grains certainly aren't soaked, sprouted or fermented.

Based on these factors alone, it is clear that the bread and pasta we are eating today is **very** different from the traditionally prepared wheat we have been eating for thousands of years.

Bottom Line: Wheat is processed and prepared differently these days, which makes it less nutritious and more harmful than traditionally prepared wheat.

Today's Wheat Is Genetically and Biologically Different

The plants that wheat is made from are not all the same.

There are different breeds of wheat . . . just like there are many different breeds of dogs (a Chihuahua is very different from a German Shepherd, for example).

Back in the day, we used to consume ancient varieties like Emmer, Einkorn and Kamut.

However, almost *all* of the wheat eaten today is high-yield dwarf wheat, which was developed by cross-breeding and crude genetic manipulation around the year 1960.

Dwarf wheat has shorter stems and a much greater yield. Therefore it is much, much cheaper than the older varieties and more economically feasible.

The benefits of a high-yield crop are obvious, but we are now learning that there were some major downsides to this as well.

Specifically, modern wheat has some subtle but important differences in its nutrient and protein composition.

Bottom Line: Modern wheat was introduced around the year 1960. It was developed via cross-breeding and crude genetic manipulation, which changed the nutrient and protein composition of the plant.

Modern Wheat Is Less Nutritious

The Broadbalk Wheat Experiment is one of the longest running scientific studies in history.

Since the year 1843, the scientists have grown different strains of wheat and analyzed various factors, including nutrient composition.

From 1843 until about 1960, the nutrients in wheat didn't change much.

However, from the year 1960, which coincides with the introduction of modern wheat, the nutrient content starts trending downwards.

Concentrations of Zinc, Copper, Iron and Magnesium were **19–28% lower** in the years 1968–2005, compared to 1845–1967.

At the same time, there was no evidence that the soil had changed. So it is clearly something about the nature of modern wheat that makes it less nutritious than the older varieties.

Another study that also compared different strains of wheat found that the older varieties contained significantly more Selenium.

Given how **incredibly** widespread wheat consumption really is, it is easy to see how this may have contributed to nutrient deficiencies.

Bottom Line: Modern wheat is less nutritious than old wheat. The amount of minerals like Zinc, Copper, Iron and Magnesium has decreased by 19–28%.

Modern Wheat Is Much More Harmful to Celiac Patients

Celiac disease is the most severe form of gluten intolerance.

When people with this disease eat wheat, the immune system in the gut mistakenly assumes that the gluten proteins are foreign invaders and mounts an attack.

However . . . the immune system doesn't only attack the gluten proteins, it also attacks the gut lining itself, leading to degeneration of the intestinal lining, leaky gut, massive inflammation and various harmful effects.

Celiac disease is serious business . . . it has been on the rise for decades, increasing about fourfold in the past 45 years. Right now, about 1% of people have celiac disease.

Another condition, called non-celiac gluten sensitivity, is believed to be much more common, perhaps afflicting around 6–8% of people.

Gluten is actually not a single protein, it is a family of different proteins and only some of them are recognized by the immune system of celiac patients.

One of the gluten proteins that seems to be problematic is called Glia-α9. One study found that the amount of this protein is significantly higher in modern wheat.

Therefore . . . many researchers have speculated that modern wheat, due to its higher amount of problematic glutens, may be worse for celiac patients than older varieties of wheat.

Interestingly, this has been tested in several studies.

One study compared the effects of Einkorn (old) and modern wheat on intestinal cells from celiac patients. Compared to modern wheat, Einkorn didn't have any harmful effects.

In another study in 12 celiac patients, gluten from Einkorn caused significantly less adverse reactions than modern gluten and was **even better tolerated than rice**—a gluten-free grain!

The way wheat is prepared may also be important. In one study, sourdough bread (bread made from fermented wheat) did not cause a reaction in celiac patients in the same way as regular bread.

Of course, these studies do not suggest that celiac patients should start buying Einkorn wheat or sourdough bread instead. This needs to be studied a lot more before any recommendations can be made.

But what these studies DO suggest is that *modern* wheat has a unique ability to trigger an auto-immune reaction in the gut and is probably the main reason why celiac disease and gluten sensitivity are on the rise.

Bottom Line: Modern wheat contains more of the problematic glutens and there are some studies showing that older wheat varieties don't cause a reaction in celiac patients.

Studies Show That Modern Wheat Is More Harmful to Healthy People as Well

Pretty much everyone agrees that wheat can be a problem . . . for celiac patients.

Awareness and acceptance of non-celiac gluten sensitivity has been increasing as well.

But one thing that most skeptics **refuse** to accept is the possibility that wheat can be harmful for other people as well. That is, people who *don't* have celiac disease or gluten sensitivity.

Well . . . I also found a couple of studies in healthy people.

One of them was published in early 2013. This study compared Kamut (an older variety of wheat) against modern wheat. It was a randomized controlled cross-over trial with 22 healthy participants.

The participants consumed either Kamut or modern wheat, for 8 weeks each.

This is what happened to their cholesterol levels and blood mineral content:

As you can see, Kamut wheat caused a reduction in both Total and LDL cholesterol compared to modern wheat. It also increased blood concentrations of potassium

and magnesium, while these minerals decreased with the modern wheat.

Kamut also caused a mild reduction in fasting blood sugars (3 mg/dL), but that isn't shown on the graph.

Here is what happened to inflammatory markers. Excess inflammation in the body is linked to almost every modern disease, including heart disease, diabetes, metabolic syndrome, stroke, Alzheimer's, arthritis and many more.

As you can see, Kamut led to a major decrease in some important inflammatory markers (IL-6, IL-12 and TNF-α), while modern wheat did not. In the case of TNF-α,

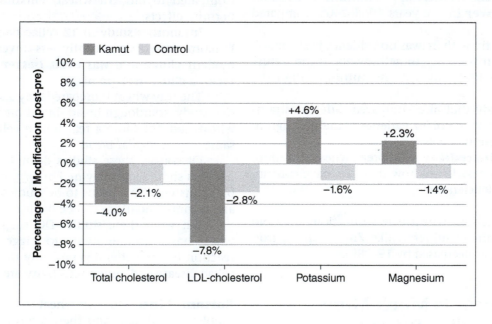

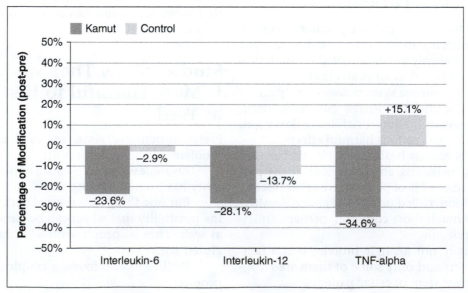

modern wheat caused an **increase**, although it was not statistically significant.

What this study implies is that Kamut wheat is, at the very least, much "less bad" than modern wheat.

There was also another study that tested an old Italian variety of wheat and noticed significant improvement in blood cholesterol and inflammatory markers compared to modern wheat.

Bottom Line: Relative to older wheat varieties, modern wheat has adverse effects on cholesterol, blood mineral content and inflammatory markers, potentially contributing to disease.

Is There Such a Thing as Healthy Wheat Bread?

If you can get your hands on whole grain bread made with Einkorn or some of the older varieties of wheat, then perhaps it can be a part of a healthy diet.

Another way is to make it yourself.

You can dig around and find someone who sells whole wheat grains of the old breed, then you can grind and ferment the wheat and bake your own healthy bread.

Or you could just save yourself the trouble and skip the wheat altogether. There's no nutrient in it that you can't get in greater amounts from other foods.

Modern Wheat Should Be Avoided

Even though wheat may have been healthy in the past, the wheat people are eating today is completely different.

It's the same as with many other modern foods . . . when scientists try to "enhance" what nature has already provided us with, things tend to go wrong.

In the case of wheat, this ancient diet staple was accidentally turned into a modern health nightmare.

If you care about your health and can't get your hands on the older varieties of wheat, then do yourself a favor and avoid wheat like the plague.

Kris Gunnars is CEO, editor-in-chief, and founder of Nutrition Authority—An Evidence-Based Approach website. He is a nutrition researcher with a BS in medicine and has spent years reading books, blogs, and scientific studies on nutrition. Evidence-based nutrition is his passion and he plans to devote his career to informing people about it.

Donald D. Kasarda

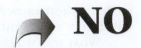 **NO**

Can an Increase in Celiac Disease Be Attributed to an Increase in the Gluten Content of Wheat as a Consequence of Wheat Breeding?

Introduction

There is recent evidence that the incidence of celiac disease has increased during the second half of the 20th century.[1–3] These studies provide evidence that the incidence is changing based on the presence of tissue transglutaminase antibodies (a marker for celiac disease) in selected sets of serum samples, although there are no continuous data relating to the incidence of celiac disease in the U.S. population on a year-by-year basis. In addition, there is increasing interest in other gluten-related disorders: wheat allergy and nonceliac gluten sensitivity.[4] It has been speculated that the increase in celiac disease may have occurred because of changes in wheat proteins that resulted from wheat breeding—mainly an increase in the gluten content,[4] which is directly proportional to protein content. Here, I will focus on conventional breeding carried out for various purposes: to increase or decrease gluten proteins or modify them in other ways, to increase yield, to change kernel size or shape, or to improve disease or insect resistance. My focus will be on the United States, and because there are no GMO-type (genetically engineered) wheats used commercially in the United States, direct genetic modification of the wheat genome to increase protein content need not be considered. I will discuss briefly the history of wheat from its domestication to modern times and some factors that may have a bearing on the question of whether or not the increase in celiac disease can be attributed to an increase in the gluten content of modern wheats.

Wheat History

Diploid Wheat

Man first domesticated a diploid and tetraploid wheats about 10000 years ago[5] (see timeline of Figure 1). One

Figure 1

Events in evolution in relation to the appearance of wheat (approximate dates).

Evolution of Wheat	
4,000,000,000 years BP* →	Origins of life
400,000,000 years BP →	Complex organisms living in the seas invade the land (B cells and T cells already present in sharks)
200,000,000 years BP →	Flowering plants begin to evolve
100,000,000 years BP →	Grasses begin to evolve
20,000,000 years BP →	Divergence of the common line that gives rise to wheat and barley
500,000 years BP →	Early man (*Homo sapiens*)
10,000 years BP →	Diploid wheat domesticated by man

*BP = Before Present

of the wheat forms originally domesticated, sometimes called "einkorn," had only one genome, usually designated the A genome. Because the vegetative tissues of plants contain two copies of the genome (hence, diploid), the plant designation is AA. The diploid wild wheat that was first domesticated is thought to have been *Triticum urartu*, but other diploid wheat species may have been involved as well. These diploid species are likely to have evolved from a common line that included oats, barley, and rye (Figure 2). In the centuries following domestication, the genome changed as a consequence of breeding and selection, which would have introduced and fixed

Kasarda, Donald D. "Can an Increase in Celiac Disease Be Attributed to an Increase in the Gluten Content of Wheat as a Consequence of Wheat Breeding?" *Journal of Agricultural and Food Chemistry,* February, 2013. Published by American Chemical Society.

Figure 2

Divergence of a common line leading to the diploid progenitors of wheat.

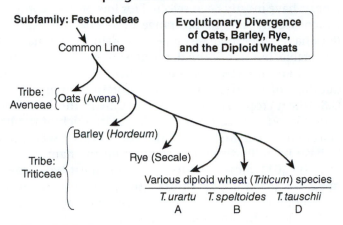

some new genes and/or controlling sequences into the genome. Consequently, the domesticated modern diploid wheat took on a significantly different character from the wild wheat. Wild wheat species usually have tiny grains, often needle-like in appearance, compared to the larger grains of modern wheats. When grown today, the grains of these wild species usually have high protein contents, in the 16–28% range.[6] Early farmers and breeders probably selected for seed size (among other traits)—larger grains being easier to recover from the plant during threshing. In doing so, they inadvertently increased the starch content relative to protein content; thus, the apparent seed protein percentage decreased. The domesticated diploid wheat, (einkorn) was designated *Triticum monococcum* (genus *Triticum*, species *monococcum*) by Linnaeus in the 18th century. The small amount of *T. monococcum* that is grown today is used mostly for animal feed. In the early millennia following domestication, the protein content of domesticated wheat was most likely steadily declining because of selection for traits that had an inverse relationship to protein percentage, such as seed size and starch content.

Throughout most of the 10000 years of wheat domestication it was not possible to measure the protein content of wheat grain. The concept of protein as a unique substance was developed only about 250 years ago, and it was not until 1883 when Johan Kjeldahl developed his method for organic nitrogen determination that the stage was set for the development of an accurate and moderately convenient method for determining the protein content of wheat. Even so, the proper factor for converting the nitrogen content of wheat grain to protein content

was a subject of debate throughout the early part of the 20th century. In the late 20th century, with the development of the near-infrared reflectance (NIR) spectroscopy method for the determination of wheat protein content, measurement of this quantity was greatly simplified. The gluten content of wheat is approximately proportional to the protein content and usually ranges between 70 and 75% of total protein content. Statements in the literature, such as, "Since the first farmers, strains of wheat have been selectively bred for their gluten content, and the gluten content has progressively increased through time"[7] and ". . . the selection of wheat varieties with higher gluten content has been a continuous process during the past 10,000 years . . ."[4] are therefore not correct. The earliest farmers were selecting for many traits, but protein content was not one of them. However, with the development of yeast-fermented (leavened) bread baking about 2000–5000 years ago (the date is not known with any precision), farmers may have indirectly begun to select for protein content because leavened bread requires a relatively high protein content (at present 11% is considered somewhat minimal for bread making in the United States).

Polyploid Wheats: Tetraploids and Hexaploids

It is likely that tetraploid wheat was domesticated about the same time as diploid wheat.[5] The tetraploid wheats

Figure 3

Combinations of diploid wheats leading to the polyploid forms.

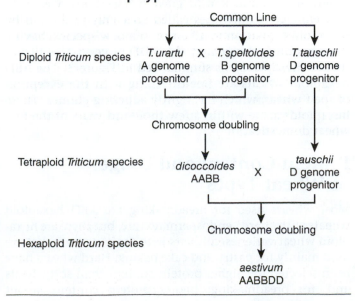

have two genomes that, for vegetative tissues, are designated AABB (hence, tetraploid) (Figure 3). Wheats with more than one genome are known as polyploid wheats. (I will not attempt a discussion of polyploid formation[8] here.) The A genome of the tetraploid wheats is closely similar to that of *T. monococcum*, and the B genome is related to *Triticum speltoides*. When grown today, wild tetraploids usually have protein contents in the range of 16–27%,[6] whereas domesticated tetraploids usually have lower protein contents of about 10–12%. The wild tetraploids are often designated *Triticum dicoccoides*, and the domesticated equivalents are classified as *Triticum turgidum* (sometimes *Triticum dicoccum*). *T. turgidum* has two sub-species/varieties, one with the common name *emmer* and the other called *durum*. Emmer wheat is not free-threshing, which means that there is a tightly adhering husk, or glume, that is difficult to remove from the grains. Durum wheat is free-threshing, that is, the seeds are readily released from the glumes. The main wheat of the Roman empire was emmer, and its current form, now somewhat in vogue for gourmet cooking, is usually known as *farro*. Durum wheats are now used mainly for pasta, although bread can be made from durum wheat, and such bread is common in parts of Italy, such as the Puglia region.

The next step up in complexity was to hexaploid wheat, which, for *Triticum aestivum*, consists of three genomes designated A, B, and D. The A and B genomes of hexaploid wheats are nearly identical to the A and B genomes of tetraploid wheat. The hexaploid wheats have no wild equivalents, and the ABD hexaploids resulted from hybridization of a cultivated (domesticated) emmer and a wild grass species known as *Triticum tauschii*[9] (sometimes called goat grass) followed by polyploid formation to give rise to a new species having three genomes designated AABBDD in vegetative tissues (hence, hexaploid), as summarized in Figure 3. The ABD hexaploid wheats are free-threshing with the exception of spelt wheat, which has tightly adhering glumes. These hexaploids arose within a few thousand years of the first wheat domestication.

Protein Content and Usage of Wheat Types

Most wheats used for breadmaking are ABD hexaploid wheats with "hard" endosperm texture, but there are hexaploid wheat varieties/cultivars with "soft" texture that are used mainly for pastry and cake baking. Hard wheats have been selected for higher protein content than soft wheats and, for breadmaking, higher protein content (about

12–14%) is usually desirable. For the soft wheats, low protein is usually desirable, because it is the starch rather than the protein that plays the more important role in determining desirable pastry characteristics. Consequently, soft wheats have mostly been selected for low protein content, which usually falls in the range of 7–11%. All purpose flour has an intermediate range of protein, which makes it acceptable, but not optimal, for most uses.

There are few pertinent papers that address the question of whether or not the protein content of the U.S. wheat crop has increased over time in the 20th century. Although adequate data may exist, much of the literature from the first half of the 20th century seems not to have been digitized. Information on the Kansas crops of 1949–2011 shows that for the main wheat type grown in Kansas (hard winter wheat, used primarily for breadmaking), many crops fell within a protein content range of 11–13%, with an unusual high of 14.1% in 1956 and an unusual low of 10.7 in 1961.[10] Some papers from the first half of the 20th century[11] indicated protein contents ranging from 8.77 to 14.26% for various samples of hard winter wheats. The 8.77% number appeared to be an outlier, and there was no obvious deviation from the results for protein content in the second half of the 20th century.[10]

The hard spring wheats, grown mostly in the Northern Plains, are considered to be highly desirable for bread baking and tend to have protein contents that in general exceed the usual protein contents of winter wheats by about 2 percentage points. The protein contents of hard spring wheats vary on average over a range of about 3–4 percentage points from year-to-year, usually falling in the 12–16% range as exemplified by the data in Table 1 (extracted from Table 42 of Bailey[12]). The basis for the higher protein content of the spring wheat from the Northern Plains is probably related partly to genetics and partly to growing conditions (environment). In the late 1920s, the protein contents of the Northern Plains wheats were relatively low (about 13%), presumably due to normal to high levels of rainfall,[12] but increased to average levels of about 15% in the 1930s, presumably due to drought conditions[12] (Table 1). The North Dakota Wheat Commission reported[13] that, in 2009, the hard red spring wheat crop ". . . yielded an average of 13.1 percent (which) was well below the traditional level of more than 14%," and these protein contents are fairly typical of late 20th century crops for the hard spring wheat region. Various studies have compared the protein contents of wheat varieties from the early part of the 20th century with those of recent varieties.[14,15] When grown under comparable conditions, there was no difference in the protein

Table 1

Average Percentages of Protein in Spring Wheat Marketed through Minneapolis, MN, by Crop Years (Data Excerpted from Table 42 of Reference 12)

crop year	no. of samples	av protein (%)	standard deviation (σ)	av moisture content (%)
1925	33246	12.49	1.34	
1926	26145	13.28	1.55	13.7
1927	63944	11.96	0.78	13.2
1928	49964	12.42	0.77	13.4
1929	37202	13.70	1.41	13.4
1930	52041	14.85	1.47	13.1
1931	17182	15.00	1.22	
1932	45027	14.21	0.99	11.7
1933	28829	15.03	0.89	11.5
1934	12900	14.80	1.04	11.4
1935	28544	15.30	1.71	11.8
1936	16698	15.92	1.64	
1937	12185	14.83	1.28	11.6
1938	13169	18.78	1.04	11.5

contents. Although nitrogen fertilization can have strong effects on protein content for some wheat varieties,[16] the data do not seem to be in accord with the likelihood that recent fertilization protocols have had a strong effect on the protein contents of wheat grown in the United States.

Interpretation of protein data is complicated by occasional major deviations from the more usual range. In 1938, the protein content of spring wheat was exceptionally high (Table 1), averaging close to 19%; these years of exceptionally high protein (or low protein) occur occasionally and are likely to result mainly from environmental factors, rather than nitrogen fertilization or wheat breeding. To maintain a uniformity of quality characteristics from year to year, flour mills usually blend wheat flour that is intended for commercial use by specific customers, for example, bakeries. Very high protein content would usually be unsuitable for direct use, and so high-protein wheat flours would usually be blended with lower protein grain to achieve a more normal protein level before reaching the consumer. The connection between celiac disease and wheat ingestion was not made until 1950,[17] so that any variations in the incidence of celiac disease prior to that would not have been distinguished from gastrointestinal diseases in general. Even today, data for the incidence of celiac disease that could be used to recognize short-term variations are not available.

With acknowledgment that the data that are available were not suitable for rigorous statistical interpretation, I found no evidence of any obvious trend toward higher protein content for either winter or spring wheats since the early part of the 20th century when the key ancestral varieties of current bread wheats (of both winter and spring habits) were introduced to the United States from Europe and Asia. Hard winter and spring wheats are the predominant types grown in the United States, mostly for bread baking, and these wheats will have the highest protein contents. Soft wheats have significantly lower protein contents because high protein contents are undesirable for many of the products made from soft wheats.

Diet, Gluten Consumption, and Celiac Disease

Bread is the most common wheat-based food in the United States, although pastries and pasta are also widely consumed. Because bread wheats in the United States range in protein content from about 11 to about 16% and pastry wheats from about 7 to 11%, the amounts of gluten ingested might vary considerably from individual to individual depending on diet choices. Economic Research Service (USDA-ARS-ERS) statistics[18] indicate that the per person per year intake of wheat flour (from all classes of wheat) reached a high of 220 lb (100 kg) per person in about 1900, declining steadily to a low of about 110 lb (50 kg) per person in 1970 and then gradually rising to about 146 lb (66 kg) per person in 2000, with a slight decrease

Figure 5

U.S. per capita wheat flour use (figure redrawn from ref 18 and data supplied by G. Vocke).

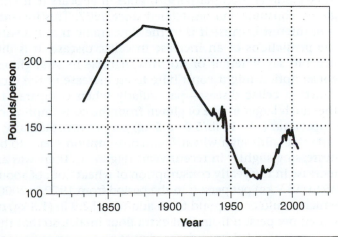

occurring since 2000 to about 134 lb (61 kg) per person in 2008 (Figure 5). The per capita numbers of Figure 5 do not include U.S. wheat that is exported or used for animal feed, but presumably include wheat flour used to produce vital gluten. If I arbitrarily suggest that the average protein content of the wheat crop (all types of wheat) would be around 11%, the gluten equivalent of this U.S. grain/flour would be about 11.1 lb (5 kg) per person (assuming a per capita intake of 134 lb of wheat flour and that 75% of total flour protein would be gluten protein); if the average protein content was closer to 12%, the gluten equivalent would be about 12.1 lb (5.1 kg) per capita.

Vital Gluten

Gluten fractionated from wheat flour by washing starch granules from a dough (sometimes called vital gluten) is often added to food products to achieve improved product characteristics. About 80% of the gluten used in the United States is imported—mainly from Australia, the European Union, Canada, and China. The question of how much vital gluten contributes to the total consumption of gluten (wheat flour and wheat grain + vital gluten) is complicated by a lack of accessible information about gluten production and imports for the United States in recent years and by indications that imports are rising rapidly. I make a crude estimate of what both factors might be as follows: Gluten imports were 177×10^6 lb (80×10^6 kg)[19] in 1997 and 386×10^6 lb (175×10^6 kg) in 2007.[20] imports would currently be 490×10^6 lb (222×10^6 kg). I assumed that the population of the United States is 330×106, that vital gluten is 75% protein, and that 80% of vital gluten is used for human food, to obtain a per person (per year) intake of gluten of 0.9 lb (408 g). Following the same approach, I estimate the gluten intake in 1977 to be 0.3 lb (136 g) per person. Thus, it appears that vital gluten consumption has tripled since 1977. This increase is of interest because it is in the time frame that fits with the predictions of an increase in celiac disease. It is difficult to say whether or not this increase in vital gluten consumption might contribute to an increase in the incidence of celiac disease—particularly when compared to the much larger intake of gluten from the consumption of wheat flour (11−12 lb/5.0−5.5 kg) per person). Similarly, I note that, although wheat flour consumption seems to be decreasing slightly in recent years (Figure 5), there was an increase in the yearly consumption of wheat flour of about 35 lb (15.9 kg) per person in the period from 1970 to 2000, which would correspond to an additional 2.9 lb (1.3 kg) of gluten per person from that extra flour intake, so that the 1970 intake of 9.1 pounds (4.1 kg) of gluten (from flour or grain) had increased to 12 pounds (5.4 kg) in 2000. It may be noted that whole wheat products, which are increasing in consumption for health reasons (especially the higher fiber content), often have vital gluten added to them to compensate for the negative effects of the ground whole grain on quality factors, such as loaf volume in breadmaking. This increase amounts to about 1.5–2.0 percentage points in product protein content, but the significance (if any) of this increase is not known—it must be considered in the context of other factors.

There is evidence that the D genome of bread wheat has more epitopes active in celiac disease than the A and B genomes,[21] and some of these might be the most active epitopes. Consequently, tetraploid wheats (mainly durum wheats used for pasta) and diploid wheats, such as *T. monococcum*, are likely to be less toxic to celiac patients than bread wheats. However, given that all of these wheats, even *T. monococcum*,[22,23] have proteins with several of the potentially active sequences that have been defined as being toxic for people with celiac disease, the significance of the decreased number of epitopes in tetraploids and diploids needs additional investigation.

The estimates that celiac disease is increasing in the United States are based on studies that cover approximately the last half of the 20th century. Could this increase be attributed to the increased consumption of wheat during that period, or to an increased use of vital gluten in food products, rather than any systematic increase in the protein content of wheat in the United States? Some diagnosed celiac patients in remission exhibit changes to the intestinal epithelium characteristic of celiac disease with a daily intake of 50–100 mg of gluten, generally considered the minimal toxic dose of gluten.[24] The average slice of bread weighs approximately 40 g and contains about 2.4 g of protein—of that protein, about 1.8 g (1800 mg) would be gluten. It might seem, intuitively, that the variations in protein content of wheat would not be a key factor in the sensitization of potential celiac patients, given the seemingly large excess of gluten in most wheat-containing products over the minimum allowable intake. Nevertheless, one cannot rule out that the process by which the immune system switches from tolerance of wheat gluten protein to intolerance (celiac disease) might be dependent on the total amount of gluten encountered.[25] Development of immune system tolerance to food proteins in general is an as yet imperfectly understood process—as is the loss of immune system tolerance to gluten proteins that is characteristic of celiac disease.[26]

In summary, I have not found clear evidence of an increase in the gluten content of wheat in the United States during the 20th century, and if there has indeed been an increase in celiac disease during the latter half of the century, wheat breeding for higher gluten content does not seem to be the basis. Changes in the per capita intake of wheat and gluten might play a role; both increased during the period in question, but there is a lack of suitable data on the incidence of celiac disease by year to test those possibilities. The normal fluctuation of wheat crop protein content from year-to-year, being equivalent to or larger than the intake of fractionated gluten, is a complicating factor, but one that would be diminished by the practice of flour blending. Other factors, such as per capita vital gluten intake, variations in individual diets with regard to the amount and types of wheat consumed, wheat genetics, and agronomic practices (such as nitrogen fertilization), that affect protein content might contribute to determining the "toxicity" of wheat for people with the appropriate genetic susceptibility for celiac disease (mainly those carrying the genes for particular proteins of the major histocompatibility complex, DQ2 and DQ8); further research would be needed to evaluate such factors.

References

(1) Rubio-Tapia, A.; Kyle, R. A.; Kaplan, E. L.; Johnson, D. R.; Page, W.; Erdtmann, F.; Brantner, T. L.; Kim, W. R.; Phelps, T. K.; Lahr, B. D.; Zinsmeister, A. R.; Melton, L. J., 3rd; Murray, J. A. Increased prevalence and mortality in undiagnosed celiac disease. *Gastro-enterology* **2009**, 137, 88–93.

(2) Catassi, C.; Kryszak, D.; Bhatti, B.; Sturgeon, C.; Helzlsouer, K.; Clipp, S. L.; Gelfond, D.; Puppa, E.; Sferruzza, A.; Fasano, A. Natural history of celiac disease autoimmunity in a USA cohort followed since 1974. *Ann. Med.* **2010**, *42*, 530–538.

(3) Lohi, S.; Mustalahti, K.; Kaukinen, K.; Laurila, K.; Collin, P.; Rissanen, H.; Lohi, O.; Bravi, E.; Gasparin, M.; Reunanen, A.; Maki, M. Increasing prevalence of coeliac disease over time. *Aliment. Pharmacol. Ther.* **2007**, *26*, 1217–1225.

(4) Sapone, A.; Bai, J. C.; Ciacci, C.; Dolinsek, J.; Green, P. H.; Hadjivassiliou, M.; Kaukinen, K.; Rostami, K.; Sanders, D. S.; Schumann, M.; Ullrich, R.; Villalta, D.; Volta, U.; Catassi, C.; Fasano, A. Spectrum of gluten-related disorders: consensus on nomenclature and classification. *BMC Med.* **2012**, *10*, 13.

(5) Harlan, J. R.; Zohary, D. Distribution of wild wheats and barley. *Science* **1966**, *153*, 1074–1080.

(6) Ciaffi, M.; Dominici, L.; Lafiandra, D.; Porceddu, E. Seed storage proteins of wild wheat progenitors and their relationships with technological properties. *Hereditas* **1992**, *116*, 315–322.

(7) Cronin, C. C.; Shanahan, F. Why is celiac disease so common in Ireland? *Perspect. Biol. Med.* **2001**, *44*, 342–352.

(8) Harlan, J. R.; deWet, J. M. J. On Ö Winge and a prayer: The origins of polyploidy. *Bot. Rev.* **1975**, *41*, 361–390.

(9) Kihara, H. Origin of cultivated plants with special reference to wheat. Seiken Ziho, *Report of the Kihara Institute for Biological Research* **1975**, *25–26*, 1–24.

(10) Kansas Wheat History, Kansas Agricultural Statistics, U.S. Department of Agriculture, National Agricultural Statistics Service, Kansas Field Office (http://www.nass.usda.gov/Statistics_by_State/Kansas/Publications/Crops/whthist.pdf), 2012.

(11) Bulletin 289. A comparison of hard red winter and hard red spring wheats. Agricultural Experiment Station, Kansas College of Agriculture and Applied Science, Manhattan, KS, 1940; pp 57 (www.ksre.ksu.edu/historicpublications/pubs/SB289.PDF).

(12) Bailey, C. H. *Constituents of Wheat and Wheat Products;* ACS Monograph Series 96; American Chemical Society: Washington, DC, 1944; pp 332.

(13) North Dakota Wheat Commission, Annual Report to Producers, 2009–2010 (http://www.ndwheat.com/uploads/resources/764/annual-report-09-10.pdf).

(14) Khalil, I. H.; Carver, B. F.; Krenzer, E. G.; MacKown, C. T.; Horn, G. W.; Rayas-Duarte, P. Genetic trends in winter wheat grain quality with dual-purpose and grain-only management systems. *Crop Sci.* **2002**, *42*, 1112–1116.

(15) Fufa, H.; Baenziger, P. S.; Beecher, B. S.; Graybosch, R. A.; Eskridge, K. M.; Nelson, L. A. Genetic improvement trends in agronomic performances and end-use quality characteristics among hard red winter wheat cultivars in Nebraska. *Euphytica* **2005**, *144*, 187–198.

(16) Godfrey, D.; Hawkesford, M. J.; Powers, S. J.; Millar, S.; Shewry, P. Effects of crop nutrition on wheat grain composition and end-use quality. Effects of crop nutrition on wheat grain composition and end use quality. *J. Agric. Food Chem.* **2010**, *58*, 3012–3021.

(17) Dicke, W. K. *Coeliac Disease: Investigation of the Harmful Effects of Certain Types of Cereal on Patients Suffering from Coeliac Disease.* M.D. Thesis, 2nd English translation; Utrecht University, The Netherlands, **1950**; pp 97.

(18) Vocke, G. Wheat's role in the U.S. diet has changed over the decades. ERS/USDA Briefing Room (http://www.ers.usda.gov/ topics/crops/wheat/wheats-role-in-the-us-diet.aspx), 2009.

(19) United States—Definitive Safeguard Measures on Imports of Wheat Gluten from the European Communities. Report of the Panel, World Trade Organization, July 31, 2000; pp 98 (www.worldtradelaw.net/reports/wtopanels/us-wheatgluten(panel).pdf).

(20) Neufeld, J. Quoted by Roxanna Hegeman, "Imports decimate industry", Topeka Capitol-Journal (cjonline.com), 2007 (cjonline.com/stories/050307/bus_167236241.shtml).

(21) van Herpen, T. W. J. M.; Goryunova, S. V.; van der Schoot, J.; Mitreva, M.; Salentijn, E.; Vorst, O.; Schenk, M. F.; van Veelen, P. A.; Koning, F.; van Soest, L. J. M.; Vosman, B.; Bosch, D.; Hamer, R. J.; Gilissen, L. J. W. J.; Smulders, M. J. M. α-Gliadin genes from the A, B, and D genomes of wheat contain different sets of celiac disease epitopes. *BMC Genomics* **2006**, *7*, 1 DOI: 10.1186/1471-2164-7-1.

(22) Kasarda, D. D. Letter to the editor: *Triticum monococcum* and celiac disease. *Scand. J. Gastroenterol.* **2007**, *42*, 1141–1142.

(23) Vaccino, P.; Becker, H. A.; Brandolini, A.; Salamini, F.; Kilian, B. A catalogue of *Triticum monococcum* genes encoding toxic and immunogenic peptides for celiac disease patients. *Mol. Gen. Genomics* **2009**, *281*, 289–300.

(24) Catassi, C.; Fabiani, E.; Iacono, G.; D'Agate, C.; Francavilla, R.; Biagi, F.; Volta, U.; Accomando, S.; Picarelli, A.; De Vitis, I.; Pianelli, G.; Gesuita, R.; Carle, F.; Mandolesi, A.; Bearzi, I.; Fasano, A. A prospective, double-blind, placebo-controlled trial to establish a safe gluten threshold for patients with celiac disease. *Am. J. Clin. Nutr.* **2007**, *85*, 160–166.

(25) Koning, F. Celiac disease: quantity matters. *Semin. Immunopathol.* **2012**, *34* (DOI: 10.1007/s00281-012–0321-0).

(26) Depaolo, R. W.; Abadie, V.; Tang, F.; Fehiner-Peach, H.; Hall, J. A.; Wang, W.; Marietta, E. V.; Kasarda, D. D.; Waldmann, T. A.; Murray, J. A.; Semrad, C.; Kupfer, S. S.; Belkaid, Y.; Guandalini, S.; Jabri, B. Co-adjuvant effects of retinoic acid and IL-15 induce inflammatory immunity to dietary antigens. *Nature* **2011**, 220–225.

DONALD D. KASARDA has a PhD in physical chemistry from Princeton. He was a research chemist with the USDA's Western Regional Research Center until his retirement in 1999. He is an associate in the Experiment Station at UC Davis. His research focuses on the structure of grain storage proteins, especially the gluten proteins of wheat, and, for the past 40 years, has collaborated with various medical research groups in attempts to define the basis for the activity of these proteins in celiac disease.

EXPLORING THE ISSUE

Is Modern Wheat Unhealthy?

Critical Thinking and Reflection

1. Using various celiac resources, describe the problems that may arise in people who have untreated celiac.
2. Describe the differences in the following types of flour: spelt, kamut, diploid, polyploid, durum, soft, hard, winter, and spring.
3. Using the USDA Nutrient database (http://ndb.nal.usda.gov/ndb/foods), compare the protein content of 1 cup of the following types of flour: spelt, kamut, hard red winter, soft red winter, industrial white, bread, and cake.
4. Find and summarize a recent peer-reviewed article that examines the symptoms, causes, and/or treatment of non-celiac gluten sensitivity.
5. In the United Kingdom, gluten-free foods are covered by many insurance companies for people who have "coeliac" disease if they have a physician's prescription. Describe the pros and cons of a government requiring gluten-free foods to be paid for by insurance. (Suggested site: www.coeliac.org.uk)

Is There Common Ground?

Both Gunnars and Kasarda agree that celiac disease and gluten sensitivity are problems in many individuals and that some people should avoid wheat because of these health conditions. Their differences begin with the wheat itself. Gunnars insists that there are genetic changes in modern wheat. He claims that the wheat that was introduced in 1960 was developed by "cross-breeding and crude genetic manipulation, which changed the nutrient and protein composition of the plant." He also concludes that wheat is processed differently and contains less nutrients than wheat that was grown years ago. He describes why he believes that the new wheat is the root of a variety of health problems.

With decades of experience as a cereal chemist for the USDA and UC Davis, Donald Kasarda concludes that the speculation that today's wheat is the cause of celiac disease or gluten sensitivity is unfounded. He reports that today's wheat has the same level of protein and gluten it had hundreds of years ago and believes modern wheat is not the cause of celiac disease or gluten sensitivity. He supports his position with documentation that the protein content of wheat has remained relatively constant since 1925.

Additional Resources

Allen PJ. Gluten-related disorders: Celiac disease, gluten allergy, non-celiac gluten sensitivity. *Pediatr Nurs.* 2015 May–June;41(3):146–50.

Fasano A, Sapone A, Zevallos V, Schuppan D. Nonceliac gluten sensitivity. *Gastroenterology.* 2015 May; 148(6):1195–204. doi: 10.1053/j.gastro.2014.12.049.

Nijeboer P, Bontkes HJ, Mulder CJ, Bouma G. Non-celiac gluten sensitivity. Is it in the gluten or the grain? *J Gastrointestin Liver Dis.* 2013 December;22(4):435–40.

Internet References . . .

Celiac Disease Foundation

www.celiac.org

National Association of Wheat Growers

www.wheatworld.org

National Foundation of Celiac Awareness

www.celiaccentral.org

United States Department of Agriculture (USDA)

www.usda.gov

US Wheat Associates

www.uswheat.org

Selected, Edited, and with Issue Framing Material by:
Janet M. Colson, *Middle Tennessee State University*

ISSUE

Should Infant Formulas Contain Synthetic ARA and DHA?

YES: Haley C. Stevens and Mardi K. Mountford, from "Infant Formula and DHA/ARA," International Formula Council (IFC) Statement on DHA/ARA and Infant Formula (http://www.infantformula.org/news-room /press-releases-and-statements/infant-formula-and-dha/ara) (2008)

NO: Ari LeVaux, from "Dangerous Hype: Infant Formula Companies Claim They Can Make Babies 'Smarter,' " *AlterNet* (http://www.alternet.org/health/143369) (2009)

Learning Outcomes
After reading this issue, you will be able to:
• Explain why infant formulas contain added docosahexaenoic acid (DHA) and arachidonic acid (ARA).   • List comments from various health and consumer agencies about DHA and ARA added to formulas.   • Outline the health concerns surrounding lab-grown DHA and ARA.

ISSUE SUMMARY

YES: Haley Stevens and Mardi Mountford, representing the International Formula Council (IFC), point out "the available evidence strongly supports benefits of adding DHA and ARA to infant formula." They point out that "a large database exists concerning not only the safety but also the efficacy of infant formula containing both ARA and DHA. These facts, together, support the addition of both ARA and DHA when LC-PUFAs [long-chain polyunsaturated fatty acids] are added to formula."

NO: Ari LeVaux is more skeptical. He says the oils are produced from lab-grown algae and fungi and extracted with the neurotoxin hexane. He also is concerned that some "parents and medical professionals believe these additives are causing severe reactions in some babies, and it has been repeatedly shown that taking affected babies off DHA/ARA formula makes the problems go away almost immediately."

Infant formulas have come a long way since they became popular after World War II. Federal regulations for making infant formulas went into effect in 1941. The first formulas consisted of a simple base of modified cow's milk protein. In 1959, iron-fortified formulas were introduced; a few years later, formulas made with isolated soy protein became available. Each time significant changes are made, the formula manufacturer must notify the Food and Drug Administration (FDA), the federal agency that monitors the safety of America's food supply.

The American Academy of Pediatrics considers human milk to be the "gold standard" when it comes to infant feeding. Formula companies continue to examine nutrients in breastmilk and try to imitate them in their artificially made products. In the 1990s, many studies reported that the intellectual and visual superiority of infants who were breastfed are linked to the long-chain fatty acids DHA and ARA that are abundant in human milk. European countries and Australia were quick to add the fatty acids to infant formula. Some Europeans ones began in 1994; Australia and New Zealand began in about 1998. According to a 2003 Food Standards Australia and New Zealand report, in 2001, DHA and ARA were being added to about 17 percent of formula intended for term infants up to 6 months of age, and about 87 percent of pre-term formula. In 2002, Mead Johnson Nutritionals, a leading U.S. infant formula manufacturer, introduced Enfamil LIPIL™ to the American market. Subsequently, other companies began adding the fatty acids to their infant formulas.

So why are the two fatty acids added to formula? Mead Johnson claims DHA and ARA *"may* help to support babies' mental and visual development." In her June 9, 2010, *Food Politics* blog, Marion Nestle says that DHA is added to formula as a marketing ploy. She writes:

> DHA (an omega-3 fatty acid) came first. As I discuss in my book, *What to Eat,* infant formula companies could not wait to add it. They knew they could market it on the basis of preliminary evidence associating DHA with visual and cognitive benefits in young infants. Although evidence for long term benefits is scanty, the companies also knew that they could charge higher prices for formulas containing DHA.
>
> The FDA approved the use of DHA in infant formulas on the grounds that it is safe, but did not require the companies to establish that DHA makes any difference to infant health after the first year. Because of its marketing advantage, virtually all infant formulas now contain DHA. Surprise! They also cost more.

But more importantly, are they safe for the infants who consume them? The Cornucopia Institute, a farming advocacy group from Wisconsin, says "No." They question the safety and value of adding synthetically made DHA and ARA to infant formula. The group also wonders if the addition is a "risky marketing gimmick" by the formula industry. Their 2008 report points out that the DHA and ARA are "extracted from laboratory-grown fermented algae and fungi and processed utilizing the toxic chemical, hexane." DHASCO® (DHA-rich Single Cell Oil) is extracted from the algae *Crypthecodinium cohnii* and ARASCO® (ARA-rich Single Cell Oil) is extracted from the fungus *Mortierella alpina*. Cornucopia also cites evidence from laboratory studies that link the synthetic fat to increases in liver weight in lab animals and diarrhea in children. (Many baby food manufacturers use tuna oil for their source of added DHA.)

To answers common questions parents have about infant formulas, the FDA posts answers to some questions about DHA and ARA in their "Questions & Answers for Consumers Concerning Infant Formula" page on the FDA website. Some of the questions/answers are below:

- **I see formulas on the market that contain ingredients called DHA and ARA. What foods contain the fatty acids DHA (docosahexaenoic acid) and ARA (arachidonic acid)?**
  DHA is contained in varying amounts in fish oils, with oils from cold-water fish containing higher amounts. DHA and ARA are also found in some algae and fungi, eggs, and in human breast milk. Some manufacturers make dietary supplements containing DHA and ARA.
- **Why is there interest in adding DHA and ARA to infant formulas?**
  While infants can make these fatty acids from other ("essential") fatty acids in their diet, including the fatty acids in infant formulas, some studies suggest that some infants, such as premature infants, may benefit from direct consumption. Other studies suggest no benefit. It is known that long-chain polyunsaturated fatty acids (DHA in particular) accumulate in brain and eye of the fetus, especially during the last trimester of pregnancy. These fatty acids are also found in the fat of human breast milk. Blood levels of DHA and ARA are typically higher in breast-fed infants than in infants fed formulas not containing these fatty acids. For these reasons, some infant formula manufacturers and consumers are interested in providing DHA and ARA directly to infants. These manufacturers and consumers argue that adding oils containing these fatty acids to the fats and oils already in infant formula will provide an infant with both pre-formed DHA and ARA and the essential fatty acids an infant needs to make its own DHA and ARA.
- **What is the evidence that addition of DHA and ARA to infant formulas is beneficial?**
  The scientific evidence is mixed. Some studies in infants suggest that including these fatty acids in infant formulas may have positive effects on visual function and neural development over the short term. Other studies in infants do not confirm these benefits. There are no currently available published reports from clinical studies that address whether any long-term beneficial effects exist.
- **I understand that oils containing DHA and ARA have been added to infant formulas for several years in other countries. Isn't there information from those countries on any long-term benefits or adverse consequences of formulas containing these fatty acids?**
  Systematic monitoring efforts are not in place to collect and analyze information on effects of infant formulas containing DHA and ARA in countries where these formulas are in use.
- **Why has FDA asked manufacturers to do post-market surveillance of infants consuming formulas containing ARA or DHA?**

These are new ingredients that were not used in infant formulas in this country before early 2002, and infant formulas containing ARASCO (ARA Single Cell Oil) and DHASCO (DHA Single Cell Oil) have been marketed in other countries for only a few years. FDA views any evaluation of the safety of use of new food ingredients such as DHASCO and ARASCO as a time-dependent judgment that is based on general scientific knowledge as well as specific data and information about the ingredient. Therefore, scientific data that become available after specific products containing a new ingredient enter the market must be considered as a part of the totality of information about the ingredient. Pre-market clinical studies evaluating the effects of infant formulas containing DHASCO and ARASCO on physical growth and some aspects of development are short-term studies, while some studies suggest that feeding of infant formulas with oils containing DHA and ARA to infants may have long-term effects on growth and development. For all these reasons, manufacturers have been asked to closely monitor these new infant formulas in the marketplace.

After reading the two selections, decide what you think about the safety of added DHA and ARA to formulas. Haley Stevens and Mardi Mountford speak for the Infant Nutrition Council for America and point out "the available evidence strongly supports benefits of adding DHA and ARA to infant formula." Ari LeVaux is more skeptical and agrees with Cornucopia's concern about the toxic potential of the hexane used to manufacture the oils.

DEFINITIONS

Arachidonic Acid (ARA)   The 20-carbon, omega-6 fatty acid that is involved in brain and visual development.

Crypthecodinium cohnii   Algae used to produce DHA.

Docosahexaenoic acid (DHA)   The 22-carbon, omega-3 fatty acid that is involved in brain and visual development.

Hexane   A known neurotoxin and possible carcinogen used as an organic solvent in DHA/ARA production.

Long-chain polyunsaturated fatty acid (LC-PUFA)   A fatty acids with 12 or more carbons and two double bonds.

Mortierella alpina   Fungus used to produce ARA.

YES ↵

**Haley C. Stevens and
Mardi K. Mountford**

Infant Formula and DHA/ARA

U.S. infant formula manufacturers currently offer formulas containing docosahexaenoic acid (DHA) and arachidonic acid (ARA). Formulas containing DHA and ARA have been shown to provide visual and mental development similar to that of the breastfed infant. The decision to supplement formulas with these nutritional long-chain polyunsaturated fatty adds (LCPUFAs) was made following years of research studying the clinical effects of both DHA and ARA in infants. The use of LCPUFAs in infant formulas has been reviewed and supported by the U.S. Food and Drug Administration, the European Food Safety Authority, the Food and Agriculture Organization and World Health Organization, the Codex Alimentarius Commission, the Agence Francaise De Securite Sanitaire Des Aliments, the American Dietetic Association and the Dietitians of Canada, the European Society for Paediatric Gastroenterology and Nutrition, the World Association of Perinatal Medicine and Child Health Foundation, the Commission of European Communities and the National Academy of Sciences.

DHA and ARA are considered to be "building blocks" for the development of brain and eye tissue. Research has demonstrated that DHA and ARA, both present in human milk, are physiologically important in prenatal and post-natal life during the period of rapid brain and eye development and throughout life as well. DHA and ARA have been shown to rapidly accumulate in the brain during the last trimester prenatally and the first two years postnatally, and preclinical studies have also demonstrated their importance in visual and neural systems.

The IFC supports breastfeeding and the position of the World Health Organization, the American Academy of Pediatrics and other leading health organizations that breastfeeding is ideal, and offers specific child and maternal benefits. However, for those mothers who cannot or choose not to breastfeed, infant formula is recommended. Years of product development and careful clinical research have resulted in commercially available infant formulas that provide the appropriate levels of protein, fat, carbohydrate, vitamins, and minerals for a baby to sustain a rapid rate of growth and development without stressing the infant's delicate and developing organ systems. With the addition of DHA and ARA to infant formulas, the industry continues its commitment to provide the best nutrition for infants whose mothers cannot or choose not to breastfeed.

After reviewing the recent literature and current recommendations regarding LC-PUFA for term infant nutrition during the first months of life, a 2008 international expert working group on LC-PUFAs in perinatal practice led by B. Koletzko concluded that "the available evidence strongly supports benefits of adding DHA and ARA to infant formula." The panel stated that the addition of DHA and ARA to infant formula "appears appropriate." Furthermore, the authors stated that, "a large database exists concerning not only the safety, but also the efficacy, of infant formula containing both ARA and DHA. These facts, together, support the addition of both ARA and DHA when LC-PUFAs are added to formula."

Parents and health professionals can be assured infant formula is safe and nutritious. Worldwide Regulatory Bodies Who Support DHA and ARA for Infants.

U.S. Food and Drug Administration (FDA)

In May 2001, following [is] an extensive review of the available scientific data supporting the safety of DHA and ARA, the FDA agreed that oils containing DHA and ARA are generally recognized as safe (GRAS) for use in infant formula. Additionally, in accordance with the requirements of the Infant Formula Act of 1980 and its subsequent amendments, any manufacturer wishing to add these oils to a specific infant formula was required to notify the FDA 90 days prior to the introduction of such a new formula, so that the agency could conduct an appropriate review of the scientific literature and testing that has been assembled by the manufacturer to demonstrate the formula's ability to support growth as a substitute for breast milk.

European Food Safety Authority (EFSA)

In March 2010, the scientific opinion of the EFSA Panel on Dietetic Products, Nutrition, and Allergies (NDA) regarding Dietary Reference Values (DRVs) for fats, including saturated fatty acids, polyunsaturated fatty acids, monounsaturated fatty acids, trans fatty adds, and cholesterol was published. The opinion set an Adequate Intake (AI) level for DHA for infants and young children, and stated "small amounts of DHA may be needed for optimal growth and development of infants and children," including 20–50 mg/day for infants 0–6 months of age.

Food Agriculture Organization (FAO) and the World Health Organization (WHO)

FAO and WHO have recommended the addition of DHA and ARA to infant formula at the levels found in human breast milk. In October 1993, a joint expert consultation concluded: "In view of the evidence on the higher efficiency of long-chain polyunsaturated fatty acids for neural development . . . and the data on premature infants . . . the long-chain polyunsaturated fatty acids should be included in infant formula." Additionally, in 2008 the WHO restated its views about the importance of DHA and ARA for infants.

Codex Alimentarius Commission (CAC)

The CAC, a global body formed by the FAO and the WHO, adopted in July 2007 the Revised Standard for Infant Formula and Formula for Special Medical Purposes Intended for Infants, which upholds the safety and provides for the optional addition of LCPUFAs to infant formulas.

Agence Francaise De Securite Sanitaire Des Aliments (AFSSA)

In March 2010, AFSSA published Dietary Reference Intakes (DRIs) for Fatty Acids, including DRIs for infants 0–6 months and infants and young children 6–36 months.

AFSSA also recognized DHA as an essential fatty acid for its role in structure and function of the brain and eye.

American Dietetic Association (ADA) and the Dietitians of Canada (DC)

The ADA and the DC have recommended the inclusion of DHA and ARA in infant formula and have highlighted the importance of DHA and ARA to infant health. In their position statement on dietary fatty acids, the ADA/DC note "no adverse effects of feeding marketed infant formula containing both ARA and DHA in amounts found in human milk are known. Because of possible benefits and lack of adverse effects, it is recommended that all infants who are not breastfed be fed a formula containing both ARA and DHA through at least the first year of life."

European Society for Pediatric Gastroenterology, Hepatology and Nutrition (ESPGHAN)

ESPGHAN recommends the addition of LCPUFAs to infant formulas. In 2005, an ESPGHAN-coordinated International Expert Group supported the addition of DHA and ARA to infant formulas. In 2006, the ESPGHAN Committee on Nutrition concluded that preterm infants, when formula fed, should receive infant formula with provision of LCPUFAs.

World Association of Perinatal Medicine (WAPM) and the Child Health Foundation

In 2001, the Child Health Foundation, under guidance from the WAPM, asked investigators in the field of LCPUFAs to review available scientific data and form a recommendation. That working group supported the addition of DHA and ARA to infant formulas for term and premature infants. Further, a recommendation from the 2001 workshop was that investigators update its recommendation as additional data became available. Therefore, in 2008, the same group of investigators reviewed the available scientific literature and endorsed its previous position.

Commission of the European Communities (EC)

The EC states that DHA and ARA are considered safe for use as an optional ingredient for infant formulas.

National Academy of Sciences (NAS)

In 2005, a panel organized by NAS developed a report on dietary reference intakes for various macronutrients, including dietary fatty acids like LCPUFAs, and supports the addition of DHA to infant formula in the amounts found in breast milk. According to NAS, "n-3 polyunsaturated fatty acids provide DHA that is important for developing brain and retina."

Background

DHA is particularly required for the development of the cerebral cortex, the region of the brain responsible for language development and information processing, and plays a vital function in developing visual sharpness (acuity). ARA is an important precursor for modulators/mediators of a variety of essential biological processes (e.g., the inflammatory response, regulation of blood pressure, regulation of sleep/wake cycle). DHA and ARA are synthesized in the body from the precursor essential fatty acids, α-linolenic acid (ALA) and linoleic acid (LA), respectively, that are also present in human milk and infant formula.

Evidence that blood levels of DHA and ARA are typically higher in breastfed infants than in infants fed formulas not containing these LCPUFAs provided a basis for investigating the addition of DHA and ARA to infant formulas. Studies suggest that premature infants may benefit the most from direct consumption of DHA and ARA. Throughout the third trimester, a mother passes DHA and ARA to the baby through the placenta. Postnatally, these nutrients are passed through human milk.

In the event that a baby is born prematurely, placental transport of DHA and ARA is interrupted, thereby reducing the baby's total accumulation of ARA and DHA prior to birth. Addition of the GRAS sources of DHA and ARA to preterm formula provides these important nutrients safely. Studies show that formulas containing added DHA and ARA are safe and support visual and cognitive development.

U.S. infant formula manufacturers continue to evaluate the potential benefits of adding nutritional fatty acids to infant formulas. They also take very seriously their responsibility to provide safe and nutritious infant formulas to the millions of infants fed infant formula, often as the sole source of nutrition. Millions of infants in the U.S. and worldwide have safely been fed infant formula with DHA and ARA and millions more continue to be fed every day. The addition of DHA and ARA to infant formula is modeled on the levels present in breast milk. Clinical studies did not find more adverse events in subjects fed DHA and ARA containing infant formulas. There has not been an increase in diarrhea and vomiting complaints, as alleged by recent media reports, since introduction of these ingredients into infant formulas.

HALEY C. STEVENS is the scientific affairs specialist for the Infant Nutrition Council of America (formerly International Formula Council, IFC).

MARDI K. MOUNTFORD is the executive vice president of the Infant Nutrition Council of America (formerly the International Formula Council, IFC).

Ari LeVaux   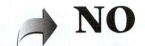 **NO**

Dangerous Hype: Infant Formula Companies Claim They Can Make Babies 'Smarter'

If you believed a certain baby formula would make your child smarter, would you buy it?

Infant formula manufacturers are banking that you would. That's why, since 2002, several companies have fortified their products with synthetic versions of DHA and ARA, long-chain fatty acids that occur naturally in breast milk and have been associated with brain development.

The oils are produced by Martek Biosciences Corp. from lab-grown algae and fungus and extracted with hexane, according to the company's patent application. Hexane is a neurotoxin.

A growing number of parents and medical professional believe these additives are causing severe reactions in some babies, and it has been repeatedly shown that taking affected babies off DHA/ARA formula makes the problems go away almost immediately. The FDA has received hundreds of letters to this effect by upset parents, even as products containing the additives are being marketed as better than breast milk.

Karen Jensen says that due to health complications she was unable to breastfeed her daughter, and so fed her daughter Neocate, a formula with DHA/ARA.

"At two weeks, my daughter would often stop breathing in her sleep and was having various other serious health conditions. She cried constantly and couldn't sleep due to gastrointestinal upset."

After many trips to the hospital, a CT scan, an EEG, time on an apnea monitor and thousands of dollars in bills, "we tried the Neocate without the DHA/ARA in it. Within 24 hours, we had a brand-new, entirely different baby. She had no abdominal distress, no gas, she smiled and played, and for the first time ever we heard her laugh."

Jensen's story is echoed many times over in similar letters urging the FDA to ban DHA and ARA from baby foods, or at the very least to put warning labels on the product advising that some babies may experience adverse reactions like bloating, gastrointestinal distress, vomiting, and diarrhea.

While only a fraction of babies seem to react in this way, it's a common enough occurrence to have earned DHA/ARA baby formula the nickname "the diarrhea formula" in the neonatal unit of an Ohio hospital.

In 2001, the FDA expressed concerns about the safety of adding DHA and ARA to infant-formula additives and notified Martek of the agency's plans to convene a group of scientists to study these concerns.

Martek wrote back: ". . . convening a group of scientific experts to answer such hypothetical concerns would not be productive." Within months, the FDA wrote to Martek that it would allow DHA and ARA in infant formula, without any scientific review of its own.

While quick to protest hypothetical safety concerns about DHA/ARA, Martek was ready to pounce on the hypothetical benefits of its oils.

In a 1996 investment brief, Martek explained, "Even if [the DHA/ARA blend] has no benefit, we think it would be widely incorporated into formulas as a marketing tool and to allow companies to promote their formula as 'closest to human milk.'"

Mead Johnson Nutritionals took this opportunity to heart, drawing the ire of breastfeeding advocates when it began promoting its DHA/ARA Enfamil Lipil as "The Breast Milk Formula."

Mead Johnson was also involved with a report in current issue of the journal *Child Development*, in which a Dallas team of scientists provided evidence that DHA and ARA in baby food improves brain development. Several members of the team have received Mead Johnson money in the form of research funding, as well as the coveted currency known as "consulting fees."

The report claims that infants fed DHA/ARA baby formula (supplied for free by Mead Johnson) showed greater ability to solve certain problems, like pulling a blanket with a ball on it toward them. The researchers say this problem-solving ability correlates with enhanced IQ and vocabulary development.

"New evidence favors baby formula," announced the *Los Angeles Times*, in an ambiguously worded headline that begs the question: Over what is baby formula favored?

Breastfeeding advocates went on the warpath over the suggestion that formula could be better for babies than breast milk.

"Parents will be encouraged to forgo breastfeeding in favor of a hyped-up infant formula," complained Barbara Moore, president and CEO of Shape Up America. "Breast milk has other benefits not related to mental development. It confers protection against infection, including viral infections, and the CDC promotes breastfeeding to confer maximal protection against swine flu and other infections."

Charlotte Vallaeys, a researcher for the Cornucopia Institute, wrote a substantial report on the risks and benefits of DHA/ARA in baby formula. She says the Mead Johnson-funded team behind the *Child Development* story is "the only group that has found real differences in cognitive development" resulting from the addition of DHA and ARA to formula.

Not that other research teams haven't looked. To make sense of the growing body of research on the subject, a team of scientists led by Karen Simmer compiled a review, published in January 2008, of all available literature. The team found "feeding term infants with milk formula enriched with [DHA and ARA] had no proven benefit regarding vision, cognition or physical growth."

A March 2009 review by the European Food Safety Authority also found the available data "insufficient to establish a cause-and-effect relationship" between DHA, ARA and brain development.

Nonetheless, the use of DHA and ARA has grown, and has even won approval for use in organic baby formula, as well as in organic milk.

In an article for the *Washington Post* on the eroding integrity of the "certified organic" label, Kimberly Kindy described how these laboratory produced oils received organic approval.

> . . . in 2006, [USDA] staff members concluded that the fatty acids could not be added to organic baby formula because they are synthetics that are not on the standards board's approved list. . . . Barbara Robinson, who administers the organics program and is a deputy USDA administrator, overruled the staff decision after a telephone call and an e-mail exchange with William J. Friedman, a lawyer who represents the formula makers.

While the FDA has raised serious questions regarding the safety of DHA/ARA, the issue remains in limbo, with concerned parents, medical professionals and advocacy groups pushing one way, and the deep-pocketed corporations pushing the other.

The FDA did instruct Martek and the formula companies to conduct post-market surveillance of its DHA and ARA products, but after seven years none has been submitted.

Until conclusive proof emerges on the safety and/or benefit of DHA and ARA in baby formula, it's buyer beware for parents of newborns. And last I checked, breast milk—the product of millions of years of evolutionary shaping into the perfect food for babies—remains widely available and free of charge. . . .

ARI LEVAUX writes "Flash in the Pan," a syndicated weekly food column and is contributor to *AlterNet*. He received his master's from the University of Montana.

EXPLORING THE ISSUE

Should Infant Formulas Contain Synthetic ARA and DHA?

Critical Thinking and Reflection

1. List the benefits that DHA and ARA may provide to growing infants.
2. List two reasons why formula manufacturers add DHA and ARA to infant formulas.
3. Prepare a table that includes the positions of various infant and health care agencies around the world regarding LC-PUFA added to infant formula. Include the date of the statement, the type of oils mentioned, and their rationale behind their positions.
4. Write a letter to the FDA requesting that they develop a warning label for infant formula about the risk of added ARA and DHA. The letter should be limited to one page in length.
5. Your best friend has decided to formula feed the infant she is expecting in a month. She asks for your opinion on which type of formula she should use. What advice would you give her and why would you give her this advice?

Is There Common Ground?

The main debate is if the synthetically derived ARA and DHA are safe for human infants and questions the safety of the processing technique which includes use of hexane. It is interesting to point out that babies thrived on infant formulas for 70 years and most of the people, who are now adults, are normal and reasonably intelligent human beings. However, the formula industry modifies the formulation for infant formulas rather frequently. Do the formula companies make the modifications to improve the nutritional profile of the formula or to increase sales—and profits?

Ari LeVaux is more skeptical of ARA and DHA added to formula. His argument focuses on the hexane used in processing. He also is concerned that some "parents and medical professionals believe these additives are causing severe reactions in some babies, and it has been repeatedly shown that taking affected babies off DHA/ARA formula makes the problems go away almost immediately. He concludes, "Until conclusive proof emerges on the safety and/or benefit of DHA and ARA in baby formula, it's buyer beware for parents of newborns."

Obviously, the common ground is that all want infants to be healthy, and they do support infant use of infant formula, but the question is should laboratory-grown ARA and DHA be allowed in the formula.

Additional Resources

Kent G. Regulating fatty acids in infant formula: Critical assessment of U.S. policies and practices. *Int Breastfeed J.* 2014;9(1):2.

Lapillonne A, Pastor N, Zhuang W, Scalabrin DM. Infants fed formula with added long chain polyunsaturated fatty acids have reduced incidence of respiratory illnesses and diarrhea during the first year of life. *BMC Pediatr.* 2014;14:168.

Ryan AS, Astwood JD, Gautier S, Kuratko CN, Nelson EB, Salem N. Effects of long-chain polyunsaturated fatty acid supplementation on neurodevelopment in childhood: A review of human studies. *Prostaglandins Leukot Essent Fatty Acids.* 2010;82(4):305–14.

Internet References . . .

The American Academy of Pediatrics

www.aap.org

Cornucopia

www.cornucopia.org

The Food and Drug Administration (FDA)

www.fda.gov

Mead Johnson Nutrition

www.meadjohnson.com

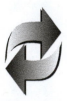

Unit 4

Nutrition and Food Policy

*T*he government is heavily involved in food and nutrition laws and policies that influence matters as diverse as the amount we pay for junk foods to the level of caffeine children should consume. Because food is such a big business, the food industry reacts to almost any action taken by local, state, and federal governments that might affect their profits. In this unit, debates focus on policies that relate to government control of our food supply. Some of the food controversies focus on food processors such as limiting the sugar in food or reducing the sodium in savory snacks, whereas others question the way foods are grown such as the use of pesticides.

Government regulation of food policies begins with the Executive Office of the President of the United States— and the Office of the First Lady. People of the United States should recognize First Lady Michelle Obama, and her interest in the health and nutritional status of American youth, as a leading force in nutrition reform during this decade. Other government offices that monitor nutrition are the Food and Drug Administration (FDA) and the Environmental Protection Agency (EPA). FDA has the main responsibility to ensure the safety of our food supply by writing and enforcing regulations based on laws passed by Congress. The FDA, housed under the U.S. Department of Health and Human Services, is the oldest federal consumer protection agency. FDA's current mission is to "protect consumers and enhance public health by maximizing compliance of FDA-regulated products and minimizing risk associated with those products." Under the direction of FDA's Center for Food Safety and Applied Nutrition, the nation's food supply is monitored. EPA was created in 1970 to protect human health and the environment. The FDA and EPA work hand-in-hand to protect our food and water supply.

Several other government, or government-sponsored, agencies investigate food and nutrition matters. For example, the General Accounting Office conducts research in response to congressional queries. In 2010, they investigated the safety of herbal dietary supplements and provided the report to Congress. The Institute of Medicine of the National Academies is a private, non-profit group; the government contracts with them to conduct research related to health and formulate recommendations for dietary intake levels.

As is true for all of the issues, be sure to consider who is writing the selection and what they have to gain as you read and critique the selections.

Selected, Edited, and with Issue Framing Materials by:
Janet M. Colson, *Middle Tennessee State University*

ISSUE

Should Government Control Sodium Levels in the Food Supply?

YES: Institute of Medicine, from "Strategies to Reduce Sodium Intake in the United States: Brief Report," *The National Academies Press* (2010)

NO: Michael Moss, from "The Hard Sell on Salt," *The New York Times* (2010)

Learning Outcomes

After reading this issue, you will be able to:

- Outline the Institute of Medicine's recommendation to the FDA about sodium.
- List the stakeholders that need to be involved to reduce sodium content of the American food supply and the steps each stakeholder should take to accomplish the task.
- List and describe the barriers the food industry will encounter if it attempts to reduce sodium levels in its products.

ISSUE SUMMARY

YES: The Institute of Medicine's report on sodium recommends for the FDA to set mandatory national standards for the sodium content of foods and require the food industry (including manufacturers and restaurants) to gradually lower the amount of sodium they add to processed foods and prepared meals.

NO: Writer Michael Moss describes the numerous problems that food giants such as Kellogg, Frito-Lay, and Kraft claim to face if they attempt to lower sodium in the foods they make.

For years, Americans have been advised to eat less sodium, and many people think they are consuming less. They claim that they never use a salt shaker at the table or salt when cooking. (And some people don't even have a box of Morton's salt in the kitchen.) What most people do not realize is that close to 80 percent of the sodium we consume is added by the food industry in packaged foods purchased at the grocery store and salt added by cooks in restaurants. People are so concerned about calories and fat grams that they seldom look at the sodium content listed on food labels. A cup of canned spaghetti sauce is packed with 1,154 mg of sodium, and Subway's 6" meatball sub has 920 mg, and that is without adding chips or a cookie. So, unless you are a Martha Stewart or Rachel Ray and make everything from scratch—including breads, crackers, soup, pizza, taco sauce, and salad dressing—it is hard to eat less salt.

For the last 40 years, dietitians, physicians, and the government have been warning people to cut back on salt. (Regular table salt is about 40 percent sodium and 60 percent chloride.) Because of our increasing dependence on cheap, processed foods and the convenience of eating out, our sodium intake has steadily increased. Michael Jacobson, executive director of the Center for Science in the Public Interest reports, "Salt is the single most harmful element in our food supply, silently killing about 100,000 people each year." Excessive sodium not only raises blood pressure, but also increases risk for stroke, coronary heart disease, kidney disease, and osteoporosis. Recent evidence shows the adverse effects begin during childhood.

Cutting back on sodium has been a part of the *Dietary Guidelines for Americans* since it was introduced in 1980. Every five years, as a new advisory committee reviews the latest scientific data, changes evolve. These changes have largely been based on the escalating rate of hypertension (HTN) and death rates associated with the disease.

In 1980, when 17 percent of Americans had HTN, the recommendation was simply to "avoid too much sodium." Even though HTN rate climbed to 25 percent, the 1985 message did not change.

In 1990, when 33 percent of the nation had HTN, the message changed to "Use salt and sodium only in moderation." Finally, in 1995, the *Dietary Guidelines* put a number with the recommendation. It advised us to eat less than 2,400 mg each day. This continued in 2000.

In 2005, when it was predicted that 90 percent of Americans would develop HTN at some time in their lives, the recommended amount was lowered to 2,300 mg. And for people with HTN, blacks, and middle-aged and older adults, the aim was to consume no more than 1,500 mg. At that time, the committee realized that it would be hard to change people's taste preferences for salt, but cited studies that showed it is possible to kick the salt habit after eating low salt foods for 8 to 12 weeks.

Finally, the 2010 committee, after realizing that the majority of Americans, including children, need to consume less sodium, changed the goal to 1,500 mg per day for the majority of the population. In its summary report, it concludes:

> Reduce daily sodium intake to less than 2,300 milligrams (mg) and further reduce intake to 1,500 mg among persons who are 51 and older and those of any age who are African American

or have hypertension, diabetes, or chronic kidney disease. The 1,500 mg recommendation applies to about half of the U.S. population, including children, and the majority of adults.

The 2015 Dietary Guidelines Advisory Committee also concludes that there is "strong evidence" that cutting back to 1,500 mg per day will help control blood pressure, and if that is not possible "reducing sodium intake by at least 1,000 mg/d lowers blood pressure."

Sodium recommendations throughout the world are similar. Australia recommends that the adequate intake (AI) for adults is 460 to 920 mg per day with an upper limit (UL) of 2,300 mg. Both the United States and Canada set the AI by age category, with adults aged 50 or less set at 1,500 mg, those aged 51 to 70 years limited to 1,300, and adults over 70 years only 1,200 mg per day. The UL is also 2,300 mg. The World Health Organization simply recommends that adults limit sodium to 2,000 mg per day, or 5 g of salt.

The two selections on the following pages look at sodium from the food industry's standpoint. Food manufacturers and restaurants dictate what we eat, because they make the vast majority of foods that are available. After reading the selections, you decide if it is possible for Americans to slash sodium intake to the recommended 1,500 mg per day, or at least to reduce intake by 1,000 mg per day. The Institute of Medicine says it is possible, but it will require a coordinated approach including cooperation by the food industry. Journalist Michael Moss is realistic and points out the problems those food manufacturers will encounter if they cut salt out of their recipes and the influence it will have on their sales, and on profit.

YES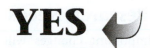

Institute of Medicine

Strategies to Reduce Sodium Intake in the United States: Brief Report

Americans consume unhealthy amounts of sodium in their food, far exceeding public health recommendations. Consuming too much sodium is a concern for all individuals, as it increases the risk for high blood pressure, a serious health condition that is avoidable and can lead to a variety of diseases. Analysts estimate that population-wide reductions in sodium could prevent more than 100,000 deaths annually.

While numerous stakeholders have initiated voluntary efforts to reduce sodium consumption in the United States during the past 40 years, they have not succeeded. Challenges arise because salt—the primary source of sodium in the diet—and other sodium-containing compounds often are used to enhance the flavor of foods, and high amounts are found in processed foods and foods prepared in restaurants. Sodium also is added to enhance texture or to serve as a preservative or thickener. In fact, very little of the sodium in foods is naturally occurring most of it is added as it is being processed or prepared by the food industry. The actual sodium levels in food may surprise consumers, especially if the food does not taste salty.

In 2008, Congress asked the Institute of Medicine (IOM) to recommend strategies for reducing sodium intake to levels recommended in the Dietary Guidelines for Americans—currently no more than 2,300 mg per day for persons 2 or more years of age. This amounts to about 1 teaspoon of salt per day, while the average American consumes about 50 percent more than that—more than 3,400 mg of sodium per day. The IOM committee that authored this report concludes that a new, coordinated approach is needed to reduce sodium content in food, requiring new government standards for the acceptable level of sodium. Manufacturers and restaurants/foodservice operators need to meet these standards so that all sources in the food supply are involved and so that the consumer's taste preferences can be changed over time to the lower amounts of salt in food. The goal is to slowly, over time, reduce the sodium content of the food supply in a way that goes unnoticed by most consumers as individuals' taste sensors adjust to the lower levels of sodium.

Identifying the Problem

Despite efforts to reduce sodium intake in the United States, consumption levels remain high. [There is] an upward trend in sodium intake since the early 1970s. Further, in recent years, consumers have not focused nearly as much on reducing sodium intake as they have on other nutrients of concern such as fat. One reason for high sodium consumption is that consumers have become accustomed to high levels of sodium in processed and restaurant foods and have difficulty adjusting to foods with healthier levels of sodium. However, the preference for salty taste can be changed. What is needed is a coordinated effort to reduce sodium in foods across the board by manufacturers and restaurants—that is, create a level playing field for the food industry. All segments of the food industry would be carrying out the same reductions and none would be at a disadvantage.

No one is immune to the adverse health effects of excessive sodium intake. While some may have the impression that sodium reduction is only necessary for individuals with hypertension or for groups with a higher risk of developing hypertension (for example, African Americans and older adults), in reality, it is necessary for all populations in order to avoid high blood pressure and cardiovascular disease.

Recommended Strategies to Reduce Sodium Intake

As its primary strategy for sodium reduction, the committee recommends that the FDA set mandatory national standards for the sodium content in foods—not banning outright the addition of salt to foods but beginning the process of reducing excess sodium in processed foods and menu items to a safer level. It is important that the reduction in sodium content of foods be carried out gradually, with small reductions instituted regularly as part of a carefully monitored process. Evidence shows that a decrease in sodium can be accomplished successfully without affecting consumer enjoyment of food products if it is done in a stepwise process that systematically and gradually lowers sodium levels across the food supply.

The Food, Drug, and Cosmetic Act specifies that substances added to foods by manufacturers must be proven safe under the conditions of their intended use, unless the substance is generally recognized as safe, known in the industry as GRAS. Currently, the manufacturers' addition of salt and a number of other sodium-containing compounds to foods is considered a GRAS use of the substance, but no standard level that constitutes a "safe use" has been set. Therefore, the committee recommends that the FDA modify the GRAS status of such compounds added to processed foods—that is, change the level to which the use of such compounds is considered safe. This change, when carried out in a stepwise manner, will reduce the sodium content of the food supply slowly, in a way that should avoid making food unpalatable to consumers.

A range of stakeholders, including public health and consumer organizations and the food industry, will need to work together in order to successfully reduce sodium intake among Americans. In order to implement these new food standards, leadership and coordination at the national level [are] essential. Specifically, the Secretary of Health and Human Services (HHS) should act in cooperation with other government and non-government groups to design and implement a nation-wide campaign to reduce sodium intake and should set a timeline for achieving the sodium intake levels established by the *Dietary Guidelines for Americans.* Consumers do not have direct control over how much sodium is added to foods, but they have an important role to play in reducing their sodium intake by making healthy food choices and selecting lower-sodium foods. In addition, government agencies, public health and consumer organizations, health professionals, the health insurance industry, the food industry, and public–private partnerships should support the implementation of the sodium standards for foods and also support consumers in reducing their sodium intake. Finally, better monitoring of sodium intake and of the progress toward changing salt taste preference are essential so that the reduction efforts can be tracked cand evaluated, and improvements can be made as needed.

Implementation and Research Needs

The implementation of these important changes will require preliminary data-gathering, dialogue among stakeholders, and careful analysis of food supply data. Further, if carried out in a stepwise manner, the process can be informed by the continual monitoring of the impact of the steps. In other areas, the committee identified three topics that require research:

- Understanding how salty taste preferences develop throughout the life span
- Developing innovative methods to reduce sodium in foods while maintaining palatability, physical properties, and safety
- Enhancing current understanding of factors that impact consumer awareness and behavior relative to sodium reduction

Conclusion

In the face of chronic disease risks associated with sodium intake, the current level of sodium in the food supply—added by food manufacturers, foodservice operators, and restaurants—is too high to be "safe." The recommended strategies in this report set a new course for reducing sodium intake with an innovative and unprecedented approach to gradually reducing sodium levels in foods. The patchwork of voluntary approaches that have been implemented over the years [has] not worked and [has] not created the level playing field deemed critical to any successful effort to reduce the sodium content of the overall food supply. While these efforts are laudable, they are not sustainable. The current focus on instructing consumers to select lower-sodium foods and making available reduced-sodium "niche" products cannot result in intakes consistent with public health recommendations. Without major change, hypertension and cardiovascular disease rates will continue to rise, and consumers, who have little choice, will pay the price for inaction.

Report at a Glance

Released: 4/20/2010

Primary Strategies

Recommendation 1: The Food and Drug Administration (FDA) should expeditiously initiate a process to set mandatory national standards for the sodium content of foods.

- FDA should modify the generally recognized as safe (GRAS) status of salt added to processed foods in order to reduce the salt content of the food supply in a stepwise manner.

- FDA should likewise extend its stepwise application of the GRAS modification, adjusted as necessary, to encompass salt added to menu items offered by restaurant/foodservice operations that are sufficiently standardized so as to allow practical implementation.
- FDA should revisit the GRAS status of other sodium-containing compounds as well as any food additive provisions for such compounds and make adjustments as appropriate consistent with changes for salt in processed foods and restaurant/foodservice menu items.

Interim Strategies

Recommendation 2: The food industry should voluntarily act to reduce the sodium content of foods in advance of the implementation of mandatory standards.

- Food manufacturers and restaurant/foodservice operators should voluntarily accelerate and broaden efforts to reduce sodium in processed foods and menu items, respectively.
- The food industry, government, professional organizations, and public health partners should work together to promote voluntary collaborations to reduce sodium in foods.

Supporting Strategies

Recommendation 3: Government agencies, public health and consumer organizations, and the food industry should carry out activities to support the reduction of sodium levels in the food supply.

- FDA and the U.S. Department of Agriculture (USDA) should revise and update—specifically for sodium—the provisions for nutrition labeling, related sodium claims, and disclosure or disqualifying criteria for sodium in foods, including a revision to base the Daily Value for sodium on the Adequate Intake.
- FDA should extend provisions for sodium content and health claims to restaurant/foodservice menu items and adjust the provisions as needed for use within the restaurant/foodservice sector.
- Congress should act to remove the exemption of nutrition labeling for food products intended solely for use in restaurant/foodservice operations.
- Food retailers, governments, businesses, institutions, and other large-scale organizations that purchase or distribute food should establish sodium specifications for the foods they purchase and the food operations they oversee.

- Restaurant/foodservice leaders in collaboration with other key stakeholders, including federal, state, and local health authorities, should develop, pilot, and implement innovative initiatives targeted to restaurant/foodservice operations to facilitate and sustain sodium reduction in menu items.

Recommendation 4: In tandem with recommendations to reduce the sodium content of the food supply, government agencies, public health and consumer organizations, health professionals, the health insurance industry, the food industry, and public-private partnerships should conduct augmenting activities to support consumers in reducing sodium intake.

- The Secretary of Health and Human Services (HHS) should act in cooperation with other government and non-government groups to design and implement a comprehensive, nationwide campaign to reduce sodium intake and act to set a timeline for achieving the sodium intake goals established by the *Dietary Guidelines for Americans*.
- Government agencies, public health and consumer organizations, health professionals, the food industry, and public–private partnerships should continue or expand efforts to support consumers in making behavior changes to reduce sodium intake in a manner consistent with the *Dietary Guidelines for Americans*.

Recommendation 5: Federal agencies should ensure and enhance monitoring and surveillance relative to sodium intake measurement, salt taste preference, and sodium content of foods, and should ensure sustained and timely release of data in user-friendly formats.

- Congress, HHS/CDC (Centers for Disease Control and Prevention), and USDA authorities should ensure adequate funding for the National Health and Nutrition Examination Survey (NHANES), including related and supporting databases or surveys.
- CDC should collect 24-hour urine samples during NHANES or as a separate nationally representative "sentinel site" type activity.
- CDC should, as a component of NHANES or another appropriate nationally representative survey, begin work immediately with the National Institutes of Health (NIH) to develop an appropriate assessment tool for salt taste preference, obtain baseline measurements, and track salt taste preference over time.
- CDC in cooperation with other relevant HHS agencies, USDA, and the Federal Trade Commission should strengthen and expand its activities

to measure population knowledge, attitudes, and behavior about sodium among consumers.

- FDA should modify and expand its existing Total Diet Study and its Food Label and Package Survey to ensure better coverage of information about sodium content in the diet and sodium-related information on packaged and prepared foods.
- USDA should enhance the quality and comprehensiveness of sodium content information in its tables of food composition.
- USDA in cooperation with HHS should develop approaches utilizing current and new methodologies and databases to monitor the sodium content of the total food supply.

THE INSTITUTE OF MEDICINE is a division of the National Academies of Sciences, Engineering, and Medicine. The Academies are private, nonprofit institutions that provide independent, objective analysis and advice to the nation and conduct other activities to solve complex problems and inform public policy decisions related to science, technology, and medicine.

Michael Moss   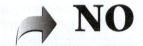 **NO**

The Hard Sell on Salt

With salt under attack for its ill effects on the nation's health, the food giant Cargill kicked off a campaign last November to spread its own message.

"Salt is a pretty amazing compound," Alton Brown, a Food Network star, gushes in a Cargill video called Salt 101. "So make sure you have plenty of salt in your kitchen at all times."

The campaign by Cargill, which both produces and uses salt, promotes salt as "life enhancing" and suggests sprinkling it on foods as varied as chocolate cookies, fresh fruit, ice cream and even coffee. "You might be surprised," Mr. Brown says, "by what foods are enhanced by its briny kiss."

By all appearances, this is a moment of reckoning for salt. High blood pressure is rising among adults and children. Government health experts estimate that deep cuts in salt consumption could save 150,000 lives a year.

Since processed foods account for most of the salt in the American diet, national health officials, Mayor Michael R. Bloomberg of New York and Michelle Obama are urging food companies to greatly reduce their use of salt. [The] Institute of Medicine went further, urging the government to force companies to do so.

But the industry is working overtly and behind the scenes to fend off these attacks, using a shifting set of tactics that have defeated similar efforts for 30 years, records and interviews show. Industry insiders call the strategy "delay and divert" and say companies have a powerful incentive to fight back: they crave salt as a low-cost way to create tastes and textures. Doing without it risks losing customers, and replacing it with more expensive ingredients risks losing profits.

When health advocates first petitioned the federal government to regulate salt in 1978, food companies sponsored research aimed at casting doubt on the link between salt and hypertension. Two decades later, when federal officials tried to cut the salt in products labeled "healthy," companies argued that foods already low in sugar and fat would not sell with less salt.

Now, the industry is blaming consumers for resisting efforts to reduce salt in all foods, pointing to, as Kellogg put it in a letter to a federal nutrition advisory committee, "the virtually intractable nature of the appetite for salt."

The federal committee is finishing up recommendations on nutrient issues including salt. While its work is overseen by the Department of Agriculture, records released to *The New York Times* show that the industry nominated a majority of its members and has presented the panel with its own research. It includes two studies commissioned by ConAgra suggesting that the country could save billions of dollars more in health care and lost productivity costs by simply nudging Americans to eat a little less food, rather than less salty food.

Even as it was moving from one line of defense to another, the processed food industry's own dependence on salt deepened, interviews with company scientists show. Beyond its own taste, salt also masks bitter flavors and counters a side effect of processed food production called "warmed-over flavor," which, the scientists said, can make meat taste like "cardboard" or "damp dog hair."

Salt also works in tandem with fat and sugar to achieve flavors that grip the consumer and do not let go— an allure the industry has recognized for decades. "Once a preference is acquired," a top scientist at Frito-Lay wrote in a 1979 internal memorandum, "most people do not change it, but simply obey it."

In recent months, food companies, including Kellogg, have said they were redoubling efforts to reduce salt. But they say they can go only so far, so fast without compromising tastes consumers have come to relish or salt's ability to preserve food. "We have to earn the consumer's trust every day," said George Dowdie, a senior vice president of Campbell Soup. "And if you disappoint the consumer, there is no guarantee they will come back."

Case Study: The Cheez-It

The power that salt holds over processed foods can be seen in an American snack icon, the Cheez-It.

At the company's laboratories in Battle Creek, Mich., a Kellogg vice president and food scientist, John Kepplinger, ticked off the ways salt makes its little square cracker work.

Salt sprinkled on top gives the tongue a quick buzz. More salt in the cheese adds crunch. Still more in the dough blocks the tang that develops during fermentation. In all, a generous cup of Cheez-Its delivers one-third of the daily amount of sodium recommended for most Americans.

As a demonstration, Kellogg prepared some of its biggest sellers with most of the salt removed. The Cheez-It fell apart in surprising ways. The golden yellow hue faded. The crackers became sticky when chewed, and the mash packed onto the teeth. The taste was not merely bland but medicinal.

"I really get the bitter on that," the company's spokeswoman, J. Adaire Putnam, said with a wince as she watched Mr. Kepplinger struggle to swallow.

They moved on to Corn Flakes. Without salt the cereal tasted metallic. The Eggo waffles evoked stale straw. The butter flavor in the Keebler Light Buttery Crackers, which have no actual butter, simply disappeared.

"Salt really changes the way that your tongue will taste the product," Mr. Kepplinger said. "You make one little change and something that was a complementary flavor now starts to stand out and become objectionable."

Salt started out more than 5,000 years ago as a simple preservative. But salt and dozens of compounds containing sodium—the element in salt linked to hypertension—have become omnipresent in processed foods from one end of the grocery store to the other.

For example, salt makes 10 appearances on the label for the Hungry-Man roasted turkey dinner, made by the Pinnacle Foods Group, with nine additional references to sodium compounds. The label for Roasted Chicken Monterey, a ConAgra Healthy Choice product, has five references to salt. It makes its most surprising cameo in the accompanying peach dessert, which is flavored with whiskey mixed with salt.

"Without adding the salt, we would be required to carry a liquor license," explained a ConAgra spokeswoman, Teresa Paulsen.

The food industry releases some 10,000 new products a year, the Department of Agriculture has reported, and processed foods, along with restaurant meals, now account for roughly 80 percent of the salt in the American diet. The rest comes from the kitchen saltshaker or occurs naturally in food. In promoting cooking with salt, Cargill and its star chef, Mr. Brown, said they recognized the health concerns and recommended "smarter salting."

Making deep cuts in salt can require more expensive ingredients that can hurt sales. Companies that make low-salt pasta sauces improve the taste with vine-ripened tomatoes and fresh herbs that cost more than dried spices and lower grade tomatoes.

Food companies say that reducing salt by 10 percent or so is easy, but that going further is difficult.

Take smoked ham sold by Kraft Foods under its Oscar Mayer label. Three slices have 820 milligrams of sodium, more than half of the daily intake recommended for most Americans. Kraft said it was releasing a version with 37 percent less sodium, but when it tried to eliminate an additional 3 percent, consumer testers failed it on flavor, texture and aroma. "We often fall off a cliff, and that's what we did here," said Russell Moroz, a Kraft vice president.

Campbell says it has reduced salt in over 100 soups through a variety of changes, including using a sea salt with half the normal sodium. But some soups present bigger challenges.

"It feels unfinished," Dr. Dowdie, the Campbell vice president and scientist, said while tasting vegetable beef soup that the company prepared with less sodium for *The Times*. "The sweetness of the carrots isn't pronounced. The broth, you don't get an explosion of flavors."

Chicken noodle soup has been especially vexing, he said. With only 150 calories, a single can of the condensed soup has more than a whole day's recommended sodium for most Americans.

"It's a very unique recipe," Dr. Dowdie said. "Consumers of chicken noodle, they love it and they know it and they have a strong bond with it. And any slight change they will recognize."

Dr. Howard Moskowitz, a food scientist and consultant to major food manufacturers, said companies had not shown the same zeal in reducing salt as they had with sugars and fat. While low-calorie sweeteners opened a huge market of people eager to look better by losing weight, he said, salt is only a health concern, which does not have the same market potential.

"If all of a sudden people would demand lower salt because low salt makes them look younger, this problem would be solved overnight," he said.

Diversionary Tactics

In 1978, Michael F. Jacobson, an M.I.T.-trained microbiologist, was studying food additives when he noticed the growing research linking sodium to hypertension. "I realized that conventional ingredients like salt were probably far more harmful," said Dr. Jacobson, who directs the Center for Science in the Public Interest, a consumer group.

He petitioned the Food and Drug Administration to reclassify salt from an ingredient like pepper or vinegar posing no health concerns to a food additive that the agency could regulate by mandating limits or warning labels.

The broadside on the food industry was taken seriously by the F.D.A. and touched off a scramble by producers to head off regulation, confidential company records and interviews show.

Robert I-San Lin, who was then overseeing research and development at Frito-Lay, said in an interview that he had been caught between corporate and public interests.

"The public's concern over high sodium intake is justifiable," Dr. Lin wrote in a 1978 memo. A handwritten memo titled "Salt Strategy" shows that his staff worked on ways to reduce sodium, including adjusting the fat in potato chips as a way of lowering the need for salt and using a finer salt crystal.

But the company adopted few of his recommendations and joined the industry's resistance.

Scientists testifying for the snack industry at a government hearing warned that lower salt consumption could pose certain health risks to children and pregnant women. The food industry also challenged the link between salt and hypertension, emphasizing studies that found no significant correlation.

In what Dr. Lin says was an attempt to divert attention from salt, records show, Frito-Lay also financed research on whether calcium might negate the harmful effects of salt, even though Dr. Lin said he doubted it would really absolve salt. "An effective promotion of 'Calcium Antihypertension Theory' may release the pressure on sodium for the time being," Dr. Lin wrote in a memo at the time.

In 1982, Campbell sponsored an American Heart Association symposium that included a study on calcium, which is now seen as having only a small role in reducing hypertension, and another that asserted that only some people were susceptible to hypertension from salt.

That same year, the F.D.A. finally responded to Dr. Jacobson's petition. An advisory panel had concluded that salt should no longer have a blanket designation as safe, which "would normally trigger F.D.A. action," Michael R. Taylor, a current deputy commissioner at the agency wrote last year in analyzing salt regulation. But the agency decided to rely on consumer education and voluntary efforts by companies.

Sanford A. Miller, then director of the F.D.A.'s Center for Food Safety and Applied Nutrition, said agency officials had recognized the health effects of salt, but had believed that they did not have enough data to justify mandating sodium levels. "The salt people, especially, were constantly badgering us on that," Dr. Miller said. "There were little tidbits that people could challenge us on."

Dr. Lin, who works for a nutrition supplement producer, said Frito-Lay's response back then was a "macho show of force" by an otherwise responsible company. "I was employed at a time I couldn't do much about it," he said.

A Frito-Lay spokeswoman, Aurora Gonzalez, says the company has aggressively searched for solutions to nutrition issues. In March, its parent company, PepsiCo, announced it would cut on average 25 percent of the salt in its products. "We are proactive," Ms. Gonzalez said. One solution it recently embraced takes a page from Dr. Lin's old research: using a finer grade of salt.

Back in the 1980s, some companies began offering low-sodium products, but few sold well. Surveys by the Center for Science in the Public Interest have found little change in salt levels in processed foods.

Sugar and fat had overtaken salt as the major concern in processed foods by the 1990s, fueling the "healthy" foods market. When the F.D.A. pressured companies to reduce salt in those products, the industry said that doing so would ruin the taste of the foods already low in sugar and fat. The government backed off.

"We were trying to balance the public health need with what we understood to be the public acceptability," said William K. Hubbard, a top agency official at the time who now advises an industry-supported advocacy group. "Common sense tells you if you take it down too low and people don't buy, you have not done something good."

The Battle Broadens

On April 26, Mayor Bloomberg stood before a microphone at City Hall to announce an initiative to prod food companies to cut salt in earnest, with an initial target of 25 percent by 2014. The industry's resistance was readily apparent.

After two years of planning, nearly 30 other jurisdictions joined New York, which said it was acting because federal officials had not. But only 16 manufacturers and restaurants had signed on to the initiative, and records released to *The Times* through the state's Freedom of Information Law reveal a shift in industry strategy.

Rather than challenging salt's link to hypertension, industry representatives, in the private planning meetings with city officials, cited financial objections: the higher cost of other seasonings and the expense of new product labels and retooled production lines. In a Feb. 1 letter to a city health official, the Grocery Manufacturers Association wrote that "aggressive, short-term sodium reduction has the potential to further raise food prices."

Companies also warned that reducing salt might force them to increase sugar in foods like peanut butter, meeting minutes show.

Among those declining to join the initiative was Campbell. Chor-San Khoo, its vice president for global nutrition and health, said that the company would continue its own reduction plan, but that the city's pace "was overly aggressive."

In April, the independent Institute of Medicine said food companies were moving too slowly on their own and called on federal officials to set firm salt levels for food.

Dr. Margaret A. Hamburg, the F.D.A. commissioner, said in an interview that salt was a serious concern her agency would address in concert with other issues, like obesity. "We will use a variety of strategies, including education, voluntary reduction and potentially regulation," she said, adding that "we are really at the beginning of the process of shaping our blueprint for action."

One glaring issue before the F.D.A. concerns nutrient labels, which for years have overstated the amount of salt the government says is safe to consume. In calculating the percent of the daily recommended sodium intake in each serving, companies use the standard for healthy adults below middle age, a teaspoon of salt, or about 2,300 milligrams. But the recommendation for the vast majority of Americans—children, adults of middle age or older, all blacks and anyone with hypertension—is less than 1,500 milligrams a day.

The F.D.A. announced in 2007 that it was aware of that problem, but it has taken no action. The federal Dietary Guidelines Advisory Committee is considering adopting the lower standard for everyone as part of its review of nutrition standards.

The food industry has identified the guidelines as a battleground. The panel needs "to include expertise and perspective related to food product development," the Grocery Manufacturers Association wrote to the Agriculture Department in nominating 7 of the panel's 13 members.

Food companies then peppered the committee with their perspective on salt. In a letter, Kellogg said that lower salt guidelines were "incompatible with a palatable diet."

ConAgra, whose brands include Chef Boyardee and Orville Redenbacher, made a different argument to the panel. It submitted a study it commissioned that asserted that far more savings in health care costs—about $58 billion—could be generated if people simply cut 100 calories from their daily diets than if they consumed less salt.

The study put the savings from salt reduction at just $2.3 billion, compared with the $18 billion to $24 billion in savings cited by other analysts, including the Rand Corporation, the research giant. One scientist involved in the research, David A. McCarron, a longtime food industry consultant, said ConAgra's lower estimate stemmed from its more judicious use of hypertension data.

How the industry will fare in the fight over nutrition standards will not be clear until they are finalized later this year. But in committee meetings, some members nominated by the industry have voiced concerns about cutting salt.

Joanne L. Slavin, a committee member and nutrition professor at the University of Minnesota, told her colleagues that reducing salt in bread was difficult and warned of unintended consequences. It is an argument also made by food companies.

"Typically, sodium, sugar bounces around," she said. "So you take sodium down in a product and then sugar a lot of times has to go up just for taste."

MICHAEL MOSS is a reporter with *The New York Times*. In 2010, he won the Pulitzer Prize for Explanatory Reporting for his investigation of the dangers of contaminated meat. He has been an adjunct professor at the Columbia's Graduate School of Journalism and attended San Francisco State University.

EXPLORING THE ISSUE

Should Government Control Sodium Levels in the Food Supply?

Critical Thinking and Reflection

1. Describe the recommended steps that FDA will take to gradually reduce sodium in the American food supply.
2. Identify stakeholders that must be involved to successfully reduce the sodium content of the American diet and the role that each will have.
3. Who do you think will have the greater challenge in reducing sodium content of foods they prepare, the food processors or chefs and cooks in restaurants? Explain your answer.
4. Prepare your favorite "from-scratch" baked product (cake, cookies, or bread) without using any sodium-containing ingredients such as salt, baking soda, baking powder, or any prepared mixed. Describe how it looks, feels, and tastes compared to a product made using the traditional recipe.
5. Using a nutrient analysis program such as SuperTracker, analyze the sodium content of the foods you consumed in the last 24 hours. If the amount was greater than 1,500 mg, determine which foods could be changed to meet the 1,500 mg recommendation.

Is There Common Ground?

Both the Institute of Medicine (IOM) and journalist Michael Moss are concerned about the nation's health and acknowledge that the American diet is not perfect. Both recognize that processed foods are the main source of sodium and to reduce sodium in the U.S. food supply means that the entire food industry must alter the way foods have been prepared for the last 60 years.

The mission of the IOM report is to focus on sodium, therefore reducing the mineral is the emphasis of their report. IOM concludes that voluntary attempts over the years to lower sodium in foods have been unsuccessful and it proposes five strategies to reduce sodium in American diets:

1. FDA should set a mandatory national standard for the sodium content of foods.
2. The food industry should voluntarily lower sodium content of foods before FDA mandates it.
3. Various agencies and organizations plus the food industry should work to update food labels and include sodium content on restaurant menus.
4. Government agencies and health organizations and groups should educate the public on benefits of sodium reduction and how to select lower sodium foods.
5. Federal agencies should monitor sodium status and intake of the public.

Michael Moss is one of the leading investigative reporters in the United States and author of the book *Salt, Sugar, Fat: How the Food Giants Hooked Us*. His job is to investigate all sides of a topic, and that is what he accomplished in his investigative article. Moss reports about how the food industry has been fighting back against FDA and other groups who have tried to convince companies to produce lower sodium foods. He presents a variety of barriers the food industry claims it will encounter if it lowers the sodium content of processed foods. And he considers that sugar and fat in the American diet are bigger problems than salt.

Additional Resources

Ahuja JK, Pehrsson PR, Haytowitz DB, et al. Sodium monitoring in commercially processed and restaurant foods. *Am J Clin Nutr*. 2015;101(3):622–31.

Macgregor GA, He FJ, Pombo-rodrigues S. Food and the responsibility deal: How the salt reduction strategy was derailed. *BMJ*. 2015;350:h1936.

Niebylski ML, Redburn KA, Duhaney T, Campbell NR. Healthy food subsidies and unhealthy food taxation: A systematic review of the evidence. *Nutrition*. 2015;31(6):787–95.

Internet References . . .

Dietary Guidelines for Americans 2015

http://health.gov/dietaryguidelines/2015/

The Salt Institute

www.saltinstitute.org

Strategies to Reduce Sodium Intake in the United States

www.nap.edu/catalog.php?record_id=12818

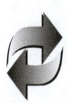

Selected, Edited, and with Issue Framing Materials by:
Janet M. Colson, *Middle Tennessee State University*

ISSUE

Should Government Levy a "Fat Tax"?

YES: Kelly D. Brownell, et al., from "The Public Health and Economic Benefits of Taxing Sugar-Sweetened Beverages," *The New England Journal of Medicine* (2009)

NO: Daniel Engber, from "Let Them Drink Water! What a Fat Tax Really Means for America," *Slate* (2009)

Learning Outcomes
After reading this issue, you will be able to:
• Explain why sugar-sweetened beverages are targeted for a "fat tax."
• Describe the different methods used to calculate a "sugar tax," as suggested by Brownell and colleagues.
• List the properties of junk foods that make them addictive.
• Discuss the influence that a "fat tax" will have on poor, nonwhite people.

ISSUE SUMMARY

YES: Kelly Brownell and colleagues propose a "fat tax" targeting sugar-sweetened beverages. They feel a tax will decrease the amount of sugary drinks people consume and ultimately help reduce obesity. They also suggest that the tax has the "potential to generate substantial revenue" to help fund health-related initiatives.

NO: Daniel Engber disagrees with a fat tax on sugary beverages since it will impact poor, nonwhite people most severely and they would be deprived of the pleasures of palatable foods. He says that the poor would be forced to "drink from the faucet" while the more affluent will sip exotic beverages such as POM Wonderful, at about $5 a pop.

Throughout history, governments have levied taxes on people and businesses. Revenues generated are used to support the government and various programs. We typically pay taxes on income, property, and purchases. Businesses pay an excise tax on the products they produce, and some of the taxes are pretty hefty. Tobacco manufacturers pay $1.01 per pack for cigarettes in federal taxes. On top of that, states and cities add sales tax on tobacco products. As of 2015, anyone who buys cigarettes in New York City pays about $13 per pack. [Tax breakdown: $1.01 to the fed, $4.35 to the state, and $1.50 to the city.] Recently, Chicago surpassed the Big Apple with a pack averaging $14, because in addition to the city and state taxes, Cook County imposes a $3 per pack tax. These taxes are often called "sin taxes" since the products being taxed are not necessities of life and are considered to be "sinful" by many.

Sin taxes have a two-fold purpose. First is to discourage use of the products, and at $13 to $14 per pack, fewer New Yorkers and Chicagoans are smoking. The second is to generate revenue; some of it may be used to cover health care costs related to tobacco- or alcohol-induced conditions and the other is used to help balance the government's budget.

Many health and economic experts have proposed various forms of "fat taxes" to help pay for obesity-related health problems. Some actually have proposed to tax fat people based on their body weight. Daniel Engber, author of the YES article, describes a fat tax proposed by A.J. Carlson during World War II. Carlson's idea was to charge the nation's largest citizens a fee for every pound of overweight. He thought proceeds from the taxes could have been used to help feed soldiers who were overseas, while helping to reduce obesity at home. His proposal did not become a reality.

More recently, economist Adam Creighton designed a similar "fat-*person* tax," which was published in *The American,* August 8, 2007. His tongue-in-check proposal calls for a "fat-*person* tax" to be administered by the IRS. He suggests that everyone would submit a self-reported BMI with their annual tax returns. Creighton describes that it would be:

> a progressive tax: the fatter the taxpayer, the higher the tax. The top of the "normal" range for BMI is 24. A BMI above 25 would pay a small surtax, say 5 percent, BMI 30s would pay 10 percent, etc. The brilliance of Art Laffer's flat income tax notwithstanding, a flat *fat* tax simply would not work, since it would not encourage weight-control once the taxpayer's BMI was well above the taxation threshold.

> To deter falsified BMIs, IRS doctors could offer a second opinion. BMI audits might be required at three or six-month intervals to get an accurate reading of each taxpayer's average BMI during the year, and to prevent unhealthy fasting during the tax season. And given the latest research showing obesity spreads socially, the IRS could even demand friendship data (cross-checked) to ensure individual friendship networks don't exceed a particular fat-friends quota.

We as Americans may find Creighton's satire about taxation humorous, but Japan does impose a penalty based on the girth of its citizens. They are among the thinnest nations in the world with only 5 percent of Japanese people obese, but this is double what it was 30 years ago. To put the brakes on this increasing trend, in 2008, the government passed a law requiring businesses and local governments to measure the waist circumferences of all employees over age 40. The upper limit for men is 33.5 inches (85 cm). (In the United States, we don't consider a man "fat" until his waist reaches 40.) If the overweight employee does not reduce his/her girth, the Japanese government recommends dieting advice. To encourage compliance, the business or local government is fined if their employees do not lose weight.

Most Americans feel that this type of tax would infringe upon their freedom and right to privacy. (Of course, some insurance companies charge higher rates for the obese in the United States) Therefore, taxing fattening foods is more realistic. In this issue's NO article, Daniel Engber points out that about 40 states already have a tax on junk foods or soda, but there is no federal tax. Kelly Brownell, lead author of the YES article, began his crusade for a "Twinkie tax" in the 1990s. He wrote an article for the *New York Times* (December 15, 1994) proposing that

Americans can "Get Slim with Higher Taxes." He called for a "sin tax" on unhealthy foods similar to what had been done for years on cigarettes and alcohol. However, a challenge with taxing "junk foods" is how do you define what should be taxed? Surely high-calorie foods would be the target, but how does one decide if a bag of Reese's Pieces, with 230 kcalories and 11 grams of fat, should be taxed while a bag of "natural and healthy" peanuts, with their 280 kcalories and 25 grams of fat, be exempt? Due to the complexity of such labeling, most proponents of taxing calorie-laden foods are targeting sugar-sweetened beverages.

In 2006, Barry Popkin (one of the authors of the YES article) led a team that developed a guidance system for beverages as outlined in the table below. The system divides beverages into six levels with plain water rated the best choice (Level 1) to drink since it provides no calories. The least preferred choice is any sugar-sweetened beverage (Level 6), with no nutritional value such soft drinks are the least preferred choice. Levels 2 through 5 are progressively less desirable because of their calorie-to-nutrient ratios.

Beverage Guidance System

Level 1	Water
Level 2	Tea or coffee, with no added sweeteners
Level 3	Skim and low-fat milk and soy beverages
Level 4	Non-calorically sweetened beverages (such as diet soft drinks)
Level 5	Caloric beverages with some nutritional benefit (i.e., fruit and vegetable juices, sports drinks for rehydration of athletes, whole fat milk, and alcoholic beverages, in moderation)
Level 6	Any sugar-sweetened beverage

Source: B. Popkin and others, from "A New Proposed Guidance System for Beverage Consumption in the United States," *The American Journal of Clinical Nutrition* (March 2006)

Kelly Brownell and colleagues propose a "fat tax" targeting beverages rated at Level 6, the sugar-sweetened ones. They feel a tax will decrease the amount of sugary drinks people consume and ultimately help reduce obesity. Daniel Engber disagrees since he believes the tax will impact poor, nonwhite people most severely and they would be deprived of the pleasures of palatable foods. What are your thoughts on the topic? Do you think a "fat tax" on sugar-sweetened beverages will decrease our consumption, while raising dollars to spend on obesity-related conditions? After reading both selections, decide for yourself if a fat tax is fair and will help reduce obesity.

YES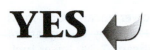

Kelly D. Brownell, et al.

The Public Health and Economic Benefits of Taxing Sugar-Sweetened Beverages

The consumption of sugar-sweetened beverages has been linked to risks for obesity, diabetes, and heart disease[1-3]; therefore, a compelling case can be made for the need for reduced consumption of these beverages. Sugar-sweetened beverages are beverages that contain added, naturally derived caloric sweeteners such as sucrose (table sugar), high-fructose corn syrup, or fruit-juice concentrates, all of which have similar metabolic effects.

Taxation has been proposed as a means of reducing the intake of these beverages and thereby lowering health care costs, as well as a means of generating revenue that governments can use for health programs.[4-7] Currently, 33 states have sales taxes on soft drinks (mean tax rate, 5.2%), but the taxes are too small to affect consumption and the revenues are not earmarked for programs related to health. This article examines trends in the consumption of sugar-sweetened beverages, evidence linking these beverages to adverse health outcomes, and approaches to designing a tax system that could promote good nutrition and help the nation recover health care costs associated with the consumption of sugar-sweetened beverages.

Consumption Trends and Health Outcomes

In recent decades, intake of sugar-sweetened beverages has increased around the globe; for example, intake in Mexico doubled between 1999 and 2006 across all age groups.[8] Between 1977 and 2002, the per capita intake of caloric beverages doubled in the United States across all age groups[9] (Fig. 1). The most recent data (2005–2006) show that children and adults in the United States consume about 172 and 175 kcal daily, respectively, per capita from sugar-sweetened beverages.

Figure 1

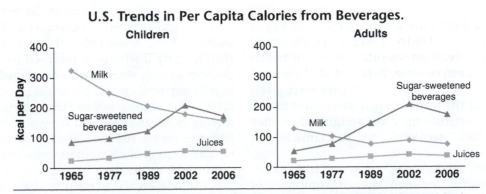

U.S. Trends in Per Capita Calories from Beverages.

Data are for U.S. children 2 to 18 years of age and adults 19 years of age or older. Data have been weighted to be nationally representative, with the use of methods that generate measures of each beverage that are comparable over time. Data for 1965–2002 are from Duffey and Popkin[9]; data for 2005–2006 have not been published previously.

The relationship between the consumption of sugar-sweetened beverages and body weight has been examined in many cross-sectional and longitudinal studies and has been summarized in systematic reviews.[1,2] A meta-analysis showed positive associations between the intake of sugar-sweetened beverages and body weight—associations that were stronger in longitudinal studies than in cross-sectional studies and in studies that were not funded by the beverage industry than in those that were.[2] A meta-analysis of studies involving children[10]—a meta-analysis that was supported by the beverage industry—was interpreted as showing that there was no evidence of an association between consumption of sugar-sweetened beverages and body weight, but it erroneously gave large weight to several small negative studies; when a more realistic weighting was used, the meta-analysis summary supported a positive association.[11] A prospective study involving middle-school students over the course of 2 academic years showed that the risk of becoming obese increased by 60% for every additional serving of sugar-sweetened beverages per day.[12] In an 8-year prospective study involving women, those who increased their consumption of sugar-sweetened beverages at year 4 and maintained this increase gained 8 kg, whereas those who decreased their intake of sugar-sweetened beverages at year 4 and maintained this decrease gained only 2.8 kg.[13]

Short-term clinical trials provide an experimental basis for understanding the way in which sugar-sweetened beverages may affect adiposity. Tordoff and Alleva[14] found that as compared with total energy intake and weight during a 3-week period in which no beverages were provided, total energy intake and body weight increased when subjects were given 530 kcal of sugar-sweetened beverages per day for 3 weeks but decreased when subjects were given noncaloric sweetened beverages for the same length of time. Raben et al.[15] reported that obese subjects gained weight when they were given sucrose, primarily in the form of sugar-sweetened beverages, for 10 weeks, whereas they lost weight when they were given noncaloric sweeteners for the same length of time.

Four long-term, randomized, controlled trials examining the relationship between the consumption of sugar-sweetened beverages and body weight have been reported; the results showed the strongest effects among overweight persons. A school-based intervention to reduce the consumption of carbonated beverages was assessed among 644 students, 7 to 11 years of age, in the United Kingdom with the use of a cluster design.[16] After 1 year, the intervention group, as compared with the control group, had a nonsignificantly lower mean body-mass index (the weight in kilograms divided by the square of the height in meters) and a significant 7.7% lower incidence of obesity. In a study involving 1140 Brazilian schoolchildren, 9 to 12 years of age, that was designed to discourage the consumption of sugar-sweetened beverages, no overall effect on body-mass index was observed during the 9-month academic year.[17] Among students who were overweight at baseline, the body-mass index was nonsignificantly decreased in the intervention group as compared with the control group; the difference was significant among overweight girls. In another clinical trial, 103 high-school students in Boston were assigned to a control group or to an intervention group that received home delivery of noncaloric beverages for 25 weeks. The body-mass index was nonsignificantly reduced in the overall intervention group, but among students in the upper third of body-mass index at baseline, there was a significant decrease in the body-mass index in the intervention group, as compared with the control group (a decrease of 0.63 vs. an increase of 0.12).[18] The effects of replacing sugar-sweetened beverages with milk products were examined among 98 overweight Chilean children.[19] After 16 weeks, there was a nonsignificantly lower increase in the percentage of body fat in the intervention group than in the control group (0.36% and 0.78% increase, respectively), whereas there was a significantly greater increase in lean mass in the intervention group (0.92 vs. 0.62 kg).

Three prospective, observational studies—one involving nurses in the United States, one involving Finnish men and women, and one involving black women—each showed positive associations between the consumption of sugar-sweetened beverages and the risk of type 2 diabetes.[13,20,21] Among the 91,249 women in the Nurses' Health Study II who were followed for 8 years, the risk of diabetes among women who consumed one or more servings of sugar-sweetened beverages per day was nearly double the risk among women who consumed less than one serving of sugar-sweetened beverages per month[13]; about half the excess risk was accounted for by greater body weight. Among black women, excess weight accounted for most of the excess risk.

Among 88,520 women in the Nurses' Health Study, the risk of coronary heart disease among women who consumed one serving of sugar-sweetened beverages per day, as compared with women who consumed less than one serving per month, was increased by 23%, and among those who consumed two servings or more per day, the risk was increased by 35%.[3] Increased body weight explained some, but not all, of this association.

Mechanisms Linking Sugar-Sweetened Beverages with Poor Health

A variety of behavioral and biologic mechanisms may be responsible for the associations between the consumption of sugar-sweetened beverages and adverse health outcomes, with some links (e.g., the link between intake of sugar-sweetened beverages and weight gain) better established than others. The well-documented adverse physiological and metabolic consequences of a high intake of refined carbohydrates such as sugar include the elevation of triglyceride levels and of blood pressure and the lowering of high-density lipoprotein cholesterol levels, which would be expected to increase the risk of coronary heart disease.[22] Because of the high glycemic load of sugar-sweetened beverages, consumption of these beverages would be expected to increase the risk of diabetes by causing insulin resistance and also through direct effects on pancreatic islet cells.[23] Observational research has shown that consumption of sugar-sweetened beverages, but not of noncalorically sweetened beverages, is associated with markers of insulin resistance.[24]

Intake of sugar-sweetened beverages may cause excessive weight gain owing in part to the apparently poor satiating properties of sugar in liquid form. Indeed, adjustment of caloric intake at subsequent meals for energy that had been consumed as a beverage is less complete than adjustment of intake for energy that had been consumed as a solid food.[25] For example, in a study involving 323 adults, in which 7-day food diaries were used, energy from beverages added to total energy intake instead of displacing other sources of calories.[26] The results of a study of school-age children were consistent with the data from adults and showed that children who drank 9 oz or more of sugar-sweetened beverages per day consumed nearly 200 kcal per day more than those who did not drink sugar-sweetened beverages.[27]

Short-term studies of the effect of beverage consumption on energy intake support this mechanism. Among 33 adults who were given identical test lunches on six occasions but were given beverages of different types (sugar-sweetened cola, noncaloric cola, or water) and amounts (12 oz [355 ml] or 18 oz [532 ml]),[28] the intake of solid food did not differ across conditions; the result was that there was significantly greater total energy consumption when the sugar-sweetened beverages were served.

Sugar-sweetened beverages may also affect body weight through other behavioral mechanisms. Whereas the intake of solid food is characteristically coupled to hunger, people may consume sugar-sweetened beverages in the absence of hunger, to satisfy thirst or for social reasons. Sugar-sweetened beverages may also have chronic adverse effects on taste preferences and food acceptance. Persons—especially children—who habitually consume sugar-sweetened beverages rather than water may find more satiating but less sweet foods (e.g., vegetables, legumes, and fruits) unappealing or unpalatable, with the result that their diet may be of poor quality.

Economic Rationale

Economists agree that government intervention in a market is warranted when there are "market failures" that result in less-than-optimal production and consumption.[29,30] Several market failures exist with respect to sugar-sweetened beverages. First, because many persons do not fully appreciate the links between consumption of these beverages and health consequences, they make consumption decisions with imperfect information. These decisions are likely to be further distorted by the extensive marketing campaigns that advertise the benefits of consumption. A second failure results from time-inconsistent preferences (i.e., decisions that provide short-term gratification but long-term harm). This problem is exacerbated in the case of children and adolescents, who place a higher value on present satisfaction while more heavily discounting future consequences. Finally, financial "externalities" exist in the market for sugar-sweetened beverages in that consumers do not bear the full costs of their consumption decisions. Because of the contribution of the consumption of sugar-sweetened beverages to obesity, as well as the health consequences that are independent of weight, the consumption of sugar-sweetened beverages generates excess health care costs. Medical costs for overweight and obesity alone are estimated to be $147 billion—or 9.1% of U.S. health care expenditures—with half these costs paid for publicly through the Medicare and Medicaid programs.[31]

An Effective Tax Policy and Projected Effects

Key factors to consider in developing an effective policy include the definition of taxable beverages, the type of tax (sales tax or excise tax), and the tax rate. We propose an excise tax of 1 cent per ounce for beverages that have any added caloric sweetener. An alternative would be to tax beverages that exceed a threshold of grams of added caloric sweetener or of kilocalories per ounce. If this approach were used, we would recommend that the threshold be set at 1 g of sugar per ounce (30 ml) (32 kcal per 8 oz [237 ml]). Another option would be a tax assessed per gram of added sugar, but such an approach would be difficult to administer. The advantage of taxing beverages that have any added sugar is that this kind of tax is simpler to administer and it may promote the consumption of no-calorie beverages, most notably water; however, a threshold approach would also promote calorie reductions and would encourage manufacturers to reformulate products. A consumer who drinks a conventional soft drink (20 oz [591 ml]) every day and switches to a beverage below this threshold would consume approximately 174 fewer calories each day.

A specific excise tax (a tax levied on units such as volume or weight) per ounce or per gram of added sugar would be preferable to a sales tax or an ad valorem excise tax (a tax levied as a percentage of price) and would provide an incentive to reduce the amount of sugar per ounce of a sugar-sweetened beverage. Sales taxes added as a percentage of retail cost would have three disadvantages: they could simply encourage the purchase of lower-priced brands (thus resulting in no calorie reduction) or of large containers that cost less per ounce; consumers would become aware of the added tax only after making the decision to purchase the beverage; and the syrups that are used in fountain drinks, which are often served with multiple refills, would remain untaxed. A number of states currently exempt sugar-sweetened beverages from sales taxes along with food, presumably because food is a necessity. This practice should be eliminated, whether or not an excise tax is enacted.

Excise taxes could be levied on producers and wholesalers, and the cost would almost certainly be passed along to retailers, who would then incorporate it into the retail price; thus, consumers would become aware of the cost at the point of making a purchase decision. Taxes levied on producers and wholesalers would be much easier to collect and enforce than taxes levied on retailers because of the smaller number of businesses that would have to comply with the tax; in addition, the sugar used in syrups could be taxed—a major advantage because of the heavy sales of fountain drinks. Experience with tobacco and alcohol taxes suggests that specific excise taxes have a greater effect on consumption than do ad valorem excise taxes and can also generate more stable revenues because they are less dependent on industry pricing strategies.[32] In addition, tax laws should be written with provisions for the regular adjustment of specific excise taxes to keep pace with inflation, in order to prevent the effect of the taxes on both prices and revenues from eroding over time.

A tax of 1 cent per ounce of beverage would increase the cost of a 20-oz soft drink by 15 to 20%. The effect on consumption can be estimated through research on price elasticity (i.e., consumption shifts produced by price). The price elasticity for all soft drinks is in the range of −0.8 to −1.0.[33] (Elasticity of −0.8 suggests that for every 10% increase in price, there would be a decrease in consumption of 8%, whereas elasticity of −1.0 suggests that for every 10% increase in price, there would be a decrease in consumption of 10%.) Even greater price effects are expected from taxing only sugar-sweetened beverages, since some consumers will switch to diet beverages. With the use of a conservative estimate that consumers would substitute calories in other forms for 25% of the reduced calorie consumption, an excise tax of 1 cent per ounce would lead to a minimum reduction of 10% in calorie consumption from sweetened beverages, or 20 kcal per person per day, a reduction that is sufficient for weight loss and reduction in risk (unpublished data). The benefit would be larger among consumers who consume higher volumes, since these consumers are more likely to be overweight and appear to be more responsive to prices.[7] Higher taxes would have greater benefits.

A controversial issue is whether to tax beverages that are sweetened with noncaloric sweeteners. No adverse health effects of noncaloric sweeteners have been consistently demonstrated, but there are concerns that diet beverages may increase calorie consumption by justifying consumption of other caloric foods or by promoting a preference for sweet tastes.[34] At present, we do not propose taxing beverages with noncaloric sweeteners, but we recommend close tracking of studies to determine whether taxing might be justified in the future.

Revenue-Generating Potential

The revenue generated from a tax on sugar-sweetened beverages would be considerable and could be used to help support childhood nutrition programs, obesity-prevention programs, or health care for the uninsured or to help meet general revenue needs. A national tax of 1 cent per ounce on sugar-sweetened beverages would raise $14.9 billion in the first year alone. Taxes at the state level would also generate considerable revenue— for example, $139 million in Arkansas, $183 million in Oregon, $221 million in Alabama, $928 million in Florida, $937 million in New York, $1.2 billion in Texas, and $1.8 billion in California. A tax calculator that is available online can generate revenue numbers for states and 25 major cities.[35]

Objections, Industry Reaction, Public Support, and Framing

One objection to a tax on sugar-sweetened beverages is that it would be regressive. This argument arose with respect to tobacco taxes but was challenged successfully by proponents of the taxes, who pointed out that the poor face a disproportionate burden of smoking-related illnesses, that nearly all smokers begin to smoke when they are teenagers, and that both groups are sensitive to price changes.[7] In addition, some of the tobacco revenue has been used for programs developed specifically for the poor and for youth. The poor are most affected by illnesses that are related to unhealthful diets, and brand loyalties for beverages tend to be set by the teenage years. In addition, sugar-sweetened beverages are not necessary for survival, and an alternative (i.e., water) is available at little or no cost; hence, a tax that shifted intake from sugar-sweetened beverages to water would benefit the poor both by improving health and by lowering expenditures on beverages. Designating revenues for programs promoting childhood nutrition, obesity prevention, or health care for the uninsured would preferentially help those most in need.

A second objection is that taxing sugar-sweetened beverages will not solve the obesity crisis and is a blunt instrument that affects even those who consume small amounts of such beverages. Seat-belt legislation and tobacco taxation do not eliminate traffic accidents and heart disease but are nevertheless sound policies. Similarly, obesity is unlikely to yield to any single policy intervention, so it is important to pursue multiple opportunities to obtain incremental gains. Reducing caloric intake by 1 to 2% per year would have a marked impact on health in all age groups, and the financial burden on those who consumed small amounts of sugar-sweetened beverages would be minimal.

Opposition to a tax by the beverage industry is to be expected, given the possible effect on sales; opposition has been seen in jurisdictions that have considered such taxes and can be predicted from the behavior of the tobacco industry under similar circumstances.[36] PepsiCo threatened to move its corporate headquarters out of New York when the state considered implementing an 18% sales tax on sugar-sweetened beverages.[37] The tobacco industry fought policy changes by creating front groups with names that suggested community involvement. The beverage industry has created Americans Against Food Taxes.[38] These reactions suggest that the beverage industry believes that a tax would have a substantial impact on consumption.

Public support for food and beverage taxes to address obesity has increased steadily. Questions about taxes in polls have been asked in various ways, and the results are therefore not directly comparable from year to year, but overall trends are clear. Support for food taxes rose from 33% in 2001 to 41% in 2003 and then to 54% in 2004.[39] A 2008 poll of New York State residents showed that 52% of respondents support a soda tax; 72% support such a tax if the revenue is used to support programs for the prevention of obesity in children and adults. The way in which the issue is framed is essential; support is highest when the tax is introduced in the context of promoting health and when the revenues are earmarked for programs promoting childhood nutrition or obesity prevention.

Conclusions

The federal government, a number of states and cities, and some countries (e.g., Mexico[8]) are considering levying taxes on sugar-sweetened beverages. The reasons to proceed are compelling. The science base linking the consumption of sugar-sweetened beverages to the risk of chronic diseases is clear. Escalating health care costs and the rising burden of diseases related to poor diet create an urgent need for solutions, thus justifying government's right to recoup costs.

As with any public health intervention, the precise effect of a tax cannot be known until it is implemented and studied, but research to date suggests that a tax on sugar-sweetened beverages would have strong positive effects on reducing consumption.[5,33] In addition, the tax has the potential to generate substantial revenue to prevent obesity and address other external costs resulting from the consumption of sugar-sweetened beverages, as well as to fund other health-related programs. Much as taxes on tobacco products are routine at both state and federal levels because they generate revenue and they confer a public health benefit with respect to smoking rates, we believe that taxes on beverages that help drive the obesity epidemic should and will become routine.

References

1. Malik VS, Schulze MB, Hu FB. Intake of sugar-sweetened beverages and weight gain: A systematic review. *Am J Clin Nutr* 2006;84:274–88.

2. Vartanian LR, Schwartz MB, Brownell KD. Effects of soft drink consumption on nutrition and health: A systematic review and meta-analysis. *Am J Public Health* 2007;97:667–75.

3. Fung TT, Malik V, Rexrode KM, Manson JE, Willett WC, Hu FB. Sweetened beverage consumption and

risk of coronary heart disease in women. *Am J Clin Nutr* 2009;89:1037–42.

4. Brownell KD. Get slim with higher taxes. *New York Times*. December 15, 1994:A29.

5. Brownell KD, Frieden TR. Ounces of prevention—the public policy case for taxes on sugared beverages. *N Engl J Med* 2009;360:1805–8.

6. Jacobson MF, Brownell KD. Small taxes on soft drinks and snack foods to promote health. *Am J Public Health* 2000;90:854–7.

7. Powell LM, Chaloupka FJ. Food prices and obesity: Evidence and policy implications for taxes and subsidies. *Milbank Q* 2009;87:229–57.

8. Barquera S, Hernandez-Barrera L, Tolentino ML, et al. Energy intake from beverages is increasing among Mexican adolescents and adults. *J Nutr* 2008;138:2454–61.

9. Duffey KJ, Popkin BM. Shifts in patterns and consumption of beverages between 1965 and 2002. *Obesity (Silver Spring)* 2007;15:2739–47.

10. Forshee RA, Anderson PA, Storey ML. Sugar-sweetened beverages and body mass index in children and adolescents: A meta-analysis. *Am J Clin Nutr* 2008;87:1662–71. [Erratum, *Am J Clin Nutr* 2009;89:441–2.]

11. Malik VS, Willett WC, Hu FB. Sugar-sweetened beverages and BMI in children and adolescents: Reanalyses of a meta-analysis. *Am J Clin Nutr* 2009;89:438–9.

12. Ludwig DS, Peterson KE, Gortmaker SL. Relation between consumption of sugar-sweetened drinks and childhood obesity: A prospective, observational analysis. *Lancet* 2001;357:505–8.

13. Schulze MB, Manson JE, Ludwig DS, et al. Sugar-sweetened beverages, weight gain, and incidence of type 2 diabetes in young and middle-aged women. *JAMA* 2004;292:927–34.

14. Tordoff MG, Alleva AM. Effect of drinking soda sweetened with aspartame or high-fructose corn syrup on food intake and body weight. *Am J Clin Nutr* 1990;51:963–9.

15. Raben A, Vasilaras TH, Moller AC, Astrup A. Sucrose compared with artificial sweeteners: different effects on ad libitum food intake and body weight after 10 wk of supplementation in overweight subjects. *Am J Clin Nutr* 2002;76:721–9.

16. James J, Thomas P, Cavan D, Kerr D. Preventing childhood obesity by reducing consumption of carbonated drinks: Cluster randomised controlled trial. BMJ 2004;328:1237. [Erratum, *BMJ* 2004;328:1236.]

17. Sichieri R, Paula Trotte A, de Souza RA, Veiga GV. School randomised trial on prevention of excessive weight gain by discouraging students from drinking sodas. *Public Health Nutr* 2009;12:197–202.

18. Ebbeling CB, Feldman HA, Osganian SK, Chomitz VR, Ellen bogen SJ, Ludwig DS. Effects of decreasing sugar-sweetened beverage consumption on body weight in adolescents: A randomized, controlled pilot study. *Pediatrics* 2006;117:673–80.

19. Albala C, Ebbeling CB, Cifuentes M, Lera L, Bustos N, Ludwig DS. Effects of replacing the habitual consumption of sugar-sweetened beverages with milk in Chilean children. *Am J Clin Nutr* 2008;88:605–11.

20. Montonen J, Järvinen R, Knekt P, Heliövaara M, Reunanen A. Consumption of sweetened beverages and intakes of fructose and glucose predict type 2 diabetes occurrence. *J Nutr* 2007;137:1447–54.

21. Palmer JR, Boggs DA, Krishnan S, Hu FB, Singer M, Rosenberg L. Sugar-sweetened beverages and incidence of type 2 diabetes mellitus in African American women. *Arch Intern Med* 2008;168:1487–92.

22. Appel LJ, Sacks FM, Carey VJ, et al. Effects of protein, mono-unsaturated fat, and carbohydrate intake on blood pressure and serum lipids: Results of the OmniHeart randomized trial. *JAMA* 2005;294:2455–64.

23. Ludwig DS. The glycemic index: Physiological mechanisms relating to obesity, diabetes, and cardiovascular disease. *JAMA* 2002;287:2414–23.

24. Yoshida M, McKeown NM, Rogers G, et al. Surrogate markers of insulin resistance are associated with consumption of sugar-sweetened drinks and fruit juice in middle and older-aged adults. *J Nutr* 2007;137:2121–7.

25. Mourao DM, Bressan J, Campbell WW, Mattes RD. Effects of food form on appetite and energy intake in lean and obese young adults. *Int J Obes* (Lond) 2007;31:1688–95.

26. De Castro JM. The effects of the spontaneous ingestion of particular foods or beverages on the meal pattern and overall nutrient intake of humans. *Physiol Behav* 1993;53:1133–44.

27. Harnack L, Stang J, Story M. Soft drink consumption among US children and adolescents: Nutritional consequences. *J Am Diet Assoc* 1999;99:436–41.

28. Flood JE, Roe LS, Rolls BJ. The effect of increased beverage portion size on energy intake at a meal. *J Am Diet Assoc* 2006;106:1984–90.

29. Cawley J. An economic framework for understanding physical activity and eating behaviors. *Am J Prev Med* 2004;27:117–25.

30. Finkelstein EA, Ruhm CJ, Kosa KM. Economic causes and consequences of obesity. *Annu Rev Public Health* 2005;26:239–57.

31. Finkelstein EA, Trogdon JG, Cohen JW, Dietz W. Annual medical spending attributable to obesity: Payer-and-service-specific estimates. *Health Aff* (Millwood) 2009;28:w822–w831.

32. Chaloupka FJ, Peck RM., Tauras JA, Yurekli A. *Cigarette excise taxation: The impact of tax structure on prices, revenues, and cigarettes smoking.* Geneva: World Health Organization (in press).

33. Andreyeva T, Long MW, Brownell KD. The impact of food prices on consumption: A systematic review of research on price elasticity of demand for food. *Am J Public Health* (in press).

34. Mattes RD, Popkin BM. Nonnutritive sweetener consumption in humans: Effects on appetite and food intake and their putative mechanisms. *Am J Clin Nutr* 2009;89:1–14.

35. Rudd Center for Food Policy and Obesity. Revenue calculator for soft drink taxes. (Accessed September 24, 2009, at http://www.yaleruddcenter.org/sodatax.aspx.)

36. Brownell KD, Warner KE. The perils of ignoring history: big tobacco played dirty and millions died: How similar is big food? *Milbank Q* 2009;87:259–94.

37. Hakim D, McGeehan P. New York vulnerable to poaching in recession. *New York Times*. March 1, 2009.

38. Americans Against Food Taxes home page. (Accessed September 24, 2009, at http://nofoodtaxes.com.)

39. Brownell KD. The chronicling of obesity: Growing awareness of its social, economic, and political contexts. *J Health Polit Policy Law* 2005;30:955–64.

KELLY D. BROWNELL is director of the Rudd Center for Food Policy and Obesity at Yale. His research deals primarily with obesity and the intersection of behavior, environment, and health with public policy. He was named in 2006 as one of "The World's 100 Most Influential People" by *Time* magazine. His undergraduate work was at Purdue and he received his PhD in clinical psychology from Rutgers.

FRANK J. CHALOUPKA is professor of economics at the University of Illinois at Chicago and affiliate of the National Bureau of Economic Research. His research focuses on the economic analysis of substance use and abuse, and on the effect of prices and substance control policies in affecting the demands for tobacco, alcohol, and illicit drugs.

THOMAS FARLEY was New York City Health Commissioner when the article was written. His research interests include prevention of HIV/STDs, infant mortality, and obesity. He is coauthor of *Prescription for a Healthy Nation*. He received his medical degree from Tulane University.

DAVID S. LUDWIG is a pediatric endocrinologist and professor at Harvard Medical School. His research focuses on the effects of dietary intake on hormones, metabolism, and body weight regulation. He is the founding director of the Optimal Weight for Life clinic at Children's Hospital. He received his medical degree from Stanford.

BARRY M. POPKIN is a professor and head of nutrition epidemiology at the University of North Carolina, Chapel Hill. His research deals with dynamic changes in diet, physical activity and inactivity, and body composition. He received his doctorate in agricultural economics from Cornell.

JOSEPH W. THOMPSON is Surgeon General for Arkansas and professor of medicine and public health at the University of Arkansas. He earned his medical degree from UA and his MPH from the University of North Carolina at Chapel Hill.

WALTER C. WILLETT is the Fredrick John Stare Professor of Epidemiology and Nutrition, and Chair of the Department of Nutrition at Harvard. He is the principal investigator of the second Nurses' Health Study and has published over 1,000 articles regarding various aspects of diet and disease and author of *Eat, Drink and Be Healthy*. He received his medical degree from the University of Michigan Medical School and a doctorate in public health from Harvard School of Public Health.

Daniel Engber

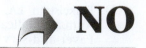 **NO**

Let Them Drink Water! What a Fat Tax Really Means for America

Not long after the attack on Pearl Harbor, in the winter of 1942, physiologist A.J. Carlson made a radical suggestion: If the nation's largest citizens were charged a fee—say, $20 for each pound of overweight—we might feed the war effort overseas while working to subdue an "injurious luxury" at home.

Sixty-seven years later, the "fat tax" is back on the table. We're fighting another war—our second-most-expensive ever—and Congress seems on the verge of spending $1 trillion on health care. Once again, a bloated budget may fall on the backs of the bloated public. Some commentators, following Carlson, have lately called for a tax on fat people themselves (cf. the *Huffington Post* and the *New York Times*); others . . . propose a hefty surcharge on soft drinks instead.

The notion hasn't generated much enthusiasm in Congress, but fat taxes are spreading through state legislatures: Four-fifths of the union now takes a cut on the sales of junk food or soda. Pleas for a federal fat tax are getting louder, too. The *New York Times* recently endorsed a penny-per-ounce soda tax, and Michael Pollan has made a convincing argument for why the insurance industry may soon throw its weight behind the proposal. Even President Obama said he likes the idea in a recent interview with *Men's Health*. (For the record, Stephen Colbert is against the measure: "I do not obey big government; I obey my thirst.")

For all this, the public still has strong reservations about the fat tax. The state-level penalties now in place have turned out to be way too small to make anyone lose weight, and efforts to pass more heavy-handed laws have so far fallen short. But proponents say it's only a matter of time before taxing junk food feels as natural as taxing cigarettes. The latter has been a tremendous success, they argue, in bringing down rates of smoking and death from lung cancer. In theory, a steep tax on sweetened beverages could do the same for overeating and diabetes.

It may take more than an analogy with tobacco to convince voters. As my colleague William Saletan points out, the first step in policing eating habits is to redefine food as something else. If you want to tax the hell out of soda, you need to make people think that it's a drug, not a beverage—that downing a Coke is just like puffing on a cigarette. But is soda as bad as tobacco? Let's ask the neuropundits.

Junk food literally "alters the biological circuitry of our brains," writes David Kessler in this summer's bestseller, *The End of Overeating*. In a previous book, Kessler detailed his role in prosecuting the war on smoking as the head of the FDA; now he's explaining what makes us fat with all the magisterial jargon of cognitive neuroscience. Eating a chocolate-covered pretzel, he says, activates the brain's pleasure system—the dopamine reward circuit, to be exact—and changes the "functional connectivity among important brain regions." Thus, certain foods—the ones concocted by industrial scientists and laden with salt, sugar, and fat—can circumvent our natural inclinations and trigger "action schemata" for mindless eating. Got that? Junk food is engineered to enslave us. Kessler even has a catchphrase to describe these nefarious snacks: They're hyperpalatable.

Try as we might, we're nearly powerless to resist these treats. That's because evolution has us programmed to experience two forms of hunger. The first kicks in when we're low on energy. As an adaptation, its purpose is simple enough—we eat to stay alive. The second, called hedonic hunger, applies even when we're full—it's the urge to eat for pleasure. When food is scarce, hedonic hunger comes in handy, so we can stock up on calories for the hard times ahead. But in a world of cheap food, the same impulse makes us fat.

That's the problem with junk food. Manufacturers have figured out how to prey on man's voluptuous nature. Like the cigarette companies, they lace their products with addictive chemicals and cajole us into wanting things we don't really need. Soda is like a designer drug, layered with seductive elements—sweetness for a burst of dopamine, bubbles to prick the trigeminal nerve.

It's hard to draw a line, though, between foods that are drugs and foods that are merely delicious. Soda and candy aren't the only stimuli that "rewire your brain," of course. Coffee does, too, and so do video games, Twitter, meditation, and just about anything else that might give you pleasure (or pain). That's what brains do—they learn, they rewire. To construe an earthly delight as hyperpalatable—as too good for our own good—we're lashing out at sensuality itself. "Do you design food specifically to be highly hedonic?" Kessler asks an industry consultant at one point in the book. What's the guy going to say? "No, we design food to be bland and nutritious. . . ."

It's ironic that so many advocates for healthy eating are also outspoken gourmands. Alice Waters, the proprietor of Chez Panisse, calls for a "delicious revolution" of low-fat, low-sugar lunch programs. It's a central dogma of the organic movement that you can be a foodie and a health nut at the same time—that what's real and natural tastes better, anyway. Never mind how much fat and sugar and salt you'll get from a Wabash Cannonball and a slice of *pain au levain*. Forget that *cuisiniers* have for centuries been catering to our hedonic hunger—our pleasure-seeking, caveman selves—with a repertoire of batters and sauces. Junk foods are *hyperpalatable*. Whole Foods is *delicious*. Doughnuts are a drug; brioche is a treat.

Some tastes, it seems, are more equal than others.

A fat tax, then, discriminates among the varieties of gustatory experience. And its impact would fall most directly on the poor, nonwhite people who tend to be the most avid consumers of soft drinks and the most sensitive to price. Under an apartheid of pleasure, palatable drinks are penalized while delicious—or even hyperdelicious—products come at no extra charge. What about the folks who can't afford a $5 bottle of POM Wonderful? No big deal, say the academics writing in the *New England Journal of Medicine*; they can always drink from the faucet. Here's how the article puts it: "Sugar-sweetened beverages are not necessary for survival, and an alternative (i.e., water) is available at little or no cost." So much for *Let them eat cake*.

We've known for a long time that any sin tax is likely to be a burden on the poor, since they're most prone to unhealthy behavior. (James Madison fought the snuff tax on these grounds way back in 1794.) But you might just as well say that poor people have the most to gain from a sin tax for exactly the same reason. It's also possible that revenues from a fat tax would be spent on obesity prevention—or go back to the community in other ways. There's a knotty argument here about the vexing and reciprocal interactions among health, wealth, and obesity. (I'll try to untangle some of these in my next column.) It's not clear whether, and in what direction, a soda tax might redistribute wealth. Whatever you think of the economics, though, raising the price on soda—and offering water in its place—will redistribute pleasure.

I don't mean to imply that any such regulation is unjust. We have laws against plenty of chemicals and behaviors that are as delightful as they are destructive. These are, for the most part, sensible measures to protect our health. What's disturbing is the thought that the degree of government control should vary according to who's using which drug. In April, the Obama administration called for an end to a long-standing policy that gives dealers of powdered cocaine 100 times more leeway than dealers of crack when it comes to federal prison sentences. Let's not repeat this drug-war injustice in the war on obesity. We may be ready to say that foods are addictive. Are we ready to judge the nature of a delicious high?

DANIEL ENGBER is science editor of *Slate* magazine and finalist for the James Beard Award for reporting on health and nutrition. He received his bachelor's in literature from Harvard and master's in neurobiology from Columbia.

EXPLORING THE ISSUE

Should Government Levy a "Fat Tax"?

Critical Thinking and Reflection

1. List health problems associated with consumption of sugar-sweetened beverages (SSB).
2. Outline the various ways to calculate a tax on SSB as proposed by Brownell and colleagues.
3. Explain why some people think that SSB are addictive.
4. New York's former Governor Paterson proposed a penny per ounce tax on SSB but it did not pass. There were several anti-tax groups that lobbied heavily against the tax proposal. What type of people do you think would be opposed to this form of "fat tax" and what arguments do you think they would have?
5. Many poor, slim people enjoy the taste, and actually benefit from the extra calories from sugar-sweetened beverages and high-fat snacks. What effect could taxation of sugary beverages have on poor, thin people? Design a strategy to ameliorate this problem.

Is There Common Ground?

There is a vast difference between the backgrounds (and writing styles) of the authors of the first selection and the sole author of the second selection. The YES selection is written by seven of the nation's leading researchers on nutrition and health. Their article takes an academic approach and begins with an overview of studies on the effect of sugar-sweetened beverages (SSB) on health. They point out that as SSB intake increases, body weight rises as do the incidences of type 2 diabetes and coronary heart disease. They outline the other problems and mechanisms that SSB have on health—elevated triglycerides, high blood pressure, lowered HDL levels, poor satiating properties, and changes in taste preferences. They also outline the economic detriment of SSB—consumption increases the chance of becoming overweight or obese, which results in higher medical costs—about $147 billion. The authors then introduce several possible federal tax structures that could be levied and the possible revenue from them.

In the NO selection, journalist Daniel Engber paints a very different picture of sugary drinks and other "hyperpalatable" foods. He begins by citing David Kessler's description of the metabolic impact of junk food on the brain, then points out the irony behind Alice Walter's call for a "delicious revolution." (He questions why a gourmet food such as brioche is considered delicious yet common donuts are junk foods—even though they may be equal

in sugar, fat, and calories and the impact on health.) He disagrees with Brownell and colleagues' proposed SSB taxation and argues that an increase in cost of SSB through taxation "discriminates among the varieties of gustatory experience. And its impact would fall most directly on the poor, nonwhite people who tend to be the most avid consumers of soft drinks."

Additional Resources

Bødker M, Pisinger C, Toft U, Jørgensen T. The rise and fall of the world's first fat tax. *Health Policy.* 2015;119(6):737–42.

Caraher M, Cowburn G. Guest commentary: Fat and other taxes, lessons for the implementation of preventive policies. *Prev Med.* 2015;77:204–6.

Ford CN, Ng SW, Popkin BM. Targeted beverage taxes influence food and beverage purchases among households with preschool children. *J Nutr.* 2015;145(8):1835–43.

Long MW, Gortmaker SL, Ward ZJ, et al. Cost effectiveness of a sugar-sweetened beverage excise tax in the U.S. *Am J Prev Med.* 2015;49(1):112–23.

Niebylski ML, Redburn KA, Duhaney T, Campbell NR. Healthy food subsidies and unhealthy food taxation: A systematic review of the evidence. *Nutrition.* 2015;31(6):787–95.

Internet References . . .

The American Beverage Association

    www.ameribev.org

Fed Up

    fedupmovie.com

Slate Magazine

    www.slate.com

Selected, Edited, and with Issue Framing Materials by:
Janet M. Colson, *Middle Tennessee State University*

ISSUE

Can Michelle Obama's "Let's Move!" Initiative Halt Childhood Obesity?

YES: White House Press Release, from "First Lady Michelle Obama Launches *Let's Move*: America's Move to Raise a Healthier Generation of Kids" (2010)

NO: Michele Simon, from "Michelle Obama's *Let's Move*—Will It Move Industry?" *AlterNet* (2010)

Learning Outcomes
After reading this issue, you will be able to:
• List the four key objectives of the Task Force on Childhood Obesity.
• Describe the public and private resources that will work to solve childhood obesity and the role each will play.
• Identify the early signs outlined by Michele Simon that indicate the initiative is more talk than action.

ISSUE SUMMARY

YES: First Lady Michelle Obama says that the Let's Move! campaign can correct the health problems of the upcoming generation and realizes that the problem cannot be solved overnight. She thinks that "with everyone working together, it can be solved." The "first ever" Task Force on Childhood Obesity was formed to help implement the campaign.

NO: Public health attorney Michelle Simon claims that Let's Move! is just another task force and there is more talk than action. She questions if it's realistic to be able to reverse the nation's childhood obesity epidemic in a generation.

One of the good things about having a healthy president and first lady is they can speak out about the problem of obesity and lead by example. In February 2010, our physically fit president issued a press release about the formation of the "first ever Task Force on Childhood Obesity" and his equally-fit wife's role in the effort. In the release he announced:

My Administration is committed to redoubling our efforts to solve the problem of childhood obesity within a generation through a comprehensive approach that builds on effective strategies, engages families and communities, and mobilizes both public and private sector resources.

Nearly one third of children in America are overweight or obese—a rate that has tripled in adolescents and more than doubled in younger children since 1980. One third of all individuals born in the year 2000 or later will eventually suffer from diabetes over the course of their lifetime, while too many others will face chronic obesity-related health problems such as heart disease, high blood pressure, cancer, and asthma. Without effective intervention, many more children will endure serious illnesses that will put a strain on our health-care system. We must act now to improve the health of our Nation's children and avoid spending billions of dollars treating a preventable disease.

Therefore, I have set a goal to solve the problem of childhood obesity within a generation so that children born today will reach adulthood at a healthy weight. The First Lady will lead a national public awareness effort to tackle the epidemic of childhood obesity.

The Task Force that he mentions is headed by the Department of Health and Human Services (HHS). The mission and functions of that group are as follows:

> The Task Force shall work across executive departments and agencies to develop a coordinated Federal response while also identifying nongovernmental actions. . . . The functions of the Task Force are . . . making recommendations to meet the following objectives:
> (a) ensuring access to healthy, affordable food;
> (b) increasing physical activity in schools and communities;
> (c) providing healthier food in schools; and
> (d) empowering parents with information and tools to make good choices for themselves and their families.

Is it possible to meet these objectives and to solve the problem of childhood obesity within a generation? First Lady Michelle Obama thinks it is and that people working together through the Let's Move! campaign is the way it can be accomplished.

Although not required, it is expected for first ladies of the United States to have a mission and make a contribution to the nation during her husband's presidency. In the article, "First Ladies' Contributions to Political Issues and the National Welfare," Betty Boyd Caroli describes the roles of the first ladies over the last 50 years. In the article, available on the Gilder Lehrman Institute of American History website, Caroli highlights Lady Bird Johnson's Highway Beautification Act. When Lyndon Johnson was elected president in 1964, American roadways were filled with unsightly billboards and littered with trash. First Lady Johnson spearheaded efforts to beautify the nation and convinced her husband to support a bill that would improve the appearance of U.S. highways. Caroli describes contributions of other first ladies:

> Every first lady after Lady Bird Johnson followed her example and campaigned actively for their husbands and led a project to improve the national welfare. Pat Nixon focused on volunteerism; Betty Ford encouraged dance and the passage of the Equal Rights Amendment; Rosalynn Carter promoted mental health; Nancy Reagan urged Americans to "Just Say No" to illegal drugs; Barbara Bush championed literacy; Hillary Rodham Clinton, health care reform; Laura Bush returned to the cause of literacy; and Michelle Obama mounted an anti-obesity campaign for juveniles . . .

So the Let's Move! anti-obesity campaign will be Michelle Obama's legacy. Each February, on the Let's Move!'s anniversary, the White House releases an update about the progress being made to fulfill the Let's Move! mission. Below are excerpts from the first anniversary (February 9, 2011) press release, "Remarks of First Lady Michelle Obama Let's Move! Launch Anniversary Speech to Parents":

> Now, we're not just here today to celebrate the first anniversary of a campaign to solve the problem of childhood obesity in a generation. We're here to celebrate a new conversation in this country about the health and well-being of our children. It's a conversation about what our kids eat and how they move. It's about how they feel and how they feel about themselves. And it's about what that means, not just for their physical and emotional health, but for their success in school and in life.
>
> And over this past year, we've seen the first signs of a fundamental shift in how we live and eat. We've seen changes at every level of our society—from classrooms, to boardrooms, to the halls of Congress.
>
> There's a reason I wanted to talk with all of you—parents from all different backgrounds with kids of all different ages. And that's because these changes are happening for one simple reason: because you asked for them. You see, that's really what Let's Move! is all about. That's how it all started—by listening to parents just like you. By working to meet your needs, by working to fulfill your hopes and dreams for your kids.
>
> You asked for more fresh, nutritious food in your communities. So we're working to bring more grocery stores into underserved areas. You wanted healthier, more affordable options on those grocery store shelves. So food manufacturers made a "Healthy Weight Commitment," pledging to cut 1.5 trillion calories a year from their products. And Walmart promised to sell products with less sugar, salt and trans-fat—and to reduce prices on healthy items like fresh fruits and vegetables.
>
> You asked for more information about the food you buy for your kids. And today, we're seeing better, clearer labels on beverage cans and many other products in our grocery stores. You asked for better food in your kids' schools—the kind of balanced meals you're trying to make at home. So we're putting salad bars in 6,000 schools across the country. Congress passed the Healthy, Hunger-Free Kids Act, historic legislation that will provide healthier school meals to millions of American children. And more than

2,000 professional chefs have signed up to help local schools develop healthier menus.

You asked for better role models for your kids. So we recruited professional athletes to encourage kids to stay active. You asked for healthier communities that can sustain healthy families. And through Let's Move Cities and Towns, 500 mayors have committed to tackling obesity in their communities. They're building bike paths, they're planting gardens, they're starting youth sports leagues and so much more.

You asked for practical, affordable, real-life advice to keep your kids healthy. So we launched a public service campaign and a website—letsmove. gov—with helpful tips on exercise and nutrition. The American Academy of Pediatrics is now urging doctors to not just screen kids for obesity, but to actually write out prescriptions for exercise and healthy eating. And under the Affordable Care Act—the health care law that Congress passed last year—these screenings will be fully covered by insurance so you won't have to pay a penny out of pocket. And all of this has happened in just one year!

So if we can do all this in the first year just imagine what we'll achieve next year, and the year after that. So we're making some real progress here. We're gaining momentum. But as far as we've come, when nearly one in three kids in this country is still overweight or obese then we've still got a long way to go . . .

In February 2012, 2013, and again in 2014, Mrs. Obama updated the nation on Let's Move!'s progress. In 2015, on its fifth anniversary, the First Lady asked Americans to tweet or post to Facebook five ways to stay fit under the hashtag #GimmeFive. Is her hard work paying off? Has Let's Move! made any strides in reducing childhood obesity?

Weight status of the nation is estimated through data from the National Health and Nutrition Survey (NHANES) and published by the Centers for Disease Control and Prevention (CDC). Weight status of children is assessed using BMI-for-age. "Obese" is defined as having excessive body fat that may have an adverse impact on health and a BMI-for-age >95th percentile. "Overweight" refers to a pre-obese state, having more body fat than is desirable, and a BMI-for-age >85th to <94.9th percentile.

Based on CDC data in the table below, the only age group that has had significant decreases in obesity is preschool-age children (aged 2 to 5) decreasing from a high of 13.9 percent in 2003/2004 to only 8.4 percent in 2011/2012. There was a slight dip in obesity among school-age children, but an increase among adolescents during the same time frame. Overall, obesity and overweight rates have remained constant since 2003/2004. Five years after the launch of Let's Move!, about one-third of children are still at an unhealthy body weight. (The table below only includes data for obesity, not overweight.)

The selections for this issue focus on Let's Move! The "YES" selection is the 2010 White House press release about Let's Move! The "NO" selection is an article by public health lawyer Michele Simon, who predicted in 2010 that the "early signs [of Let's Move!] indicate more talk than action." So what are your thoughts? Do you think that our nation has made strides in reducing childhood obesity since 2010, or do you agree with Michelle Simon, that it's been more talk than action?

Prevalence of obesity among U.S. children and adolescents aged 2–19, from 1971 through 2012					
Age (in years)	NHANES 1971–1974	NHANES 1988–1994	NHANES 1999–2000	NHANES 2003–2004	NHANES 2007–2008	NHANES 2011–2012
Total	5.0	10.0	13.9	17.1	16.9	16.9
2–5	5.0	7.2	10.3	13.9	10.4	8.4
6–11	4.0	11.3	15.1	18.8	19.6	17.7
12–19	6.1	10.5	14.8	17.4	18.1	20.9

Source: Adapted from: http://www.cdc.gov/obesity/data/childhood.html.

YES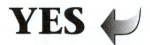

First Lady Michelle Obama Launches *Let's Move*: America's Move to Raise a Healthier Generation of Kids

The White House, Washington—First Lady Michelle Obama today announced an ambitious national goal of solving the challenge of childhood obesity within a generation so that children born today will reach adulthood at a healthy weight and unveiled a nationwide campaign—*Let's Move*—to help achieve it. The *Let's Move* campaign will combat the epidemic of childhood obesity through a comprehensive approach that builds on effective strategies, and mobilizes public and private sector resources. *Let's Move* will engage every sector impacting the health of children to achieve the national goal, and will provide schools, families and communities simple tools to help kids be more active, eat better, and get healthy. To support *Let's Move* and facilitate and coordinate partnerships with States, communities, and the non-profit and for-profit private sectors, the nation's leading children's health foundations have come together to create a new independent foundation—the Partnership for a Healthier America—which will accelerate existing efforts addressing childhood obesity and facilitate new commitments toward the national goal of solving childhood obesity within a generation.

Almost a year ago, Mrs. Obama began a national conversation about the health of America's children when she broke ground on the White House Kitchen Garden with students from Bancroft Elementary School in Washington, DC. Through the garden, she began a discussion with kids about proper nutrition and the role food plays in living a healthy life. That discussion grew into the *Let's Move* campaign announced today.

Over the past three decades, childhood obesity rates in America have tripled, and today, nearly one in three children in America are overweight or obese. One third of all children born in 2000 or later will suffer from diabetes at some point in their lives; many others will face chronic obesity-related health problems like heart disease, high

blood pressure, cancer, and asthma. A recent study put the health care costs of obesity-related diseases at $147 billion per year. This epidemic also impacts the nation's security, as obesity is now one of the most common disqualifiers for military service.

"The physical and emotional health of an entire generation and the economic health and security of our nation is at stake," said Mrs. Obama. "This isn't the kind of problem that can be solved overnight, but with everyone working together, it can be solved. So, *let's move.*"

The First Lady launched the *Let's Move* campaign at the White House where she was joined by members of the President's cabinet, including Agriculture Secretary Vilsack, HHS Secretary Sebelius, Education Secretary Duncan, HUD Secretary Donovan, Labor Secretary Solis, and Interior Secretary Salazar, Surgeon General Regina Benjamin, Members of Congress, mayors from across the nation and leaders from the media, medical, sports, entertainment, and business communities who impact the health of children and want to be part of the solution. Program participants included: Tiki Barber, NBC correspondent and former NFL football player; Dr. Judith Palfrey, President of the American Academy of Pediatrics; Will Allen, Founder and CEO of Growing Power; Mayor Curtatone of Somerville, Massachusetts; Mayor Chip Johnson of Hernando, Mississippi; and local students, including a student from DC's Bancroft elementary school, and members of the 2009 National Championship Pee-Wee football team, the Watkins Hornets.

Let's Move is comprehensive, collaborative, and community oriented and will include strategies to address the various factors that lead to childhood obesity. It will foster collaboration among the leaders in government, medicine and science, business, education, athletics, community organizations and more. And it will take into account how life is really lived in

The White House, Office of the First Lady, Press Release, February 9, 2010.

communities across the country—encouraging, supporting and pursuing solutions that are tailored to children and families facing a wide range of challenges and life circumstances.

President Barack Obama kicked off the launch by signing a Presidential Memorandum creating the first ever *Task Force on Childhood Obesity* which will include the DPC, Office of the First Lady, Interior, USDA, HHS, Education, NEC and other agencies. Within 90 days, the Task Force will conduct a review of every single program and policy relating to child nutrition and physical activity and develop a national action plan that maximizes federal resources and sets concrete benchmarks toward the First Lady's national goal. While the review is under way, Administration and public and private efforts are already moving to combat obesity and reach the First Lady's national goal.

Helping Parents Make Healthy Family Choices

Parents play a key role in making healthy choices for their children and teaching their children to make healthy choices for themselves. But in today's busy world, this isn't always easy. So *Let's Move* will offer parents the tools, support and information they need to make healthier choices for their families. The Administration, along with partners in the private sector and medical community, will:

Empower Consumers

By the end of this year, the Food and Drug Administration will begin working with retailers and manufacturers to adopt new nutritionally sound and consumer friendly front-of-package labeling. This will put us on a path toward 65 million parents in America having easy access to the information needed to make healthy choices for their children.

Already, the private sector is responding. Today, the American Beverage Association announced that its member companies will voluntarily put a clear, uniform, front-of-pack calorie label on all of their cans, bottles, vending and fountain machines within two years. The label will reflect total calories per container in containers up to 20 oz. in size. For containers greater than 20 oz., the label will reflect a 12-oz. serving size. While more work remains to be done, this marks an important first step in ensuring parents have the information they need to make healthier choices.

Provide Parents with an Rx for Healthier Living

The American Academy of Pediatrics, in collaboration with the broader medical community, will educate doctors and nurses across the country about obesity, ensure they regularly monitor children's BMI, provide counseling for healthy eating early on, and, for the first time ever, will even write a prescription for parents laying out the simple things they can do to increase healthy eating and active play.

Major New Public Information Campaign

Major media companies—including the Walt Disney Company, NBC, Universal and Viacom—have committed to join the First Lady's effort and increase public awareness of the need to combat obesity through public service announcements (PSAs), special programming, and marketing. The Ad Council, Warner Brothers and Scholastic Media have also partnered with the U.S. Department of Health and Human Services (HHS) to run PSAs featuring top professional athletes, Scholastic Media's Maya & Miguel, and Warner Brothers' legendary Looney Tunes characters.

Next Generation Food Pyramid

To help people make healthier food and physical activity choices, the U.S. Department of Agriculture will revamp the famous food pyramid. MyPyramid.gov is one of the most popular Web sites in the federal government, and a 2.0 version of the Web site will offer consumers a host of tools to help them put the Dietary Guidelines into practice.

Empower Change

USDA has created the first-ever interactive database—the Food Environment Atlas—that maps healthy food environments at the local level across the country. It will help people identify the existence of food deserts, high incidences of diabetes, and other conditions in their communities. This information can be used by parents, educators, government and businesses to create change across the country.

LetsMove.gov

To help children, parents, teachers, doctors, coaches, the non-profit and business communities and others understand the epidemic of childhood obesity and take steps to combat it, the Administration has launched a new "one-stop" shopping Web site—LetsMove.gov—to provide helpful tips, step-by-step strategies for parents, and regular updates on how the federal government is working with partners to reach the national goal.

Serving Healthier Food in Schools

Many children consume as many as half of their daily calories at school. As families work to ensure that kids eat right and have active play at home, we also need to ensure our kids have access to healthy meals in their schools. With more than 31 million children participating in the National School Lunch Program and more than 11 million participating in the National School Breakfast Program, good nutrition at school is more important than ever. Together with the private sector and the non-profit community, we will take the following steps to get healthier food in our nation's schools:

Reauthorize the Child Nutrition Act

The Administration is requesting an historic investment of an additional $10 billion over ten years starting in 2011 to improve the quality of the National School Lunch and Breakfast program, increase the number of kids participating, and ensure schools have the resources they need to make program changes, including training for school food service workers, upgraded kitchen equipment, and additional funding for meal reimbursements. With this investment, additional fruits, vegetables, whole grains, and low-fat dairy products will be served in our school cafeterias and an additional one million students will be served in the next five years.

Double the Number of Schools Participating in the Healthier US School Challenge

The Healthier US School Challenge establishes rigorous standards for schools' food quality, participation in meal programs, physical activity, and nutrition education—the key components that make for healthy and active kids—and provides recognition for schools that meet these standards. Over the next school year, the U.S. Department of Agriculture, working with partners in schools and the private sector, will double the number of schools that meet the Healthier US School Challenge and add 1,000 schools per year for two years after that.

We are bringing to the table key stakeholder groups that have committed to work together to improve the nutritional quality of school meals across the country.

New Commitments from Major School Food Suppliers

School food suppliers are taking important first steps to help meet the Healthier US School Challenge goal. Major school food suppliers including Sodexho, Chartwells School Dining Services, and Aramark have voluntarily committed to meet the Institute of Medicine's recommendations within five years to decrease the amount of sugar, fat and salt in school meals; increase whole grains; and double the amount of produce they serve within 10 years. By the end of the 2010–2011 school year, they have committed to quadruple the number of the schools they serve that meet the Healthier US School Challenge.

School Nutrition Association

The School Nutrition Association (SNA), which represents food service workers in more than 75% of the nation's schools, has joined the *Let's Move* campaign. Working with other education partners, SNA has committed to increasing education and awareness of the dangers of obesity among their members and the students they serve, and ensuring that the nutrition programs in 10,000 schools meet the Healthier US School Challenge standards over the next five years.

School Leadership

Working with school food service providers and SNA, the National School Board Association, the Council of Great City Schools and the American Association of School Administrators Council have all embraced, and committed to meeting, the national *Let's Move* goal. The Council of Great City Schools has also . . . set a goal of having every urban school meet the Healthier US Schools gold standard within five years. The American Association of School Administrators has committed to ensuring that an additional 2,000 schools meet the challenge over the next two years. These combined efforts will touch 50 million students and their families in every school district in America.

Accessing Healthy, Affordable Food

More than 23 million Americans, including 6.5 million children, live in low-income urban and rural neighborhoods that are more than a mile from a supermarket. These communities, where access to affordable, quality, and nutritious foods is limited, are known as *food deserts*. Lack of access is one reason why many children are not eating recommended levels of fruits, vegetables, and whole grains. And food insecurity and hunger among children [are] widespread. A recent USDA report showed that in 2008, an estimated 49.1 million people, including 16.7 million children, lived in households that experienced hunger multiple times throughout the year. The Administration, through new federal investments and the creation of public-private partnerships, will:

Eliminate Food Deserts

As part of the President's proposed FY 2011 budget, the Administration announced the new Healthy Food Financing Initiative—a partnership between the U.S. Departments of Treasury, Agriculture and Health and Human Services that will invest $400 million a year to help bring grocery stores to underserved areas and help places such as convenience stores and bodegas carry healthier food options. Through these initiatives and private sector engagement, the Administration will work to eliminate food deserts across the country within seven years.

Increase Farmers Markets

The President's 2011 Budget proposes an additional $5 million investment in the Farmers Market Promotion Program at the U.S. Department of Agriculture which provides grants to establish, and improve access to, farmers markets.

Increasing Physical Activity

Children need 60 minutes of active play each day. Yet, the average American child spends more than 7.5 hours a day watching TV and movies, using cell phones and computers, and playing video games, and only a third of high school students get the recommended levels of physical activity. Through public–private partnerships, and reforms of existing federal programs, the Administration will address this imbalance by:

Expanding and Modernizing the President's Physical Fitness Challenge

In the coming weeks, the President will be naming new members to the President's Council on Physical Fitness and Sports, housed at the U.S. Department of Health and Human Services. The council will be charged with increasing participation in the President's Challenge and with modernizing and expanding it, so that it is consistent with the latest research and science.

Doubling the Number of Presidential Active Lifestyle Awards

As part of the President's Physical Fitness Council, the President will challenge both children and adults to commit to physical activity five days a week, for six weeks. As part of the First Lady's commitment to solve the problem of childhood obesity in a generation, the Council will double the number of children in the 2010–2011 school year who earn a "Presidential Active Lifestyle Award" for meeting this challenge.

Safe and Healthy Schools

The U.S. Department of Education will be working with Congress on the creation of a Safe and Healthy Schools fund as part of the reauthorization of the Elementary and Secondary School Education Act this year. This fund will support schools with comprehensive strategies to improve their school environment, including efforts to get children physically active in and outside of school, and improve the quality and availability of physical education.

Professional Sports

Professional athletes from twelve leagues including the NFL, MLB, WNBA, and MLS have joined the First Lady on the *Let's Move* campaign and will promote "60 Minutes of Play a Day" through sports clinics, public service announcements, and more to help reach the national goal of solving the problem of childhood obesity in a generation.

Partnership for a Healthier America

Core to the success of this initiative is the recognition that government approaches alone will not solve this challenge. Achieving the goal will require engaging in partnerships with States, communities, and the non-profit and for-profit private sectors. To support this effort, several foundations are coming together to organize and fund a new central foundation—the Partnership for a Healthier America—to serve as a non-partisan convener across the private, non-profit and public sectors to accelerate existing efforts addressing childhood obesity and to facilitate commitments toward the national goal of solving childhood obesity within a generation. The Partnership for a Healthier America is being created by a number of leading health care foundations and childhood obesity non-profits, including the Robert Wood Johnson Foundation, The California Endowment, W.K. Kellogg Foundation, The Alliance for Healthier Generation, Kaiser Permanente, and Nemours, and will seek to add new members in the days and months ahead.

MICHELLE OBAMA is the 44th first lady of the United States and wife of U.S. President Barack Obama. Prior to her role as first lady, she was a lawyer, Chicago city administrator, and community outreach worker. She received her BS degree from Princeton and law degree from Harvard.

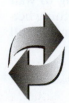

Michele Simon

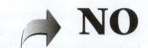

Michelle Obama's *Let's Move*—Will It Move Industry?

So what's all the fuss over Michelle Obama's *Let's Move* campaign to end childhood obesity, and will it make a difference? Of course, it's too soon to know for sure . . . , but early signs indicate more talk than action and deafening silence on corporate marketing practices.

The most obvious problem is framing the issue around obesity, which implies a couple of troubling assumptions. One, that skinny kids are just fine, no matter what garbage they are being fed, and two, that exercise, which has long been a convenient distraction, will continue to be so.

What Is *Let's Move*?

I highly recommend spending a few minutes perusing the *Let's Move* website, which is simple, but informative in describing the campaign. (For a more detailed description, read the press release.) While the name *Let's Move* implies a program all about exercise, in fact 3 of the 4 components have to do with food, which leads me to wonder why the White House wanted that to be less obvious. According to the home page:

> *Let's Move* will give parents the support they need, provide healthier food in schools, help our kids to be more physically active, and make healthy, affordable food available in every part of our country.

All laudable goals indeed, but notably absent is any criticism of the billions of dollars a year Big Food spends successfully convincing both parents and children to eat highly processed junk food and sugary beverages. Michelle Obama may be able to withstand the call of the Happy Meal, but most parents aren't so lucky to have a White House chef at their disposal.

To her credit, the First Lady is saying many good things about parents needing more support. Also, for the first time I heard the phrase "food desert" uttered on national TV. So she really does seem to understand that it's not all about education or personal responsibility.

But how exactly will Mrs. Obama and her husband attempt to end childhood obesity "within a generation." First is the formation of yet another task force. As the President's memo explains, members of the Task Force on Childhood Obesity are to include the Secretaries of the Interior, Agriculture, Health and Human Services, Education, the Director of the Office of Management and Budget, and the Assistant to the President and Chief of Staff to the First Lady. Heavy hitters yes, but might they have just a few other items already on their to-do list?

Also, in key language, the memo explains that "the functions of the Task Force are *advisory only*," meaning that this body, at the end of the day (or many months), will only make recommendations for another body (Congress?) to then maybe, someday, consider.

Do We Really Need Another Task Force?

The Obama Administration may be surprised (since they are calling it the "first ever") to learn that theirs is not the first federal task force on this issue. The previous administration had a few failed attempts. We already tried the Task Force on Media and Childhood Obesity, which the Federal Communications Commission spearheaded. Perhaps it never really went anywhere thanks to its members, who included the likes of Coca-Cola, McDonald's, and Disney.

Then there was the Food and Drug Administration's Obesity Working Group, which was broader than just childhood obesity, and whose pathetic achievement was the startling discovery (and accompanying silly web-based tool) that "calories count."

But given that we really can't count anything tried under the previous administration, I am willing to wait and see if this task force can come up with something better. It certainly can't be any worse than the lame "Small Steps" program (still online).

And let's not forget the still active Interagency Working Group on Food Marketed to Children, which is comprised of officials from four agencies: the Federal Trade Commission, the Centers for Disease Control and Prevention, the Food and Drug Administration, and the U.S. Department of Agriculture. In December [2009], this body released "tentative proposed nutrition standards" (for food products the government says are A-OK to market to kids) and is planning a final report with recommendations (for voluntary standards) to Congress this July. (Read author and fellow blogger Jill Richardson's excellent description of its public panel and proposed standards.)

This is the historical backdrop into which Michelle Obama now brings us *Let's Move*. It's not as if we haven't been here before; she's building on many failed attempts. But let's take a closer look at one of the four *Let's Move* components—school food.

How to Improve School Nutrition?

Under the "Healthier Schools" tab of the campaign's website, I recognize a few programs that have been out there for some time. For example, the underfunded Healthier US School Challenge and the ineffective Team Nutrition program, both under the U.S. Department of Agriculture, that agency whose number one mission is to prop up Big Agriculture. (The USDA also happens to be in charge of school nutrition and other food assistance programs, which has never proven to be a good combination.)

A few things are new under *Let's Move*, including doubling the number of schools that meet the Healthier US Schools Challenge and adding 1,000 schools per year for two years after that. And the President proposes to increase the federal budget by $1 billion annually to improve the quality of school meals. This sounds impressive, but as school lunch expert and Chef Ann Cooper pointed out in a recent *Washington Post* article, a mere 10 percent increase is a drop in the bucket. Currently, we feed 31 million students a day on $9.3 billion, which amounts to only $2.68 per meal. When was the last time you ate a decent lunch for less than 3 bucks? (No, the dollar menu meal doesn't count.)

And nowhere is any mention of the ongoing problem of competitive foods, which is government doublespeak for Coke and Pepsi vending machines in every school hallway, Doritos, Milky Way, and Good Humor sold in school stores, not to mention fast food like Pizza Hut that has taken over many school lunchrooms. Maybe that's because the Obama Administration has decided that

the success of *Let's Move* depends in part on "the creation of public private partnerships." That sounds familiar.

Working with Industry?

Since signing up for the *Let's Move* email updates, I haven't been too impressed. Here are two topics that landed in my in-box last week: Attention Techies! Apps for Healthy Kids Launched Yesterday and Paralympic Games Show All Athletes Can Be Champions. Now please don't send hate mail; I have nothing against apps or the Paralympics, I just don't understand how these concepts will solve childhood obesity "within a generation."

In an especially bad sign, Michelle Obama is speaking at a gathering of the Grocery Manufacturers Association this Tuesday. As I chronicled in *Appetite for Profit*, GMA, the lobbying arm of packaged foods conglomerates such as Kraft and PepsiCo has a long history of undermining school nutrition standards, among other positive policies.

As another blogger suggests, Mrs. Obama's own ties to Big Food may explain her deferential treatment of industry. She served on the board of directors of TreeHouse Foods (a spin-off of conglomerate Dean Foods) for two years until 2007, when her husband's presidential campaign became all consuming. This same blogger predicts that at the GMA meeting:

> Mrs. Obama will focus on "the pressing need to pursue comprehensive solutions to combat childhood obesity" and call upon food manufacturers to join these efforts by "providing healthier food options and better information about healthy food choices."

But Kraft, PepsiCo, Kellogg's and others have been all over that idea for several years now with their "smart choices" foods and claims of responsible marketing to children through its bogus Children's Food and Beverage Advertising Initiative.

We won't hear any scolding or warning aimed at industry. Instead, the First Lady will simply ask the major food corporations to jump on the *Let's Move* bandwagon. And they will do so gladly. With no threats looming (for example, that Congress might pass legislation to restrict marketing to kids) Big Food has nothing to fear; quite the contrary, industry gains positive PR in the process. Indeed, not missing a beat, GMA sent the White House a letter of support for the campaign on the *same day* that *Let's Move* launched.

Let's Move the Corporations Out of Washington

The bottom line for me is that while there are many things to like about *Let's Move* and it's certainly encouraging for a First Lady to talk about access to fresh, healthy food as a national priority, much of it is still rhetoric we've heard before.

To turn the talk into real action will take a ton of leadership from President Obama and even more political will from Congress. Most importantly, unless and until the ubiquitous junk food marketing stops, both in schools and out, very little of substance will change and we will be back here once again with the next administration's childhood obesity task force.

Let me know what you think.

I am a public health lawyer whose first book, *Appetite for Profit*, exposed food industry lobbying and deceptive marketing. Visit my website: www.appetiteforprofit.com.

MICHELE SIMON, a public-health attorney who teaches health policy at University of California Hastings College of the Law, is director of the Center for Informed Food Choices, a nonprofit in Oakland, California. She received her law degree from Hastings and master's from Yale.

EXPLORING THE ISSUE

Can Michelle Obama's "Let's Move!" Initiative Halt Childhood Obesity?

Critical Thinking and Reflection

1. Of the four key objectives outlined for the Task Force on Childhood Obesity, which do you think will have the greatest influence on reducing childhood obesity? Explain your answer.
2. Identify the public and private stakeholders who must work together to solve childhood obesity and summarize the role each will play.
3. Of the stakeholders, which ones do you believe will have the greatest positive influence on reducing childhood obesity? Justify your answer.
4. Identify one road block that you forecast the stakeholders will have and develop a way to overcome this road block.
5. Reflect on your own eating habits and lifestyle when you were in the 4th grade. What one thing (or person) had the greatest influence on your negative food choices or dietary practices? Who could have changed this and how?

Is There Common Ground?

Increases in childhood obesity have paralleled increases in the number of dollar items on fast food restaurant menus, the amount of junk foods allowed in schools, the number of mothers in the work force, decreases in PE teachers in schools, and the number of TVs sold by Sony and Samsung and video games sold by Walmart. At the same time, the government and some private health insurance companies are paying record amounts to care for children who already have been diagnosed with type 2 diabetes and other conditions associated with excessive weight. Who is/are responsible for these trends?

The Let's Move! campaign launched in 2010 was designed to "solve the problem of childhood obesity within a generation so that children born today will reach adulthood at a healthy weight." First Lady Michelle Obama is leading the program with a national public awareness campaign. A Google search for "Let's Move and Michelle Obama" reveals over a million hits, so the campaign has received a lot of publicity—and a government-supported website. Because the problem of childhood obesity has been steadily creeping upwards during the last 40 years, it is recognized that the problem cannot be solved overnight. The initiative garners "collaboration among the leaders in government, medicine and science, business, education, athletics, community organizations" and it has received much attention. Let's Move! claims that the campaign will "take into account how life is really lived in communities across the country—encouraging, supporting and pursuing solutions that are tailored to children and families facing a wide range of challenges and life circumstances."

Michelle Simon applauds the spirit of the campaign, but doubts that it will make a difference. She points out other government anti-obesity initiatives that have failed, such as the Federal Trade Commission's Task Force on Media and Childhood Obesity, Food and Drug Administration's Obesity Working Group, the Interagency Working Group on Food Marketed to Children, and USDA's Healthier Schools USA and TEAM Nutrition. Simon says for Let's Move! to work, it will require leadership from President Obama and willingness from Congress. Most importantly, she says that junk food marketing must stop. So there are common features—both M. Obama and M. Simon are attorneys who graduated from prestigious universities and are very strong advocates to promote the health and well-being of the nation's youth.

Additional Resources

Bumpus K, Tagtow A, Haven J. Let's Move! Celebrates 5 Years. *J Acad Nutr Diet.* 2015;115(3):338–41.

Sonntag D, Schneider S, Mdege N, Ali S, Schmidt B. Beyond food promotion: A systematic review on the influence of the food industry on obesity-related dietary behaviour among children. *Nutrients.* 2015;7(10):8565–76.

Zandian M, Bergh C, Ioakimidis I, et al. Control of body weight by eating behavior in children. *Front Pediatr.* 2015;3:89. doi:+10.3389/fped.2015.00089.

Internet References . . .

Eat Drink Politics

appetiteforprofit.com

**Gilder Lehrman Institute
of American History**

https://www.gilderlehrman.org/

**Let's Move—America's Move to Raise a
Healthier Generation**

www.letsmove.gov

Media and Childhood Obesity Website

www.fcc.gov/obesity

Small Steps

www.smallsteps.org

Partnership for a Healthier America

ahealthieramerica.org

Selected, Edited, and with Issue Framing Material by:
Janet M. Colson, *Middle Tennessee State University*

ISSUE

Do Pesticides Cause Birth Defects and Other Health Problems?

YES: Christopher Pala, from "Pesticides in Paradise: Hawaii's Spike in Birth Defects Puts Focus on GM Crops," *The Guardian* (2015)

NO: Environmental Protection Agency, from "Food and Pesticides," http://www2.epa.gov/safepestcontrol/food-and-pesticides (2015)

Learning Outcomes
After reading this issue, you will be able to:
• Explain how agrochemical companies use the islands of Hawaii to test herbicides.
• Describe the increased incidence of birth defects and other health complications that physicians suspect are linked to pesticide exposure.
• Outline the methods taken by the Environmental Protection Agency (EPA) to ensure that pesticides are safe for human health or the environment.

ISSUE SUMMARY

YES: Christopher Pala reports an increase in birth defects and pediatric morbidity in areas of Hawaii where high levels of pesticides are used for testing growth of GMO corn. He also describes the steps some Hawaiians are taking to restrict the testing of pesticides in Hawaii.

NO: The Environmental Protection Agency claims that American agricultural products are rigorously tested and the pesticide residue levels cause no health problems, especially among children.

The terms *pesticide, fungicide,* and *herbicide* are sometimes used interchangeably because they all end in the suffix *cide,* which means *killer.* The differences among the three are what they kill. *Pesticide* is a general term used to describe a substance that kills any type of pest, including fungi, weeds, insects, or rodents. Fungicides are designed to specifically kill fungi, whereas herbicides kill grass, weeds, or other vegetation.

Pesticides are used by the agricultural industry to destroy pests that would otherwise destroy crops. In turn, pesticides help increase the yield and quality of the crops—and profit for the growers. Natural pesticides, such as salt and vinegar, have been used for centuries and pose no problems to humans; however, synthetic ones are relatively new. Beginning in the late 1800s, inorganic pesticides were used extensively by farmers to control pests. Chemicals, such as arsenic, copper, lead, and sulfur mixed in varying formulations, were very effective in controlling pests.

In the early part of the 1900s, arsenic and lead were common pesticides used throughout the world. In their 2008 review, Schooley et al. describe the history of arsenic and lead use in apple orchards in the United States.

Lead arsenate ($PbHAsO_4$) was first used as an insecticidal spray in 1892 against the gypsy moth, *Lymantria dispar* (Linnaeus), in Massachusetts. . . . This inorganic pesticide was very popular among farmers because of its immediate effectiveness. It was also inexpensive, easy to mix, and very persistent. Over the next six decades, multiple applications of lead arsenate were sprayed each season to control apple pests. This increase in use eventually led to development of pesticide resistance, which in turn decreased its efficacy thus requiring growers to increase rates and application frequency to compensate. This issue eventually forced growers to switch to other methods of treatment, such as DDT.

The characteristics of the compounds that created this persistence—the basic nature of the elements in the pesticide—and the increase in application frequency and rates were key factors contributing to the contamination of thousands of acres across the United States.

Much of the arsenic remains in the soil 100 years later. In 2011, after a public scare about arsenic in apple juice, the FDA increased testing of arsenic levels in apples. Because chemicals in the soil eventually drain into streams, rivers, and lakes, water supplies are also tested for arsenic.

In the 1940s, the new synthetic pesticide was dichloro-diphenyl-trichloroethane (DDT). Originally, it was designed to destroy malaria and typhus and later used for insect control on crops. DDT's success as a pesticide, and broad use throughout the world, lead to resistance by many insect species—which in turn decreased DDT's effectiveness, thus requiring growers to increase rates and application frequency for DDT to be effective. The EPA describes the demise of DDT below:

> The U.S. Department of Agriculture, the federal agency with responsibility for regulating pesticides before the formation of the U.S. Environmental Protection Agency [EPA] in 1970, began regulatory actions in the late 1950s and 1960s to prohibit many of DDT's uses because of mounting evidence of the pesticide's declining benefits and environmental and toxicological effects. The publication in 1962 of Rachel Carson's *Silent Spring* stimulated widespread public concern over the dangers of improper pesticide use and the need for better pesticide controls.
>
> In 1972, EPA issued a cancellation order for DDT based on its adverse environmental effects, such as those to wildlife, as well as its potential human health risks. Since then, studies have continued, and a relationship between DDT exposure and reproductive effects in humans is suspected, based on studies in animals. In addition, some animals exposed to DDT in studies developed liver tumors. As a result, today, DDT is classified as a probable human carcinogen by U.S. and international authorities.

During the Vietnam War, herbicidal warfare was used to destroy the vegetation where the enemy lived. Destroying vegetation cut off the enemy's food supply and destroyed the bushes and trees that had been the hiding places of the enemy. The U.S. military spread aerial and on-ground applications of very toxic doses of herbicides, not considering the long-term effects it would have on the land, children and women who lived in the areas, or the U.S. soldiers ordered to spread the chemicals. The different types of herbicides used were identified by the color of the band painted around the drums that contained the chemicals. The herbicide in the orange barrels was known as *Agent Orange* and contained the poisonous contaminant known as *dioxin,* or *TCDD* (2,3,7,8-tetrachlorodibenzo-*p*-dioxin). Today, U.S. soldiers, Vietnamese citizens, and land still suffer the adverse effect of the toxin.

Dioxins and DDT are included on the EPA's list of banned Persistent Organic Pollutants (POPs). Although the concentrations of DDT, lead, and arsenic have decreased, the residents that still live in those areas are still concerned about contamination, especially for growing children. Today, the agrochemical industry continues to develop new pesticides to improve crop productivity. All new pesticides must be granted EPA approval prior to use. Instead of contaminating the U.S. mainland, chemical companies seek out remote locations to test their new chemicals, such as the islands of Hawaii.

This issue focuses on similar concerns related to pesticide contamination of two of the Hawaiian Islands, Kauia and Maui. Instead of the pesticides being used to increase the yield and quality of crops for the people to eat, the land is being used by agrochemical companies to test genetically modified (GM) seeds and most seeds are designed to be resistant to pesticides, such as Roundup, which contain the potentially toxic glyphosate.

The Hawaiian Island's total population is about 1.4 million with 70,000 living on the island Kauia and 163,000 on Maui; about 22 percent of the Hawaiian population are under 18 years of age. Therefore, a large percentage of the population who are being exposed to pesticides are children and teens. After reading the selections, decide for yourself if pesticides cause birth defects or other health problems among the islands' youth, and also decide what you would do if the agrochemical companies were testing their GMO seeds (and pesticides) close to your home.

YES

Christopher Pala

Pesticides in Paradise: Hawaii's Spike in Birth Defects Puts Focus on GM Crops

Local doctors are in the eye of a storm swirling for the past three years over whether corn that's been genetically modified to resist pesticides is a source of prosperity, as companies claim, or of birth defects and illnesses

Pediatrician Carla Nelson remembers catching sight of the unusually pale newborn, then hearing an abnormal heartbeat through the stethoscope and thinking that something was terribly wrong.

The baby was born minutes before with a severe heart malformation that would require complex surgery. What worried her as she waited for the ambulance plane to take the infant from Waimea, on the island of Kauai, to the main children's hospital in Honolulu, on another Hawaiian island, was that it was the fourth one she had seen in three years.

In all of Waimea, there have been at least nine in five years, she says, shaking her head. That's more than 10 times the national rate, according to analysis by local doctors.

Nelson, a Californian, and other local doctors find themselves in the eye of a storm swirling for the past three years around the Hawaiian archipelago over whether a major cash crop on four of the six main islands, corn that's been genetically modified to resist pesticides, is a source of prosperity, as the companies claim—or of birth defects and illnesses, as the doctors and many others suspect.

After four separate attempts to rein in the companies over the past two years all failed, an estimated 10,000 people marched on 9 August through Honolulu's Waikiki tourist district. Some held signs like, "We Deserve the Right to Know: Stop Poisoning Paradise" and "Save Hawaii—Stop GMOs" (Genetically Modified Organisms), while others protested different issues.

"The turnout and the number of groups marching showed how many people are very frustrated with the situation," says native Hawaiian activist Walter Ritte of the island of Molokai.

Seventeen Times More Pesticide

Waimea, a small town of low, pastel wood houses built in south-west Kauai for plantation workers in the 19th century, now sustains its economy mostly from a trickle of tourists on their way to a spectacular canyon. Perhaps 200 people work full-time for the four giant chemical companies that grow the corn—all of it exported—on some 12,000 acres leased mostly from the state.

In Kauai, chemical companies Dow, BASF, Syngenta and DuPont spray 17 times more pesticide per acre (mostly herbicides, along with insecticides and fungicides) than on ordinary cornfields in the US mainland, according to the most detailed study of the sector, by the Center for Food Safety.

That's because they are precisely testing the strain's resistance to herbicides that kill other plants. About a fourth of the total are called Restricted Use Pesticides because of their harmfulness. Just in Kauai, 18 tons—mostly atrazine, paraquat (both banned in Europe) and chlorpyrifos—were applied in 2012. The World Health Organization this year announced that glyphosate, sold as Roundup, the most common of the non-restricted herbicides, is "probably carcinogenic in humans."

The cornfields lie above Waimea as the land, developed in the 1870s for the Kekaha Sugar Company plantation, slopes gently up toward arid, craggy hilltops. Most fields are reddish-brown and perfectly furrowed. Some parts are bright green: that's when the corn is actually grown.

Both parts are sprayed frequently, sometimes every couple of days. Most of the fields lie fallow at any given time as they await the next crop, but they are still sprayed with pesticides to keep anything from growing. "To grow either seed crops or test crops, you need soil that's essentially sterile," says professor Hector Valenzuela of the

University of Hawaii department of tropical plant and soil science.

When the spraying is underway and the wind blows downhill from the fields to the town—a time no spraying should occur—residents complain of stinging eyes, headaches and vomiting.

"Your eyes and lungs hurt, you feel dizzy and nauseous. It's awful," says middle school special education teacher Howard Hurst, who was present at two evacuations. "Here, 10% of the students get special-ed services, but the state average is 6.3%," he says. "It's hard to think the pesticides don't play a role."

At these times, many crowd the waiting rooms of the town's main hospital, which was run until recently by Dow AgroSciences' former chief lobbyist in Honolulu. It lies beside the middle school, both 1,700 ft from Syngenta fields. The hospital, built by the old sugar plantation, has never studied the effects of the pesticides on its patients.

The chemical companies that grow the corn in land previously used for sugar refuse to disclose with any precision which chemicals they use, where and in what amounts, but they insist the pesticides are safe, and most state and local politicians concur. "The Hawai'i legislature has never given the slightest indication that it intended to regulate genetically engineered crops," wrote lawyer Paul Achitoff of Earthjustice in a recent court case.

As for the birth defects spike, "We have not seen any credible source of statistical health information to support the claims," said Bennette Misalucha, executive director of Hawaii Crop Improvement Association, the chemical companies trade association, in a written statement distributed by a publicist. She declined to be interviewed.

Nelson, the pediatrician, points out that American Academy of Pediatrics' report, Pesticide Exposure in Children, found "an association between pesticides and adverse birth outcomes, including physical birth defects". Noting that local schools have been evacuated twice and children sent to hospital because of pesticide drift, Nelson says doctors need prior disclosure of sprayings: "It's hard to treat a child when you don't know which chemical he's been exposed to."

Her concerns and those of most of her colleagues have grown as the chemical companies doubled to 25,000 acres in a decade the area in Hawaii they devote to growing new varieties of herbicide-resistant corn.

Today, about 90% of industrial GMO corn grown in the US was originally developed in Hawaii, with the island of Kauai hosting the biggest area. The balmy weather yields three crops a year instead of one, allowing the companies to bring a new strain to market in a third of the time.

Once it's ready, the same fields are used to raise seed corn, which is sent to contract farms on the mainland. It is their output, called by critics a pesticide delivery system, that is sold to the US farmers, along with the pesticides manufactured by the breeder that each strain has been modified to tolerate.

Corn's uses are as industrial as its cultivation: less than 1% is eaten. About 40% is turned into ethanol for cars, 36% becomes cattle feed, 10% is used by the food industry and the rest is exported.

"We Just Want to Gather Information"

At a Starbucks just outside Honolulu, Sidney Johnson, a pediatric surgeon at the Kapiolani Medical Center for Women and Children who oversees all children born in Hawaii with major birth defects and operates on many, says he's been thinking about pesticides a lot lately. The reason: he's noticed that the number of babies born here with their abdominal organs outside, a rare condition known as gastroschisis, has grown from three a year in the 1980s to about a dozen now.

"We have cleanest water and air in the world," he says. So he's working with a medical student on a study of his hospital's records to determine whether the parents of the gastroschisis infants were living near fields that were being sprayed around the time of conception and early pregnancy. He plans to extend the study to parents of babies suffering from heart defects.

"You kind of wonder why this wasn't done before," he says. "Data from other states show there might be a link, and Hawaii might be the best place to prove it."

Unbeknownst to Johnson, another two physicians have been heading in the same direction, but with some constraints. They're members of a state-county commission appointed this year to "determine if there are human harms coming from these pesticides," as its chairman, a professional facilitator named Peter Adler, tells a meeting of angry local residents in Waimea earlier this month. Several express skepticism that the panel is anything but another exercise in obfuscation.

The panel of nine part-time volunteers also includes two scientists from the chemical companies and several of their critics. "We just want to gather information and make some recommendations," Adler tells the crowd of about 60 people. "We won't be doing any original research."

But one of the two doctors, a retired pediatrician named Lee Evslin, plans to do just that. "I want see if any health trends stand out among people that might have been exposed to pesticides," he says in an interview. "It won't be a full epidemiological study, but it will probably be more complete than anything that's been done before."

The panel itself, called the Joint Fact-Finding Study Group on Genetically Modified Crops and Pesticides on Kaua'i, is the only achievement of three years of failed attempts to force the companies to disclose in advance what they spray and to create buffer zones—which they do in 11 other states, where food crops receive much less pesticides per acre.

The pushback from the expansion of the GMO acreage first emerged when Gary Hooser of Kauai, a former state senate majority leader who failed in a bid for lieutenant governor in 2010, ran for his old seat on the Kauai County council in 2012.

"Everywhere I went, people were concerned about GMOs and pesticides. They were saying, 'Gary, we gotta do something'," he recounts over coffee at the trendy Ha Coffee Bar in Lihue, the island's capital. "Some were worried about the GMO process itself and others by the threats of the pesticides, and it became one of the dominant political issues."

Once elected, Hooser, who has a ruddy complexion, piercing blue eyes and arrived in Hawaii as a teenager from California, approached the companies for information about exactly what they were spraying and in what amounts. He was rebuffed.

In the process of what he called "doing my homework," he discovered that the companies, unlike regular farmers, were operating under a decades-old Environmental Protection Agency permit to discharge toxic chemicals in water that had been grandfathered from the days of the sugar plantation, when the amounts and toxicities of pesticides were much lower. The state has asked for a federal exemption for the companies so they can avoid modern standards of compliance.

He also found that the companies, unlike regular farmers, don't pay the 4% state excise tax. Some weren't even asked to pay property taxes, worth $125,000 a year. After pressure from Hooser and the county tax office, the companies paid two years' worth of back taxes.

So with the backing of three other members of the seven-member Kauai council, he drafted a law requiring the companies to disclose yearly what they had grown and where, and to announce in advance which pesticides they proposed to spray, where and when. The law initially also imposed a moratorium on the chemical companies expanding their acreage while their environmental impact was assessed.

After a series of hearings packed by company employees and their families wearing blue and opponents wearing red, the bill was watered down by eliminating the moratorium and reducing the scope of the environmental study. The ordinance then passed, but the companies sued in federal court, where a judge ruled that the state's law on pesticides precluded the counties from regulating them. After the ruling, the state and the county created the joint fact-finding panel officially committed to conducting no new research.

Hooser is confident the ruling will be overturned on appeal: the Hawaii constitution "specifically requires" the state and the counties to protect the communities and their environment.

In his appeal, Achitoff of Earthjustice argued that Hawaii's general pesticide law does not "demonstrate that the legislature intended to force the county to sit and watch while its schoolchildren are being sent to the hospital so long as state agencies do not remedy the problem."

In the Big Island, which is called Hawaii and hosts no GMO corn, a similar process unfolded later in 2013: the county council passed a law that effectively banned the chemical companies from moving in, and it was struck down in federal court for the same reasons. A ban on genetically modified taro, a food root deemed sacred in Hawaiian mythology, was allowed to stand.

In Maui County, which includes the islands of Maui and Molokai, both with large GMO corn fields, a group of residents calling themselves the Shaka Movement sidestepped the company-friendly council and launched a ballot initiative that called for a moratorium on all GMO farming until a full environmental impact statement is completed there.

The companies, primarily Monsanto, spent $7.2m on the campaign ($327.95 per "no" vote, reported to be the most expensive political campaign in Hawaii history) and still lost.

Again, they sued in federal court, and, a judge found that the Maui County initiative was preempted by federal law. Those rulings are also being appealed.

In the state legislature in Honolulu, Senator Josh Green, a Democrat who then chaired the health committee, earlier this year attempted a fourth effort at curbing the pesticide spraying.

In the legislature, he said, it's an open secret that most heads of the agriculture committee have had "a closer relationship with the agro-chemical companies than with the environmental groups."

Green, an emergency room doctor who was raised in Pennsylvania, drafted legislation to mandate some prior disclosure and some buffer zones. "I thought that was a reasonable compromise," he says. Still, he also drafted a weaker bill as a failsafe. "If even that one doesn't pass, it's going to be obvious that the state doesn't have the political will to stand up to the chemical companies," he said in a phone interview at the time. "That would be terrible."

The chairman of the senate agricultural committee, Cliff Tsuji, didn't even bring the weaker bill to a vote, even though Hawaii's governor had pledged to sign any bill that created buffer zones.

Asked by email what he would do now, Green replied with a quip: "Drink scotch."

Christopher Pala is a freelance journalist who was living in Hawaii when his second daughter was born in 2006. Currently, Pala is based in Washington, D.C., and writes mostly about ocean issues and Kazakhstan.

Environmental Protection Agency

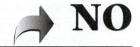

Food and Pesticides

Pesticides are widely used in producing food to control pests such as insects, rodents, weeds, bacteria, mold and fungus.

Under the Food Quality Protection Act (FQPA), EPA has the authority to ensure that all pesticides used on food in the United States meet FQPA's stringent safety standard. FQPA requires an explicit determination that a pesticide's use on food is safe for children and includes an additional safety factor, up to tenfold if necessary, to account for uncertainty in data relative to children.

The science and our understanding of chemical risk evolves and EPA continues to reevaluate each pesticide's safety every 15 years. EPA's continuous reevaluation of registered pesticides, combined with strict FQPA standards, major improvements in science, and an increase in the use of safer, less toxic pesticides, has led to an overall trend of reduced risk from pesticides.

Is Food Grown Using Pesticides Safe to Eat?

EPA is confident that the fruits and vegetables our children are eating are safer than ever. Under FQPA, EPA evaluates new and existing pesticides to ensure that they can be used with a reasonable certainty of no harm to infants and children as well as adults. EPA works continually to review and improve safety standards that apply to pesticide residues on food.

It is important to note though, that just because a pesticide residue is detected on a fruit or vegetable, that does not mean it is unsafe. Small amounts of pesticides that may remain in or on fruits, vegetables, grains, and other foods decrease considerably as crops are harvested, transported, exposed to light, washed, prepared and cooked. The presence of a detectible pesticide residue does not mean the residue is at an unsafe level. USDA's Pesticide Data Program (PDP) detects residues at levels far lower than those that are considered health risks.

What Has EPA Done to Decrease or Restrict the Amount of Pesticides in Food?

The 1996 FQPA directed EPA to completely reassess pesticide residues on food, with a special emphasis on the unique vulnerability of children. From 1996 to 2006, EPA used the improved safety standards in FQPA to cancel or restrict the use of 270 pesticides for household and food uses because they posed particular threats to children and infants. EPA also lowered the permissible pesticide residue levels for many kid's foods—for example, apples, grapes, and potatoes.

The FQPA safety standard isn't the only reason why EPA has been able to take so many steps to reduce children's exposure to pesticides in recent years. Once a pesticide is registered for its specific uses, it is not left unchecked. Starting in 2007, EPA began the systematic reevaluation of all old pesticides.

Here are some of the most notable EPA actions in recent years:

- In 2009, EPA canceled all uses of carbofuran, canceled aldicarb use on potatoes and citrus, and canceled methamidophos use on all commodities.
- In 2010, EPA canceled methomyl use on grapes and strawberries.
- In 2010, EPA canceled all products containing methyl parathion.
- In 2012 EPA canceled acephate use on green beans, oxamyl use on soybeans, and imidacloprid use on almonds.
- In 2013, EPA canceled all domestic uses of methyl parathion and canceled all uses of formetanate HCI on apples, pears, and peaches.

We have seen, through USDA's Pesticide Data Program (PDP) data, an overall decrease in the amount of pesticide residues in food, especially since the passing of FQPA in 1996. The stricter standards of FQPA and major

"Food and Pesticides," United States Environmental Protection Agency, 2015.

improvements in science and data, and an increase in the use of safer, less toxic pesticides, has led to an overall trend of reduced risk from pesticides.

For example, from 1995 to 2013, children's exposure to carbamates (a group of insecticides that affect the nervous system) fell by 70%—EPA canceled or restricted many carbamates during this time. From 1998 to 2008, tomatoes with detectable organophosphate pesticide residues fell from 37% to 9%, due to EPA canceling most organophosphates. It is important to note for some of the more recent actions, EPA expects declines will show up in future PDP data.

How Does EPA Regulate Pesticides in Food?

EPA evaluates every new pesticide for safety and every new use prior to registration. Before they may be sold, EPA must ensure that pesticides are safe for human health and the environment when used according to label directions. EPA also evaluates hundreds of different scientific studies.

Through these evaluations, EPA is ensuring the overall safety of proposed pesticide uses as required by FQPA. After pesticide registration, EPA reevaluates its safety every 15 years, taking into consideration any new data.

EPA's process for registering and re-evaluating pesticides is not a closed-door process between EPA and pesticide manufacturers. EPA relies on the best science available and places high value on transparency in decision-making. The public is invited to comment throughout the decision-making process—we request studies and data, take our findings to expert panels such as the FIFRA Scientific Advisory Panel, and consult the National Academy of Sciences on broad scientific policy questions. The agency also frequently receive hundreds or even thousands of comments from the public on our draft assessments and proposed decisions.

Public concerns about specific pesticides and food safety do not go unnoticed at EPA. We take incidents of pesticide poisoning and exposure very seriously and look at those incidents as part of our review. EPA can and has used its authority to have products removed from the market immediately when risks are imminent.

At the same time that we review dietary exposure to pesticides, we also look at worker exposure and environmental exposure. Risks to workers and the environment can lead to cancelations as well, or restrictions on how and when a pesticide can be used, including, when appropriate, establishing 'no spray' buffer zones to protect the surrounding communities and waterways.

Before allowing the use of a pesticide on food crops, EPA sets a maximum legal residue limit (called a tolerance) for each treated food. The tolerance is the residue level that triggers enforcement action. That is, if residues are found above that level, the commodity will be subject to seizure by the government. EPA receives information on how much pesticide residue remains on various foods through the PDP. Through annual sampling, PDP has collected thousands of samples on 10–15 food commodities and can detect residues at levels far lower than those that that pose health risks.

In setting the tolerance, EPA must make a safety finding that the pesticide can be used with "reasonable certainty of no harm." To make this finding, EPA considers the toxicity of the pesticide and its breakdown products, how much of the pesticide is applied and how often, and how much of the pesticide (i.e., the residue) remains in or on food by the time it is marketed. EPA ensures that the tolerance selected will be safe. The tolerance applies to food grown in the U.S. and imported food.

THE ENVIRONMENTAL PROTECTION AGENCY (EPA) is an agency of the U.S. government whose mission is to protect human health and the environment by developing and enforcing regulations.

EXPLORING THE ISSUE

Do Pesticides Cause Birth Defects and Other Health Problems?

Critical Thinking and Reflection

1. Compare the pesticide use on the various Hawaiian Islands and determine which have been affected and those that have not.
2. Discuss the effect that GMO crop and pesticide testing could have on the economic future of Hawaii. (Consider all aspects such as health status, intelligence, tourism, property values, etc.)
3. Design a study that will help the town of Waimea quantify the effect that pesticides have had on birth defects and other health problems.
4. Discuss if the EPA has fulfilled its mission of protecting the health and environment of the Island of Kauai.

Is There Common Ground?

Perhaps the common feature in this issue is that EPA's mission is to protect the health and environment by developing and enforcing policies that will protect human health and the environment; the people of Hawaii want the same—to be healthy and have healthy children and to protect their beautiful island.

A second commonality is that it appears that the fertile, and somewhat remote, land of Hawaii's islands is the ideal location to test chemical pesticides and the people of Hawaii love the lush, natural vegetation. The weather provides the ideal setting to grow corn and other crops all year long; the people of Hawaii enjoy the climate and fertile land. (But, do the native Hawaiians benefit from the agrochemical testing?)

Additional Resources

Bellinger DC. A strategy for comparing the contributions of environmental chemicals and other risk factors to neurodevelopment of children. *Environ Health Perspect.* 2012;120(4):501–7.

Center for Food Safety. *Pesticides in Paradise: Hawai'i Health and Environment at Risk.* http://www.center forfoodsafety.org/files/pesticidereportfull_86476.pdf. Published May 2015. Accessed November 13, 2015.

Handford CE, Elliott CT, Campbell K. A review of the global pesticide legislation and the scale of challenge in reaching the global harmonization of food safety standards. *Integr Environ Assess Manag.* 2015;11(4):525–36.

Landrigan PJ. Children's environmental health: A brief history. *Acad Pediatr.* 2015. doi: 10.1016/j .acap.2015.10.002.

Schooley T, Weaver MJ, Mullins D, Eick M. The history of lead arsenate use in apple production: Comparison of its impact in Virginia with other states. *J Pestic Safety Educ.* 2008;10:22–53. http://maxpond.ext.vt.edu/ojs2/index.php/jpse/article /view/1/37. Accessed November 14, 2015.

Internet References . . .

Center for Food Safety

www.centerforfoodsafety.org

Environmental Protection Agency (EPA)

www3.epa.gov

Hawai'i Department of Agriculture

hdoa.hawaii.gov

Hawai'i Seed

www.hawaiiseed.org